T0075623

Philosophy and Medicine

Founding Editors
H. Tristram Engelhardt Jr.
Stuart F. Spicker

Volume 144

Series Editors
Søren Holm, The University of Manchester, Manchester, UK
Lisa M. Rasmussen, UNC Charlotte, Charlotte, USA

Editorial Board Members
George Agich, National University of Singapore, Singapore, Singapore
Bob Baker, Union College, Schenectady, NY, USA
Jeffrey Bishop, Saint Louis University, St. Louis, USA
Ana Borovecki, University of Zagreb, Zagreb, Croatia
Ruiping Fan, City University of Hong Kong, Kowloon, Hong Kong
Volnei Garrafa, International Center for Bioethics and Humanities
University of Brasília, Brasília, Brazil
D. Micah Hester, University of Arkansas for Medical Sciences
Little Rock, AR, USA
Bjørn Hofmann, Norwegian University of Science and Technology
Gjøvik, Norway
Ana Iltis, Wake Forest University, Winston-Salem, NC, USA
John Lantos, Childrens' Mercy, Kansas City, MO, USA
Chris Tollefsen, University of South Carolina, Columbia, USA
Dr Teck Chuan Voo, Centre for Biomedical Ethics, Yong Loo Lin
School of Medicine, National University of Singapore, Singapore, Singapore

The Philosophy and Medicine series is dedicated to publishing monographs and collections of essays that contribute importantly to scholarship in bioethics and the philosophy of medicine. The series addresses the full scope of issues in bioethics and philosophy of medicine, from euthanasia to justice and solidarity in health care, and from the concept of disease to the phenomenology of illness. The Philosophy and Medicine series places the scholarship of bioethics within studies of basic problems in the epistemology, ethics, and metaphysics of medicine. The series seeks to publish the best of philosophical work from around the world and from all philosophical traditions directed to health care and the biomedical sciences. Since its appearance in 1975, the series has created an intellectual and scholarly focal point that frames the field of the philosophy of medicine and bioethics. From its inception, the series has recognized the breadth of philosophical concerns made salient by the biomedical sciences and the health care professions. With over one hundred and twenty five volumes in print, no other series offers as substantial and significant a resource for philosophical scholarship regarding issues raised by medicine and the biomedical sciences.

Christina Schües • Christoph Rehmann-Sutter
Martina Jürgensen • Madeleine Herzog
Editors

Stem Cell Transplantations Between Siblings as Social Phenomena

The Child's Body and Family
Decision-making

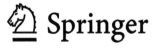 Springer

Editors

Christina Schües
Institute for History of Medicine and
Science Studies
University of Luebeck
Lübeck, Schleswig-Holstein, Germany

Christoph Rehmann-Sutter
Institute for History of Medicine and
Science Studies
University of Luebeck
Lübeck, Schleswig-Holstein, Germany

Martina Jürgensen
Institute for History of Medicine and
Science Studies
University of Luebeck
Lübeck, Schleswig-Holstein, Germany

Madeleine Herzog
Institute for History of Medicine and
Science Studies
University of Lübeck
Lübeck, Schleswig-Holstein, Germany

German Ministry of Education and Research

ISSN 0376-7418   ISSN 2215-0080   (electronic)
Philosophy and Medicine
ISBN 978-3-031-04165-5   ISBN 978-3-031-04166-2   (eBook)
https://doi.org/10.1007/978-3-031-04166-2

© The Editor(s) (if applicable) and The Author(s) 2022. This book is an open access publication.
Open Access This book is licensed under the terms of the Creative Commons Attribution 4.0
International License (http://creativecommons.org/licenses/by/4.0/), which permits use, sharing,
adaptation, distribution and reproduction in any medium or format, as long as you give appropriate credit
to the original author(s) and the source, provide a link to the Creative Commons license and indicate if
changes were made.
The images or other third party material in this book are included in the book's Creative Commons
license, unless indicated otherwise in a credit line to the material. If material is not included in the book's
Creative Commons license and your intended use is not permitted by statutory regulation or exceeds the
permitted use, you will need to obtain permission directly from the copyright holder.
The use of general descriptive names, registered names, trademarks, service marks, etc. in this publication
does not imply, even in the absence of a specific statement, that such names are exempt from the relevant
protective laws and regulations and therefore free for general use.
The publisher, the authors and the editors are safe to assume that the advice and information in this book
are believed to be true and accurate at the date of publication. Neither the publisher nor the authors or the
editors give a warranty, expressed or implied, with respect to the material contained herein or for any
errors or omissions that may have been made. The publisher remains neutral with regard to jurisdictional
claims in published maps and institutional affiliations.

This Springer imprint is published by the registered company Springer Nature Switzerland AG
The registered company address is: Gewerbestrasse 11, 6330 Cham, Switzerland

Contents

Contributors

Jutta Ecarius Faculty of Human Sciences, University of Cologne, Cologne, Germany

Tim Henning Department of Philosophy, Johannes Gutenberg University of Mainz, Mainz, Germany

Madeleine Herzog Institute for History of Medicine and Science Studies, University of Lübeck, Lübeck, Schleswig-Holstein, Germany

Martina Jürgensen Institute for History of Medicine and Science Studies, University of Lübeck, Lübeck, Schleswig-Holstein, Germany

Amy Mullin Department of Philosophy, University of Toronto, Toronto, ON, Canada

Christoph Rehmann-Sutter Institute for History of Medicine and Science Studies, University of Lübeck, Lübeck, Schleswig-Holstein, Germany

Lainie Friedman Ross Department of Pediatrics, MacLean Center for Clinical Medical Ethics, University of Chicago, Chicago, IL, USA

Christina Schües Institute for History of Medicine and Science Studies, University of Lübeck, Lübeck, Schleswig-Holstein, Germany

Margrit Shildrick Department of Ethnology, History of Religions and Gender Studies, Stockholm University, Stockholm, Sweden

Claudia Wiesemann Institute of Medical Ethics and History of Medicine, Goettingen University Medical Centre, Goettingen, Germany

Part I
Introductory and Conceptual Considerations

Chapter 1
The Child's Body and Bone Marrow Transplantation: Introduction

Christina Schües, Christoph Rehmann-Sutter, Martina Jürgensen, and Madeleine Herzog

Abstract Questions concerning the ethical status of children, and their position and their relationships within families, have been widely debated in recent moral philosophy and biomedical ethics, as well as in pedagogic sciences and sociology. This volume is intended to contribute to these interdisciplinary debates from a very specific angle. Combining philosophical, ethical and qualitative empirical research, it focuses on a medical practice that brings out a particularly challenging and complex social and familial situation, thus illuminating family responsibilities and their conflicts, children's dependency, the child's body with all its meanings, and the specific roles of family members in a transformative situation. The practice concerned is the transplantation of bone marrow between siblings who are children at the time of transplant. These renewable haematopoietic stem cells, derived from the marrow of the hip bone, can serve as a medical therapy for the sick brother or sister.

Keywords Children as donor · Stem cell transplantation · Responsibility · Family · Ethics

Questions concerning the ethical status of children, and their position and their relationships within families, have been widely debated in recent moral philosophy and biomedical ethics, as well as in pedagogic sciences and sociology. This volume is intended to contribute to these interdisciplinary debates from a very specific angle. Combining philosophical, ethical and qualitative empirical research, it focuses on a medical practice that brings out a particularly challenging and complex social and familial situation, thus illuminating family responsibilities and their conflicts,

C. Schües (✉) · C. Rehmann-Sutter · M. Jürgensen · M. Herzog
Institute for History of Medicine and Science Studies, University of Lübeck, Lübeck, Schleswig-Holstein, Germany
e-mail: c.schuees@uni-luebeck.de; christoph.rehmannsutter@uni-luebeck.de; martina.juergensen@uni-luebeck.de

© The Author(s) 2022
C. Schües et al. (eds.), *Stem Cell Transplantations Between Siblings as Social Phenomena*, Philosophy and Medicine 144,
https://doi.org/10.1007/978-3-031-04166-2_1

children's dependency, the child's body with all its meanings, and the specific roles of family members in a transformative situation. The practice concerned is the transplantation of bone marrow between siblings who are children at the time of transplant. These renewable haematopoietic stem cells, derived from the marrow of the hip bone, can serve as a medical therapy for the sick brother or sister.

Bone marrow transplantation is a standard treatment for leukaemia, Fanconi anaemia and other possibly fatal diseases of the blood system. If a person has a matching tissue type, they can act as donors (or be treated as donors) even if they are as young as 1 year old. Since it began in the 1970s, this procedure has raised ethical questions about the autonomy and welfare of the donor child, and concerns about the instrumentalization of the donor's body. For genetic reasons, the siblings of patients are often matching donors, (much less frequently, parents are suitable for donation) and if the patient has childhood cancer, sibling donors are often children as well. The extraction of bone marrow poses only a small *medical* risk to the donor but is in other ways a significant intervention into the donor's bodily integrity that carries multiple meanings and affects family interactions, both in their present lives and in the future.

Paediatric stem cell transplantation involves the healthy child who acts as a donor, and the ill child who needs the corporeal remedy for treatment. Two different sources of blood stem cells are used: the bone marrow stem cells or peripheral blood stem cell donation (less often used in children). Irrespective of precise source, stem cell transplantation constitutes a pressing ethical challenge in paediatric practice, because it lacks a direct or indirect medical benefit for the donor.[1] A sibling's stem cell transplant, however, frequently saves the life of the ill child recipient, or is at least curative.

Stem cell transplantation between young children creates a paradigm situation for biomedical ethics that needs to be studied and discussed from a variety of points

---

[1] There are two different methods of collecting haematopoietic stem cells: peripheral blood stem cell (PBSC) donation and bone marrow donation (BMD). In the case of *PBSC donation* the donor is first given medication –a growth factor (G-CSF) – for about 5 days. This hormone stimulates the growth of haematopoietic stem cells and their passage from the bone marrow into peripheral blood. A common side-effect of this treatment is the development of flu-like symptoms, which can be treated with paracetamol, for example. The cells are then collected from the donor by a procedure called stem cell apheresis. The donor's blood flows in a continuous loop from one arm vein, through a cell separator and back into the body via a vein in the other arm. This method of stem cell collection takes about 3–4 hours. In some cases it has to be repeated the following day in order to obtain the required number of stem cells. However, in most children younger than 12 years the forearm veins are too thin for the venous catheter, and a central venous catheter therefore has to be placed. For this reason, and also because they have a smaller total volume of blood, children often tolerate bone marrow donation better. In *BMD*, which is performed under general anaesthetic, no more than 20 ml per kg body weight of a mixture of bone marrow and blood is harvested from the hip bone (posterior iliac crests), with the donor lying on her stomach. The procedure takes about one to one and a half hours. Side-effects include mild pain, stiffness when walking, haematomas in the region of the collection site, and the usual potential side-effects of a general anaesthetic. The bone marrow regenerates completely within a few weeks. Sometimes iron tablets are prescribed (see Kline 2006; Müller 2015).

of view. It represents a range of conflicts of interest which are difficult to disentangle. It involves a medical intervention into the body of a healthy child, in order to help a brother or a sister who desperately needs the stem cells. This cannot easily be justified as being in the donor's own best interests. It is also debatable whether a young child can meaningfully provide informed consent to the procedure. For legal reasons, parents need to consent as proxies. Medicine that tries to save a life is in a genuine dilemma: some interests of the donors must be sacrificed in order to help the patient. This poses multiple challenges for the families who live with these transplants. This book systematically investigates these issues.

As we have learned in the nearly 9 years of work that eventually led to this book, this is an extremely rich and fascinating topic. It has many implications that reach far beyond the bioethical question of the circumstances under which it is morally permissible to take bone marrow from one child's body to save the life of another, or the question of whether selecting a matching donor child using the technique of pre-implantation diagnosis to create a "saviour sibling" is permissible. Our study focused particularly on the act of donation and its role in the overall process. Any transplantation practice, however, involves more than one person: a donor and a recipient, and it affects other people too – the rest of the family and their close social environment. We first conducted a philosophical study with the title "The best-interest of the child in conflict?" (2012–2015, led by Christina Schües and Christoph Rehmann-Sutter, funded by the Thyssen Foundation). In this theoretical phase of our work we investigated the medical-ethical and social-philosophical aspects of bone marrow donation between siblings. Special attention was paid to the frequently used formula of "child's well-being". We wanted to clarify the meaning and function of this concept in the understandings of the problem and the construction of legitimacy of the practice of transplanting haematopoietic stem cells between siblings. In parallel, three interview studies were conducted as MD dissertations. Lina Busch interviewed the leading experts in paediatric oncology and medical law in Germany, who experienced the establishment of the procedure of bone marrow transplantation in Germany over recent decades. Lilly Schwesinger interviewed leading practitioners and bioethicists in the USA, in particular about their concept of risk with regard to the donor child. Sarah Rieken conducted a pilot study of ten in-depth interviews with five parent couples who had recently experienced bone marrow transplantation between their children. This interdisciplinary work produced a theoretical and ethical framework, and led to a first round of publications.[2]

On the basis of this preliminary work, we started a larger qualitative inquiry into family experiences. We obtained funding for this from the German Ministry of Education and Research. This time we chose a long-term retrospective approach, including 17 families who had experienced a transplant up to 20 years previously. This is so far the only study with such a long-term perspective. We planned to interview every single member of the inner family. The interview study ran between

---

[2] Schües (2013), Schües and Rehmann-Sutter (2013a, b, 2014, 2015, 2017), Rehmann-Sutter et al. (2013), Rehmann-Sutter and Schües (2015), Schües (2016), Moos et al. (2016), Raz et al. (2017), Busch (2015a), and Rieken (2020).

2016 and 2019 at the Institute for the History of Medicine and Science Studies, at the University of Lübeck. Field work and interpretation was mainly conducted by Martina Jürgensen and Madeleine Herzog.[3] Christina Schües and Christoph Rehmann-Sutter regularly participated in discussing the findings against the backdrop of what was discovered during the first phase.

This book is based on the key findings of this long-term retrospective study. It presents these findings in four topical chapters, each followed by two discussion chapters, most of them written by guest authors. All the chapters emerged from an interdisciplinary workshop in February 2019 in Lübeck, where the authors had access to an extended and thematically organized selection of interview quotes, and presented the draft of their chapter. This selection of quotes has grown into the appendix of this book.

Stem cell transplantation is a practice that had its first successes about 50 years ago. Since the 1970s, increasing numbers of healthy children have served as allogeneic blood stem cell donors for their ill siblings.[4] In 1968, a child diagnosed with lymphopenic immune deficiency syndrome received the first paediatric transplant (Yeşilipek 2014). Since then, different diseases of the blood building (haematopoietic) system, such as leukaemia or Fanconi anaemia, myelodysplasia, lymphoma and thalassaemia, have been treated using stem cell transplants. Stem cell transplantation is a risky but often successful and effective therapy for a number of serious, often fatal diseases, and for some of them, it has been the only possible curative treatment. Since the introduction of the immunosuppressive drug *cyclosporine* in 1980, the chances of success have improved significantly (Weil 1984). A survey article by the European Group for Blood and Marrow Transplantation (EBMT 2019) reports that an increasing number of stem cell transplants have been carried out since the mid-1970s, but it does not specify how many involved child donations. In 2000–2002, according to one census, there were more than 31,000 child transplants throughout Europe, some of them from sibling donors (Miano et al. 2007). Siblings are often chosen as stem cell donors because in approximately 25% of casese they have a matching HLA pattern. However, unrelated donors from growing lists of potential anonymous donors can be chosen as well, if somebody is HLA compatible.

---

[3] We are grateful to Sandra Matthäus for her contributions during the first year of the project.

[4] In Europe, the number of blood stem cell therapies increases every year. In 2010 more than 30,000 transplants were carried out for the first time (autologous and allogenic added together), and this number increased by 6% between 2011 and 2012; 14,165 allogenic transplants took place in 2012. Of these, 11% were in paediatrics: 2877 allogeneic transplants were performed with a recipient under 18 years of age. The overview took into account 661 of 680 centres in 48 countries (European Society of Blood and Marrow Transplantation EBMT, Annual Report 2013). See also Antin and Raley, *Manual of Stem Cell and Bone Marrow Transplantation,* 2013. In the US, the number of allogenic blood stem cell transplants from HLA-identical siblings has remained more or less constant since 1995, ranging from about 2000 to 2500 per year, with a slight downwards tendency since around 2014, mainly due to higher numbers of haploidentical donor transplants from parents, which have increasingly been performed over the last 15 years (SIBMTR 2019).

It now seems amazing that during the first years of paediatric transplants, two opposing lines of thinking prevailed in the medical practice with children. First, up to the 1970s and still affected by the brutal medical experiments under the German National Socialist (Nazi) regime, children were explicitly excluded from medical practices that violated their fundamental right to physical and psychological integrity. Seen in this light, the twentieth century was not simply characterized by progress but also by a changing, sometimes cruel and inhuman history of medicine that also involved experiments on and the murder of many thousands of children. Yet it was also the epoch in which children's rights were explicitly formulated, which led to the child being given the moral and legal status of a subject. The years 1924 (Geneva Declaration of the Rights of the Child) and 1989 (United Nations Convention on the Rights of the Child) are particularly exemplary of these upheavals and milestones. Now, children are included in research and are allowed to donate body tissue for a sibling if it is of therapeutic use to that sibling in the event of a serious illness. Second, during the period during which transplantation practice was not yet consistently successful, when physicians still worried whether the intervention would have a healing effect on the sick child, ethical questions were rarely raised. At the forefront of the discussion were medical questions and problems such as graft-versus-host disease, which can occur after a paediatric bone marrow transplant.[5] In the 1980s, the first short-term empirical studies were conducted, focusing on the medical and social experiences of the donors and recipients of paediatric stem cell transplants (Sanders et al. 1987). It is interesting to see that at the same time that the recipients' survival rate increased, ethical concerns about the practice also became increasingly visible in the literature. Around 1990, the first articles on the ethics of this practice appeared.[6]

The ethical debate gained momentum in early 2000s. Several, mostly short-term empirical studies were undertaken by medical social scientists (Packman et al. 1997, 2004; Pentz et al. 2004, 2008; Wiener et al. 2007). Morally, psychologically and legally, the conflictual structure of sibling donation became an issue of discussion. Stem cell transplantation had become a medically established practice, but it still raises doubts that could not be easily or adequately addressed by standard decision-making models within the Western ethical tradition. The subject matter also proved difficult for classical ethical concepts, such as Aristotelian virtue ethics, Kant's ethics of duty, utilitarianism or existentialist approaches, which were developed primarily for the regulation of relationships between adults. Stem cell transplantation between siblings does not involve symmetrical relationships between responsible citizens, or obligations to persons who are not of age or unable to give their consent. As elsewhere, medical practice can be unlike ordinary life. And free and informed consent cannot resolve the matter, since small children cannot meaningfully give or withhold consent. It has become common ethical and legal practice

---

[5] GvHD means a reaction of the donated stem cells ("graft") against body cells of the recipient ("host") because they are seen as foreign ("non-self"). Symptoms vary from mild to severe, and can lead to the death of the recipient (Eisner and August 1995).

[6] Forman and Ladd (1991); Kline (2006, ch. 13).

in therapeutic decisions that those who cannot give consent are given proxies who decide on their behalf and in their best interests. This applies to children who are unable to give consent, and to people with dementia. However, these procedures cannot resolve the issues connected to actions in the field of paediatric stem cell transplantation that involve healthy children who are to act as donors and be injured simply in order to donate. Acknowledging children as subjects with their own past and future biography means recognising their specific needs and rights. It also involves giving them a voice, giving consideration to their adequate involvement in decision-making, and focusing on aspects of care for the children that are relevant.

The ethical problems of blood stem cell transplantation from donor children arise against the background of the individual rights that form the fundamental normative constitution of modern societies. They are structurally based on the formal and material recognition of every person's human rights. This set of basic rights includes the principle that every human being has a right to be protected in her or his physical integrity. If this is taken seriously as a fundamentally defensive right, it cannot be overridden by the medical need of another individual. Only a therapeutic aim that benefits the child itself can justify an intervention into the body of a child who cannot give consent. Preventing or curing the disease of *another* child *per se* are not valid reasons to infringe one child's bodily integrity. Beyond a therapeutic justification, the right to bodily integrity can only be outweighed by the principle of voluntariness, which can be met if a mature person is able to give her or his informed consent to donation. However, the law and ethics see a young minor, perhaps 5 years old or less, as being unable to freely decide about her participation in donation. Ethically and legally, teenagers are given the possibility to dissent. The standard argument is that (i) the ill child needs adequate therapeutic help, which (ii) can be provided by the sibling's stem cells, and (iii) the parents bear the responsibility to care for the sick child who may need a stem cell transplant, as much as they are committed to protecting the potential donor child; however, (iv) harvesting the stem cells is a low-risk procedure and the donor's stem cells will regenerate. Thus, in this view, (v) care for the well-being of the recipient child and care for the donor child might require and justify (mildly) injuring the donor child. This line of argument, however, is simplistic on theoretical and practical grounds. For instance, it takes for granted that there is a tight causal connection between donation and survival: if the potential donor child does not donate, the sick child will die. This is often not the case. There might be an unrelated donor who could be found, or parents could donate bone marrow for a haploidentical transplant. And equally, a stem cell transplant from a sibling is not always successful. In principle, if a matching sibling will not donate and, hence, hypothetically speaking, the sick child dies, we could also say that she has died because of her illness and not because of the sibling's refusal to donate.

This situation can be better seen as a parental *moral conflict*: parents are obliged to care for all their children, but when a stem cell transplant is an indicated treatment, they might be asked by the medical professionals looking after their sick child to agree to injuring their other child, in order to help the sibling therapeutically. If we recognize and accept the intrinsically conflicting nature of this situation and abstain from quickly resolving it by subordinating one concern under the other, in order to establish a formal justification, the moral (and legal) complexity of sibling donation can be understood in a much more nuanced way, which is also closer to the fine-tuned moral perception of the family members involved. To be specific, if blood stem cell therapy is suggested by doctors as the only therapy, and in consequence the parents are confronted with the demand to agree to the injury of their healthy child in order to fight for the life of the other, ill child, they are burdened with a decision that is conflictual at its core, even though it appears to be merely following a therapeutic imperative.

In order to better address this difficulty in the situation of decision-making, the 2010 policy statement of the American Academy of Pediatrics (AAP) states that a "donor advocate" should be appointed. This person should talk to the potential donor child, to see whether he or she understands the situation, and to help parents to see and consider the perspective of the potential donor child rather than seeing things mainly from the point of view of their sick child. According to the AAP, the donor advocate should be involved from the outset, starting with the decision about whether the minor should undergo HLA testing (American Academy of Pediatrics Committee on Bioethics 2010, 398). In Germany, the transplantation law was expanded in 1997 by a new paragraph §8a, which provides that it is permissible to extract bone marrow from the body of a minor to cure his or her sibling, if no adult donor can be found (TPG 1997, §8a) and the legal representative (i.e. the parents) have given their consent after being comprehensively informed. It does not call for a donor advocate. Before the introduction of this paragraph, stem cell transplantation from a minor donor was not mentioned in a legal document in Germany. The actual practice in Germany, however, clearly deviates from the legal provision to search for an unrelated donor first. Siblings have remained the preferred donors (Busch 2015b).

The *parental ethical conflict* of having to care for all the children and having to decide to harm the healthy in order to help the sick child, which lies at the heart of this practice, happens in a situation of extreme crisis when one child has a severe, life-threatening disease. Psychologically, the issue of stem cell transplantation between siblings concerns the whole family. Family members become involved and affected in different ways. The bioethical literature has clearly diagnosed and evaluated a conflictual situation for the parents, either on the level of the clash of norms and interests or from the perspective of proxy decision-making, the eligibility of a child as donor, and the participation of the donor child in this procedure.[7] Less attention has been given to the moral conflicts of the other siblings who are also potential donors. Some of them need to decide whether to agree to be tested, and others would be willing but are unable to donate. Non-donating siblings may be sidelined for a certain time; they may need to put aside their own demands, and may be jealous.

---

[7] Bendorf and Kerridge (2011), Bitan et al. (2016), Schües and Rehmann-Sutter (2015); see further references in AAP (2010).

Qualitative research has demonstrated a much richer complexity of donors' and other family members' moral perceptions. Rather surprisingly, as Pentz et al. (2014) found, most family members did not view sibling typing and donation as a choice. This reflects our own earlier results as well (Rehmann-Sutter et al. 2013). Donors in Pentz's study were positive about the experience, and did not express regrets. The most important lack identified was in education and psychosocial support. However, this does not mean that donors' experiences were easy. There are psychological risks to donation, which begin when parents are approached about the possibility of having one child donate haematopoietic stem cells to another (AAP 2010). As Jennifer Hoag's group recently reported from a mixed methods study, while feeling influenced by family obligations, all donors wanted to make the final decision about whether to donate. The most important factor that guided decision-making for donors was an obligation to help. However, "[m]ost of the donors felt that the decision to donate was theirs to make" (Hoag et al. 2019, 378). The role given to the donors in decision-making influenced their perception of the outcome, and their feelings of responsibility for the health of the patient sibling. Findings such as these have been included in a proposal for an improved psychosocial care pathway (Kazak et al. 2019).

So far, only short term empirical studies have been published, covering months or 1–2 years after the transplant. Long-term assessment from the point of view of all family members involved is lacking. We consider this an important omission in terms of informing the ethical and legal discussions of the norms involved, which are in conflict within this practice, yet also have a long-term meaning in retrospect. To understand the conflict from different perspectives and at different times, the families need to be investigated more comprehensively. All family members, both parents and children, donating and non-donating siblings, can provide important views, which have not yet been studied in adequate length and depth. Do family members sense this ethical conflict? Do these considerations matter to them? How do parents actually decide? How do they see their decisions in retrospect, at different timepoints afterwards, and depending on the outcome of the transplant? Do they actually feel that they decide(d)? How does a family treat the many issues of responsibility? How do families interact? How do they see the body of the donating child in the context of the emerging needs? These are a few of the questions that seem to be relevant for understanding the issues philosophically and for the ethical discussion beyond regulation and clinical decision-making.

Our long-term retrospective qualitative study included 17 families who had lived through bone marrow transplantation between siblings who were children at the time. There were about equal numbers of families at 0–5 years, 6–10 years, and 11–20 years post-transplant. One family, which we included for comparison, was just before transplant (1 week). If possible we interviewed all members of a family, if they were old enough and agreed to participate. The interviews were conducted with individuals as well as with the family as a group, and recorded and transcribed verbatim. Interpretation was based on qualitative, hermeneutic-phenomenological research methodology. In most cases, we started with the family group interview, where interactions could be recorded. This gave us insights into the particular family dynamics and the shared family narratives we heard. This was followed by a set of individual in-depth interviews with all family members. All the families that we interviewed live in Germany.[8] Thus, the context of family life and of medical practice refers to this country. For the interpretation, however, we were inspired by and included analysis and discussion from other Western countries.[9] The interview materials presented and discussed in this book cover reflections, narratives and memories of donors, recipients and other family members, as well as observations of family interactions.

We asked leading scholars from related fields such as bioethics, philosophy, and family sociology to discuss the findings from these interviews and our analysis from their perspectives. We asked them to reflect upon a broad sample of interview quotations, and gave brief introductions into our key findings. In an elaborated form, these introductions constitute the thematic introductions to the four main parts of this book. Additional quotes can be found in the appendix. For the sake of brevity we will call our own qualitative empirical study in this book the "Lübeck study".

When we started the study we defined a series of main research questions. They included: (1) What are the short- and long-term psychosocial consequences of a blood stem cell transplant between minor children? (2) How are family relationships influenced by the period of illness, the transplant practice, and the time after it? (3) How do family members perceive each other in terms of their body and its involvement in the treatment? (4) How do individual family members see the ethical questions, but also the practical concerns and emotional density connected with bone marrow transplantation? These questions inspired the interview guides. As is common in qualitative research, we chose an iterative procedure. After collecting the first interviews, we started the analysis and interpretation, and reviewed the interview guide as well as our interview strategy, continuing similarly after the next series of interviews. The guide was repeatedly revised in this cyclical procedure. There were some challenges in a few family group interviews in situations of severe tension between family members.[10] Using an inductive procedure based on systematic sentence-by-sentence coding of the interview transcripts, a series of overarching themes emerged. We have selected the main emergent themes as the topics of this book, and have organized it into four corresponding sections.

In order to introduce them, one chapter makes a link to the well-known novel and movie *My Sister's Keeper* by Jody Picoult. In this story, Anna is a young stem cell donor for her sister Kate; however, Anna has been specially conceived and selected in order to be a matching donor, using pre-implantation genetic diagnosis. Despite this obvious difference, Anna's story resonates in many ways with the stories we heard from our families. But in other respects, the fictional Anna gives a further dramatic aggravation of the family conflict. *Christoph Rehmann-Sutter and*

---

[8] We are not aware of any other qualitative study about stem cell transplantation between siblings in Germany.

[9] For further details on the stratification of the sample, the design of the interview study and the analytical methodology we used, see the introduction in the appendix.

[10] Some we discussed in Herzog et al. (2019).

Christina Schües analyse the film and make a series of comparisons between its narrative and the work of remembrance in the families. *Christina Schües* then offers a philosophical conceptual analysis of the child's well-being and the child's best interests. These ideas are central to the ethical evaluation of decision-making in paediatric medicine, and are related to the child's will and the family's well-being. How can a tragic problem be analysed and transformed so that the donor child, the recipient, and the whole family can be kept in communication with one another?

Each of the topical sections starts with a report of the relevant empirical findings, written by *Martina Jürgensen and Madeleine Herzog.*

I. *Mapping responsibilities.* How are responsibilities allocated, negotiated and understood in the complex relational network of patient, donor, other siblings, and parents, in relation to their physicians, the law and state authorities? The chapters in this section look at different types of responsibilities faced by the family members depending on their role as mother, father, donor, recipient, and other family members.

Families strongly believed that it was a shared responsibility to help the sick child and did not therefore consider donation a question to be decided, but rather a matter of course. Some even said it was a family duty. These moral understandings contributed to a dynamic differentiation of responsibilities among family members. Donors, for instance, acknowledged a responsibility for the success or failure of the transplant, and some said their duty extended over time and included more transplants later in life. In retrospect, it was also striking to see that most donors valued their donation positively.

Claudia Wiesemann comments on these findings from a medical ethics perspective. She asks how the decision to donate can be made freely and without coercion if the life of a child depends on it. She also examines whether sibling bone marrow donation can be reconciled with the moral ideal of family that is based on care. *Jutta Ecarius* introduces the perspective of education, and distinguishes a series of different dimensions of responsibility in education and family interaction within the structure of a family and with regard to the difficult situation of illness.

II. *Dealing with illness.* Which coping strategies do the families use? What does it mean for the families to be ill? Families had different attitudes, which reflected both their previous experiences and their basic attitudes toward the world.

Some families first responded by denial of the fatal diagnosis, hoping that it was a mistake. Many families suffered from a severe loss of control in several areas of their lives. The illness changed family roles. An important question is how long a child should be seen as "ill". Four different patterns of coping were identified: toughening up, resignation, ignoring, or acceptance. Families also found different things helpful in dealing with the situation and in making sense of the events around the illness: keeping or regaining control, maintaining routines, hoping that it will be all right, or making the best of bad things. In hindsight, many families felt that the experience of the disease also had a positive impact on the family as a whole, and that individual family members could learn from it.

In her response, *Amy Mullin* discusses how philosophy can help us understand family responses and decision-making. She draws on interviews and explores how a relational understanding of autonomy might help map initial decision-making, how an ethics of care can contribute to understanding the balancing of personal needs against what is wanted for a seriously ill child, and how gratitude, rather than indebtedness, is the appropriate response to sacrifices aimed at saving a sibling. *Christoph Rehmann-Sutter* searches for connections between responsibility, memory and time, in order to explain the complex meanings of "retrospective responsibilities". Story-telling within families and the emergence of family narratives is a place where responsibility is not just remembered, but also enacted. Families care about how things in the past are recounted in the present.

III. *Processes of decision-making.* How did different families and their individual members conceptualize and "make" a decision, and participate in decision-making? Do they feel they really have decided at some point? How do they evaluate the decision and the decision-making process in retrospect?

With one exception, all families said that the decision to conduct a bone marrow transplantation (BMT) was not experienced as an option but as another step in the therapeutic process, to which there was no alternative. They felt they had no other choice. The decision to have family members typed and, if they match, use them as donors, was not interpreted as a "decision" either, but was considered a matter of course for family members to do so. Families preferred a sibling donor over an unrelated one. Parents felt that they needed to talk to the (potential) donor about the donation. Most families said that the child was formally asked whether she or he agreed to the donation. However, everyone knew that a negative answer to this question was not possible.

Tim Henning takes an analytic philosophical point of view and investigates two moral pitfalls that emerge in the procedure of decision-making about stem cell donation by a child. There is a danger of violating what moral philosophers refer to as the separateness of persons, and of viewing the children as what he calls mere "value receptacles". On the other hand, there is a special danger to the child's autonomy – the danger of using the burdens of autonomy to undermine autonomy. *Lainie Friedman Ross* explores the limits of the best interest standard and the role of third-party oversight for some medical decisions even when the parents' decision is not abusive or neglectful. She argues for including a living donor advocacy team to support the potential donor child.

IV. *Familial bodies.* Body parts (tissues, cells) can become a remedy for another family member. Whose body is that of the child? How does this affect the individual's and the family's ideas of being "whole" and "integral"? Can the family itself be seen in some respects as "a body"?

After a bone marrow transplant between siblings, another family member's cells continue to live in the recipient's body. This connects family members in a variety of ways. Some families saw it as an essential change in the recipient's body and identity, while others saw it as a unification of two separate individuals. Some families described the donor's body as a "spare parts depot"; being seen as a life-saving resource then created a lasting responsibility in the donors. This relation was in fact seen by families as creating one system, one "familial body".

Margrit Shildrick explores stem cell transplantation with regard to questions of identity, of gifting, and of mortality. In looking at everything involved in the understanding of stem cell transplants – the biomedical procedure, the individual and collective experiences of the family, the data collected, the expertise and expectations of the researchers, and the varying analyses applied – what emerges, she argues, building on a Deleuzian framework, is a knowledge assemblage. *Christina Schües* investigates stem cell transplantation as a phenomenon of intercorporeality. This concept embraces the "family body" and a singular body, the sense of bodily belonging and bodily ownership, and a relationship that inheres within a transplant. She argues that even though the transplant is body material, it is always more than that: a ground for personal traits, symbols, and a particular bond between the siblings.

This interdisciplinary discussion is intended as a contribution to family research, to medical sociology, and to the understanding of ethics from the different lay perspectives involved. It also aims to be an inspiration for healthcare professionals and for bioethicists. In conclusion, perhaps two aspects elucidated in this book deserve to be especially highlighted: (1) *Family*. Today, family is predominantly seen as socially determined and fluid. In reality, however, biological kinship and parenthood still play a big role (blood relations), otherwise so much effort would not be expended in securing genetic relations to children by means of fertility treatments, in vitro fertilization, or searching for genetic parents after an adoption, or arguing for the right to know one's genetic origins. The question of a possible donorship of stem cells emphasizes the embodied similarity and dependency between,members within a "family body". What do I signify for others based on my embodied existence? What is the meaning of my body features for these others? The closeness that is realized through a transplant of tissue creates a special form of closeness – and with this, of responsibility. A family body is what we share – in a very material sense. This is not only the case for parents, but also for siblings. If families feel the wish to solve a problem using their own means, from within the family, this should be seen not only as the capability to do something tremendously important together, but also as something that has a material basis. (2) *A child's body*. Parenthood has always been a very corporeal undertaking. It involves desire, passion, sex, conception, pregnancy, birth, breastfeeding and nourishment, care, protection, touch, punishment, and so forth. The parental approach to the child is very corporeal. At first, the parents' power with regard to their access to the child's body is nearly limitless: parents decide everything (or they think they do), they have unlimited right to know what the child is eating, when it is sleeping, what clothes it wears, which hairdo it has… Is this an unquestioned prerequisite that makes it easier to use the body of the child for another, higher purpose? Is this a reason why some parents do not even realize that a donation of stem cells infringes the bodily integrity of the child? Are they just accustomed to having access to the child's body?

These are not questions that we claim to settle. But both the family narratives and the academic texts in this book flesh them out and bring a substance to them that will hopefully broaden our knowledge about the practice of paediatric transplantation and its contexts.

Acknowledgment We are immensely grateful to the participants in this study for their readiness to share their experiences with us and with the readers of this book. The 82 interviews of the Lübeck study were professionally transcribed by Monika Pohl. The selected interview quotes were translated from German to English by Monica Buckland, who also revised the English of all the chapters written by non-native English speakers. Special thanks to Jackie Leach Scully for an inspiring talk at the workshop and for helpful questions during the revision of the manuscripts. We also thank two anonymous peer reviewers for reading and commenting on the manuscript, which helped us to further clarify the text. We thank Leonie Haberer and Marina Frisman for editorial assistance. Funding was provided by the Fritz Thyssen Stiftung (grant no. AZ.10.12.2.018) and the Federal Ministry of Education and Research of Germany, as part of the research programme "ELSA stem cell research" (grant 01GP1601).

Literature

AAP – American Academy of Pediatrics. 2010. Policy statement, children as hematopoietic stem cell donors. *Pediatrics* 109 (5): 982–984.

Antin, Joseph, and Yolin Raley. 2013. *Manual of stem cell and bone marrow transplantation.* Cambridge University Press.

Bendorf, Aric and Ian H. Kerridge. 2011. Ethical issues in bone marrow transplantation in children. *Journal of Paediatrics and Child Health* 47: 614–619. https://doi.org/10.1111/j.1440-1754.2011.02165.x.

Bitan, Menachem, Suzanna M. van Walraven, Nina Worel, et al. 2016. Determination of eligibility in related pediatric hematopoietic cell donors: Ethical and clinical considerations. Recommendations from a working group of the worldwide network for blood and marrow transplantation association. *Biology of Blood and Marrow Transplantation* 22 (96–103). https://doi.org/10.1016/j.bbmt.2015.08.017.

Busch, Lina. 2015a. Zur Entwicklung der Auffassungen der ethischen Problematik der Stammzelltransplantation zwischen Geschwisterkindern in Deutschland seit ihrer Einführung bis heute: Interviews mit Klinikern und Klinikerinnen und die Regulierungsdiskussion. Med. Diss. Universität zu Lübeck.

———. 2015b. Geschwisterspender oder Fremdspender: Wer zuerst? – Diskrepanzen zwischen Gewebegesetz und klinischer Praxis hinsichtlich der Knochenmarkspende nichteinwilligungsfähiger Minderjähriger. In *Rettende Geschwister. Ethische Aspekte der Einwilligung in der pädiatrischen Stammzelltransplantation,* ed. Christina Schües and Christoph Rehmann-Sutter, 149–166. Paderborn: Mentis.

EBMT (European Group for Blood and Morrow Transplantation). 2019. *EBMT Transplant Activity Survey 2018,* 38–40. The Netherlands.

Eisner, M., and C.S. August. 1995. Impact of donor and recipient characteristics on the development of acute and chronic graft-versus-host disease following pediatric bone marrow transplantation. *Bone Marrow Transplantation* 15: 663–668.

Forman, Edwin N., and Rosalind Ekman Ladd. 1991. *Ethical dilemmas in pediatric: A case study approach.* New York: Springer.

Herzog, Madeleine, Martina Jürgensen, Christoph Rehmann-Sutter, and Christina Schües. 2019. Interviewers as intruders? Ethical explorations of joint family interviews. *Journal of Empirical Research on Human Research Ethics. Special Issue: Research Ethics in Empirical Ethics Studies: Case Studies and Commentaries* 14 (5): 458–471. https://doi.org/10.1177/1556264619857856.

Hoag, Jennifer, Eva Igler, Jeffrey Karst, Kristin Bingen, and Mary Jo Kupst. 2019. Decisionmaking, knowledge, and psychosocial outcomes in pediatric siblings identified to donate hematopoietic stem cells. *Journal of Psychosocial Oncology* 37 (3): 367–382. https://doi.org/10.108 0/07347332.2018.1489443.

Hogle, Linda. 1996. Transforming body parts into therapeutic tools: A report from Germany. *Medical Anthropology Quarterly* 10 (4): 675–682.

Joffe, Steven. 2011. Protecting the rights and interests of pediatric stem cell donors. *Pediatric Blood Cancer* 56: 517–519.

Kazak, Anne E., et al. 2019. A psychosocial clinical care pathway for pediatric hematopoietic stem cell transplantation. *Pediatric Blood & Cancer* 2019 (66): e27889.

Kesselheim, Jennifer C., et al. 2009. Is blood thicker than water? Ethics of hematopoietic stem cell donation by biological siblings of adopted children. *Archives of Pediatric and Adolescent Medicine* 163 (5): 413–416.

Kline, Ronald M., ed. 2006. *Pediatric hematopoietic stem cell transplantation*. New York: Informa Healthcare.

Lock, Margaret, and Megan Crowley-Makota. 2008. Situating the practice of organ donation in familial, cultural, and political context. *Transplantation Reviews* 22: 154–157.

Miano, Maurizio, Giorgio Dini, M. Labopin, O. Hartmann, Emanuele Angelucci, Jacqueline Cornish, Eliane Gluckman, Franco Locatelli, A. Fischer, R.M. Egeler, Reuven Or, Christina Peters, Junior Fabian Ortega, Paul Veys, P. Bordigoni, A.P. Iori, D. Niethammer, and Valdinar Rocha (for the Paediatric Diseases Working Party of the European Group for Blood and Marrow Transplantation). 2007. Haematopoietic stem cell transplantation trends in children over the last three decades: A survey by the paediatric diseases working party of the European group for blood and marrow transplantation. *Bone Marrow Transplantation* 39: 89–99.

Moos, Thorsten, Christoph Rehmann-Sutter, and Christina Schües. (eds.) 2016. Randzonen des Willens. *Entscheidung und Einwilligung in Grenzsituationen der Medizin*. Frankfurt/M.: Peter Lang (Open access).

Müller, Ingo. 2015. Klinische Praxis – Spenderfindung und Stammzelltransplantation. In *Rettende Geschwister. Ethische Aspekte der Einwilligung in der pädiatrischen Stammzelltransplantation*, ed. Christina Schües and Christoph Rehmann-Sutter. Paderborn: Mentis: 25–32.

Nuffield Council on Bioethics: Give and take? Human bodies in medicine and research. Consultation paper (2010).

Opel, Diekema. 2006. The case of a.R.: The ethics of sibling donor bone marrow transplantation revisited. *The Journal of Clinical Ethics* 17 (3): 207–219.

Packman, Wendy, Mary R. Crittenden, Jodie B. Rieger, Evonne Schaeffer Fischer, Bruce Bongar, and Morton J. Cowan. 1997. Siblings' perceptions of the bone marrow transplantation process. *Journal of Psychosocial Oncology* 15 (3/4): 81–105.

Packman, Wendy, Kimberly Gong, Kelly VanZutphen, Tani Shaffer, and Mary Crittenden. 2004. Psychosocial adjustment of adolescent siblings of hematopoietic stem cell transplant patients. *Journal of Pediatric Oncology Nursing* 21 (4): 233–248.

Parmar, Gurpreet, John W.Y. Wu, and Ka Wah Chan. 2003. Bone marrow donation in childhood: One donor's perspective. *Psycho-Oncology* 12: 91–94.

Pentz, Rebecca D., et al. 2004. Designing an ethical policy for bone marrow donation by minors and others lacking capacity. *Cambridge Quarterly of Healthcare Ethics* 13: 149–155.

———. 2008. The ethical justification for minor sibling bone marrow donation, a case study. *The Oncologist* 13: 148–151.

———. 2014. Unmet needs of siblings of pediatric stem cell transplant recipients. *Pediatrics* 133: e1156–e1162.

Raz, Aviad, Christina Schües, Nadja Wilhelm, and Christoph Rehmann-Sutter. 2017. Saving or subordinating life? Popular views in Israel and Germany of donor siblings created through PGD. *The Journal of Medical Humanities* 38: 191–207. https://doi.org/10.1007/s10912-016-9388-2.

Rehmann-Sutter, Christoph, and Christina Schües. 2015. Retterkinder. In *Rettung und Erlösung. Politisches und religiöses Heil in der Moderne*, ed. Johannes F. Lehmann and Hubert Thüring, 79–98. Fink: München.

Rehmann-Sutter, Christoph, Sarah Daubitz, and Christina Schües. 2013. Spender gefunden, alles klar! Ethische Aspekte des HLA-Tests bei Kindern im Kontext der Stammzelltransplantation. *Bioethica Forum* 6: 89–96.

Rieken, Sarah. 2020. (b. Daubitz): Wahrnehmungen und Erfahrungen von Eltern nach einer hämatopoietischen Stammzellspende ihres Kindes an ein Geschwister. Med. Diss. Universität zu Lübeck.

Ross, Lainie Friedman. 2006. A compounding of errors, the case of bone marrow donation between non-intimate siblings. *The Journal of Clinical Ethics* 17 (3): 220–226.

———. 2009. The ethics of hematopoietic stem cell donation by minors. *Archives of Pediatrics and Adolescent Medicine* 163 (11): 1065–1066.

———. 2012. My sibling's keeper, what are the ethical issues surrounding participation of minors as hematopoietic stem cell donors? *AAP News* 31 (2): 1.

Sanders, Jean E., et al. 1987. Experience with marrow harvesting from donors less than two years of age. *Bone Marrow Transplantation* 2: 45–50.

Schmidt-Recla, Adrian. 2009. Kontraindikation und Kindeswohl, die "zulässige" Knochenmarkspende durch kinder. *GesR* 11: 566–572.

Schües, Christina. 2013. Kindeswohl. In *Wörterbuch der Würde*, ed. Rolf Gröschner, Antje Kapust, and Oliver Lembcke, 354–355. Munich: Fink.

———. 2016. Epistemic injustice and the children's well-being. In *Justice, education and the politics of childhood*, ed. Johannes Drerup, Gunter Graf, Christoph Schickhardt, and Gottfried Schweiger, 155–170. Berlin: Springer.

Schües, Christina, and Christoph Rehmann-Sutter. 2013a. Hat ein Kind eine Pflicht, Blutstammzellen für ein krankes Geschwisterkind zu spenden? *Ethik Med* 25 (2): 89–102. https://doi.org/10.1007/s00481-012-0202-z.

———. 2013b. The well- and unwell-being of a child. *Topoi* 32: 197–205. https://doi.org/10.1007/s11245-013-9157-z. (Open access).

———. 2014. Retrospektive Zustimmung der Kinder? Ethische Aspekte der Stammzellentransplantation. *Frühe Kindheit*, 2: 22–27.

———, eds. 2015. *Rettende Geschwister. Ethische Aspekte der Einwilligung in der pädiatrischen Stammzelltransplantation*. Paderborn: Mentis.

———. 2016. Saranno poi d'accordo, loro, con quanto accaduto? *Rivista per le Medical Humanities* 10 (35): 30–36.

———. 2017. Has a child a duty to donate hematopoietic stem cells to a sibling? In *Ethics and oncology. New issues of therapy, care and research*, ed. Monika Bobbert, Beate Herrmann, and Wolfgang U. Eckart, 81–100. Freiburg/Munich: Alber.

SIMTR – Center for International Blood & Marrow Transplant Research: Summary Slides 2019 – HCT Trends and Survival Data. https://www.cibmtr.org/ReferenceCenter/SlidesReports/SummarySlides/pages/index.aspx. Accessed 7 November 2020.

Switzer, Galen E., Mary Amanda Dew, Victoria A. Butterworth, et al. 1997. Understanding donors' motivation: A study of unrelated bone marrow donors. *Social Science & Medicine*: 137–141.

TPG (Transplantation Gesetz). 1997. *Gesetz über die Spende, Entnahme und Übertragung von Organen*, 2631–2639. Bundesgesetzblattt Teil 1. Nr. 74. Ausgegeben 11. November 1997. Bonn.

Weil, Claude. 1984. Review of results in organ and bone-marrow transplantation in man. *Medicinal Research Reviews* 4 (2): 221–265.

Weisz, Victoria, and Jennifer K. Robbennolt. 1996. Risks and benefits of pediatric bone marrow donation: A critical need for research. *Behavioral Sciences & the Law* 14: 375–391.

Wiener, Lori S., Emilie Steffen-Smith, Terry Fry, and Alan S. Wayne. 2007. Hematopoietic stem cell donation in children: A review of the sibling experience. *Journal of Psychosocial Oncology* 25 (1): 45–66.

Yeşilipek, Mehmet Akif. 2014. Hematopoietic stem cell transplantation in children. *Turk Pediatri Ars.* 49 (2): 91–98. www.turkpediatriarsivi.com.

Open Access   This chapter is licensed under the terms of the Creative Commons Attribution 4.0 International License (http://creativecommons.org/licenses/by/4.0/), which permits use, sharing, adaptation, distribution and reproduction in any medium or format, as long as you give appropriate credit to the original author(s) and the source, provide a link to the Creative Commons license and indicate if changes were made.

The images or other third party material in this chapter are included in the chapter's Creative Commons license, unless indicated otherwise in a credit line to the material. If material is not included in the chapter's Creative Commons license and your intended use is not permitted by statutory regulation or exceeds the permitted use, you will need to obtain permission directly from the copyright holder.

Chapter 2
A Donor by Coincidence
or by Conception – *My Sister's Keeper*
Revisited

Christoph Rehmann-Sutter and Christina Schües

Abstract Thirteen-year-old Anna Fitzgerald has been conceived in order to be a matching donor for her older sister Kate, who has a rare form of leukaemia. The story in the novel "My Sister's Keeper" by Jody Picoult, and Nick Cassavetes' movie, has many striking similarities to the situations that we heard from the families we studied – despite one significant difference: Anna is created to be a saviour sibling, whereas the stem cell donors we interviewed already existed and were found to be matching. We discuss the film as an emotionally complex, multi-layered narrative that gives insight into the perspectives of different family members and into some key aspects of a paradigmatic family conflict. The temporal order of the film's story-telling using multiple flash-backs and retakes represents the entangled temporalities of experience and memory.

Keywords Film · Movies · Bioethics in movies · Saviour siblings · Organ donation · Bone marrow transplantation · Child · Child's well-being · Family narrative

> Campbell Alexander: Well, no one can force you to donate if you don't want to, can they?
> Anna Fitzgerald: They think they can. I'm under 18, they're my legal guardians.
> Campbell Alexander: They can't do that.
> Anna Fitzgerald: Well, that's I want you to tell them, because they've been doing it to me my whole life. I wouldn't even be alive if Kate wasn't sick. I'm a designer baby. I was made in a dish to be spare parts for Kate.[1]

The novel and the movie *My Sister's Keeper* (Picoult 2004; Cassavetes 2009) tell the heart-wrenching story of Anna Fitzgerald, a 13-year-old girl who was conceived to be a bone-marrow match for her older sister Kate, who suffers from a rare form

---

[1] Scene from the movie, at minute 7.

C. Rehmann-Sutter (✉) · C. Schües
Institute for History of Medicine and Science Studies, University of Lübeck,
Lübeck, Schleswig-Holstein, Germany
e-mail: christoph.rehmannsutter@uni-luebeck.de; c.schuees@uni-luebeck.de

© The Author(s) 2022
C. Schües et al. (eds.), *Stem Cell Transplantations Between Siblings as Social Phenomena*, Philosophy and Medicine 144,
https://doi.org/10.1007/978-3-031-04166-2_2

of leukaemia. This story is a showcase for the bioethical question: Should it be permissible to conceive a child using pre-implantation genetic diagnosis and selection for the purpose of generating body parts to treat a sibling with cancer?[2] But it is also so much more: an exemplar of family dynamics associated with sickness and treatment of one child in a family, and the possibility for one other sibling to help out with stem cells from her or his own body. All family members are affected, and so are their relationships. But how they are affected and the moral position they take are the issues unfolded as the story develops.

In the story, Kate had been diagnosed with acute promyelocytic leukaemia (APL) at the age of two and desperately needed a stem cell transplant. Her brother was not a match, and nor were the parents, and no unrelated donor of hematopoietic stem cells could be found. Chances to save Kate's life were fading, so the parents decided to use a novel and dramatic biotechnological procedure: pre-implantation genetic selection to find an embryo who would be a perfect match for Kate. A matching embryo is then chosen: Anna. However, blood stem cells from her umbilical cord do not work, so leukocytes, lymphocytes and bone marrow are taken from her as a little child. But Kate's cancer recurs, and her sister Anna is finally expected to donate one of her kidneys. In this situation she chooses to sue her parents for the rights to her own body. Campbell Alexander is her lawyer, representing her in court and supporting her against her parents' plan to use her as a kidney donor.

The story depicts the struggle all the members of the Fitzgerald family face, especially Anna's battle between loyalty to her dying sister and her rights to her own body (Bonk 2008; Elfarra 2018). However, it consistently avoids the individualistic stereotype of "leave me alone, my body is my own". In a surprise turn towards the end of the movie and book, we learn that Anna does not defend her individual rights to her own body *against Kate's* needs but acts in solidarity with Kate's own wishes to end being trapped in a horrific clinical odyssey that has become increasingly troublesome and burdening for her.

Superimposed on the tension between altruistic donation and the right to one's own body in this story is the conflict between two different aspects of care. One aspect is represented by the mother Sara, who organizes the family in order to obtain the stem cells as a remedy for Kate. The other is represented by Anna, who knows about Kate's deeply felt therapeutic fatigue and unwillingness to undergo further surgery. This makes the movie and the novel especially relevant and interesting for the topic of our book – despite the difference that the families in our Lübeck study did *not* conceive their donor children by IVF and did *not* select an embryo by pre-implantation genetic selection. The donors in our study were children who had already been born and *became donors by coincidence*, first, because they were a sibling and second, because their inherited HLA pattern happened to be identical to the patient.

---

[2] Vandenhouten and Groessl (2014); Trifolis (2014); Prendergast (2008). The reception of the film was also sensitive to the topic of "saviour siblings", a practice that is allowed in Israel but banned in Germany (see Raz et al. 2017). For a discussion of the ethical issues of saviour siblings see Rehmann-Sutter and Schües (2015).

2.1   Inspirations for a Multi-layered Narrative

The title "My Sister's Keeper", used for both the novel[3] and the movie after the book is certainly a biblical allusion to Genesis 4:9 – the story of Cain and Abel. We see, however, that this narrative reference does not play any role in either the novel or the film. It is a catchphrase that makes the story recognizable (and perhaps helps to sell the book and the movie). But it indicates a completely different context – a drama of jealousy, murder and guilt that is far removed from the contents of Anna Fitzgerald's story. We remember what is at the centre of this biblical text: after having murdered his brother, Cain is questioned by the Lord: "Where *is* Abel, your brother?" He then replies with a blatant lie: "I do not know," adding a remarkable counter-question: "*Am* I my brother's keeper?"[4] Cain's answer is evasive, and, given his acts and the situation, outright scandalous. The Lord was of course aware of what had happened ("The voice of your brother's blood cries out to me from the ground" Gen 4:10) and banishes Cain to a life of wandering. He protects Cain against revenge and violence by setting a mark upon him so that whoever found him will not slay him. Cain then dwells in the land of Nod, builds the city Enoch, and his wife and he have children.

In *My Sister's Keeper* we learn that Anna Fitzgerald rejects being her sister's keeper, by refusing to donate her kidney and by enforcing her decision in court. Despite this, Anna is her sister's keeper in daily life, but in a way that is resolved rather late in the film, She is her closest confidante and ally who helps her to carry through her wishes within the family. Conceptually, Anna was conceived in order to be a stem cell donor for Kate. In contrast to Cain, who was Abel's older brother, Anna was the younger sister, born with the plan to be a keeper and saviour for Kate. For Anna, this was a heavy burden that made it even more difficult to exercise her own will. By refusing to be a kidney donor, she would not only become responsible for Kate's death but would also counteract her parents' benevolent plans. She is charged with guilt herself, but would also face being viewed as guilty by others. Does she want to have a future life where others see her as a person whose body is a remedy for her sister? Is the duty to donate inscribed into her body, into her person (Schües 2017)?

There are two inspirations for Picoult's story that are more pertinent. (i) In an interview Picoult discloses a personal experience behind the novel: her youngest son Jake had a tumour in his left ear. It was benign; however, "it can get to the brain and kill you… so you've got to get rid of it. We took an experimental approach that required multiple surgeries" — 13 of them. "Had we used a more traditional approach, Jake would have been profoundly deaf."[5] Having accompanied the 5-year-old child through many operations, Picoult realized how much she was willing to do for her boy, even though he was not in a life-threatening situation. But the questions

---

[3] The German translation runs with the title "Beim Leben meiner Schwester", thus losing the biblical allusion.

[4] New King James Version.

[5] https://www.jodipicoult.com/my-sisters-keeper.html (last visited on 27 Oct. 2020).

about what it means to be a good parent, a good sister, and a good person stayed with her. Taken to the extreme, she took one question to be the guiding theme of the book: Is it morally correct to do whatever it takes to save a child's life?

From this experience she learned that it was not only Jake who was touched by the diagnosis and the treatments. The whole family was affected and its dynamics changed – by the diagnosis, the anxiety, the complicated surgeries, the sudden over-whelming importance of medicine for family life, the care relationships and so forth. "When one child gets sick, the whole family does." (Picoult 2015) As she explains, this experience provided her with a narrative perspective for writing the novel about Anna and Kate as well. She tried to tell the story from the point of view of all family members, not only the patient's and the donor's perspectives, but that of the other family members as well.

(ii) Following on from this question, she took further inspiration from a real case, which was highly publicized in the USA at the time: the story of the Nash family (Faison 2005; Hendrickson 2017). Lisa and Jack Nash found themselves at the mercy of a controversial medical procedure to save the life of their daughter Molly, who had Fanconi anaemia. They conceived Adam by IVF and PGD, to avoid the Fanconi gene and also to be able to use cord blood from the placenta. Adam Nash was born in 2000 to treat 6-year-old Molly. The media referred to him as the first "designer baby" (Franklin and Roberts 2006).

The Nash family certainly found this international media hype, with the implied questioning of their morality, difficult to endure. And Picoult's story did not intend to do justice to the Nashes. Besides, Molly could be treated without taking cells from Adam's body. For the situation of the family this certainly makes a big differ-ence. Other complications that were much more burdening for Adam and Molly, such as long-term dependence on tube feeding, are specific to Fanconi and do not appear in Picoult's scenario. In comparison with this real-life example, the novel and film both use the means of dramaturgic exaggeration, in order to highlight a dilemma: not only cord blood was donated, but also bone marrow, leukocytes and lymphocytes, and finally Anna was asked for a kidney. The novel (in contrast to the movie) has even a more dramatic turn at the end, when Anna's lawyer Campbell Alexander, driving with Anna after their success in court, is involved in a severe car crash. Anna is declared brain dead and becomes a postmortem kidney donor for Kate. In this respect Picoult's scenario does not attempt to be realistic, although representing one not very probable but still *possible escalation* (and complication) of the course of events.

Anna and Kate's story is in the centre of the play. They question each other and help each other to make sense of the events. The Nashes' story provides a real-world reference and shows how far people would go even when the situation is not about survival. The bioethical debates that were conducted in their names provide a back-ground of moral questions. The author's own son Jake's story provides a whole-family perspective on the illness and treatment of one child. All family members are affected by the child's sickness, and throughout the treatment their emotional involvement changes. The multi-layered narrative is a method for Picoult as an author to show different dimensions of meanings manifest in the family; it is therefore also a method of analysis for us as interpreters. Like the family in the film, the families in the interviews we conducted, where the members talked openly and listened to each other, also relied on a multi-layered narrative in order to understand difficult situations. The different perspectives can be used as examples that can be compared and evaluated for the given situation. The interviewees tried to make sense of and find their own story by way of other stories they knew. Or they used a collective imaginary, for instance that of the "lottery" where you can win, or of the "hero" or "saviour". Using such images and narrative tropes that seemed to be meaningful for them, interviewees tried to identify themselves and other family members with certain roles and situated the family in a complex relationality that is not in ones individual's hands.

In the analysis below, we refer to the film version of *My Sister's Keeper*, directed by Nick Cassavetes (USA 2009). It closely follows the plot of the novel – with one important exception, as already mentioned: the ending with the car crash and the postmortem kidney donation is left out. The movie ends with Kate's mother Sara finally accepting that a kidney transplant cannot happen. In the horizon where Kate and Anna have had their desires, Sara learns that she needs to let her daughter go.

2.2   Dynamic Family Perspectives

Focusing on the movie's description of the changes in family dynamics unleashed by Kate's illness and its treatment, we can distinguish three main phases.

The first phase – told in brief flashbacks, mainly in the words of mother Sara – starts with Kate becoming ill and ends with the birth of Anna. Little Kate is diagnosed with a rare form of leukaemia: this changes everything in the family. Kate's cancer is a threat to her life. The Fitzgeralds and Kate's physicians try everything possible to fight this disease but the chances fade away. Soon her only option would be a transplant of stem cells that could rebuild her damaged immune system. However, her parents and brother Jesse are not an HLA match and are therefore unable to donate. Kate's oncologist (Dr Chance) tells the parents Sara and Brian that there is one ultimate possibility, innovative but not illegal: to have another child and to make sure that it will be a 100% HLA match and a donor for cord blood. Sara immediately takes this up (Sara: "We got to do it, we got to try" Min. 14). Bearing another child is something Sara *can* do. It is in her power. With the support of modern biotechnology, the birth of this child will create an opportunity to generate healing cells for Kate. They only procedure they have talked about is using the blood from the umbilical cord, something Anna would not need once she is born, and that would otherwise be discarded.

In the second phase, Sara is the organizer of everything in the family, trying to create the best possible situation for the medical support of Kate. Both parents, however, love Anna and her elder brother Jesse as well.

The cells from the umbilical cord are used but they cannot hold back the cancer for long. They try with lymphocytes taken from Anna's blood when Anna is 5 years old, and then one year later, granulocytes, again from Anna's blood. And then a bone marrow transplant. After the bone marrow aspiration there is a complication and Anna has to be hospitalized for 6 days.

Later, doubts arise. At one point, father Brian recalls the scene when he had to hold Anna, a desperately crying, kicking and struggling little girl, down on the operating table using his whole body power until she was sedated: "Have we really pushed her too hard? … She was so little when all this started" (Min. 19). Brian, a firefighter by profession, is not as intellectual as Sara, who is a lawyer. He supports all the necessary decisions to fight for Kate's life but has a better and more balanced sense of the different feelings, needs and desires. He often just watches his children without saying much, resonating with his children's feelings. Picoult gave him the profession of a fireman and the interest in astronomy. A fireman is there to help people in a state of crisis and destruction, while astronomy is there for a scientific understanding of the positions, movements and characteristics of objects, stares, matter and radiation in the universe. A reference to Immanuel Kant's saying might help us to understand the role of the father: "Two things fill the mind with ever new and increasing admiration and reverence, the more frequently and persistently one's meditation deals with them: the starry sky above me and the moral law within me." (Kant 2002, 203) It is Brian's role to explore the moral constellations and to link them with the particular situation and position of one person. He realizes that the family is at risk of falling apart if only one perspective and one driving force prevails. Sara is the one who has such active driving force, at least in this phase of the story.

Sara's conviction that she can and must somehow save her older daughter leads her into a presumptuous attitude that she fails to ask or notice what either of her daughters actually want. Anna is regarded as a bodily remedy for her sister and a sacrifice for her mother's refusal to withdraw from her path of opting for the removal of Anna's kidney. Removing a kidney, Anna knows, is a serious operation that has long-lasting effect.

On an emotional level, Sara's care for her endangered child goes so far as to help Kate to get out of a depressive phase (Kate: "I am sick and I am tired and I am ugly" (Min. 22)) by shaving her own hair in order to look like Kate with a bald head. It works and the family has some more happy moments. Later, when Kate realizes that her end is near, she talks openly with Dr. Chance about palliative care options. Seeing that, Sara shouts at Kate: "Listen. I don't want to hear talk like that, okay, honey. You just stay strong enough for surgery!" (Min. 38). She is in denial of the situation and keeps believing that a kidney transplant could save Kate – with Anna as the donor, of course.

In this phase of the family dynamic, Jesse goes more and more off the rails. He starts having problems at school and is sent away from the family for a whole year to a special school to learn maths, a decision he accepts in tears, understanding that it is a necessary sacrifice. He plays a desperate role in the story, setting fire to things, and even watching the crises from afar and knowing that his father is part of the crew battling the flames that he has caused. Unable to help, and not being given any attention himself, he becomes involved with fire for creation and destruction, for despair and reason. Kate sees this and is sorry to have taken all the attention when Jesse needed it most (Kate: "They barely even noticed that Jesse was dyslexic" Min. 25). Nevertheless Jesse loves Kate; at one point he brings her a beautiful watercolour portrait of her that he has painted.

At the point when it is decided that she should donate her kidney, Anna starts to act on her own. She refuses to be a donor ("I don't want to do it any more, Mom" Min. 15). This action of Anna's turns the plot around. She now becomes the protagonist of the story, as she introduced herself right at the beginning of the film as "a designer baby" (Min. 7) who wants to sue her parents because they want to make her a kidney donor against her will. She finds a well-known lawyer (Campbell Alexander) with an advertised "91% success rate" in court, and mandates him as guardian *ad litem* to sue her parents for her right to refuse a live organ donation, which involves a limited termination of parental rights.

This move by Anna – the start of a third phase in the family drama – creates an additional tension for the other family members and also for the film audience: How could the 11-year-old Anna, who loves Kate so much, refuse to donate and sue her parents for her personal rights to decide about her own body? One part of her motif is easily understandable: she does need her own kidney, and she has suffered enough already (8 hospitalizations in 11 years, 6 catheterizations, 2 bone marrow aspirations, 2 stem cell purgations, and the necessary accompanying drugs with their side effects, as Campbell Alexander enumerates them in his plea). She does not want to "be careful" in her life and she wants to have children herself, all of which could be problematic with only one kidney. But is that sufficient to explain her emphatic demand and her willingness to stand for her rights in court – against her parents?

In the same period Kate's health deteriorates; she realizes that she is going to die (Kate: "I am ok with it. … I don't mind my disease killing me. But it's killing my family too" Min. 24). It is also the time of Kate's love story with the fellow terminal cancer patient Taylor, which revives her. After some intimate moments, when they run away from the prom party, Taylor dies and leaves Kate devastated.

Jesse's situation deteriorates as well. He is often seen on the streets in town. Once when he misses the last bus and comes home late in the middle of the night, he tells the audience off-screen, in a narrator's position: "When I got home, I wondered how much trouble I'd been in" (Min. 60). Dad was still up – not worrying about Jesse not yet being at home but because of worrying about Kate. He realizes how far out of his parents' main considerations he is.

The couple Sara and Brian as parents increasingly run into difficulties in their relationship. At one point, when Brian, with support of Dr. Chance, wants to take Kate out of hospital to the beach close to where they live, in order to let her see the Pacific for one last time with Anna and Jesse, Sara shouts: "You are killing her!" He yells: "I want a divorce!" (Min. 65). However, the situation brightens up again after Sara gives way and joins them on the beach, together with her sister Kelly. She sees how Kate enjoys the happy moment in the roar of the ocean waves and the sun. Facing the present moment makes a difference, and again Sara's sister and friend Kelly acts as counsellor, telling her that she does not see the big picture: "Sooner or later, you got to stop. You got to let go" (Min. 62).

During this third phase the family becomes most disconnected, close to breaking point. Brother Jesse comes back into the centre of attention, and of reasoning, when in court he breaks the secret that Kate had asked Anna to refuse to donate her kidney because she, Kate, did not want to go on with the surgeries (Kate said to Anna, asking her to refuse to donate: "You can release me" Min. 82).

Compared to Jesse, Anna, the child born to be a saviour, seems not to be at the weakest end of the family. Campbell Alexander asks Dr. Chance in court: "Can you tell us one single benefit that Anna has received from any of these procedures?" Dr. Chance replies: "Yes, she got to save her sister's life" (Min. 71). Jesse lacks this. His task is to live off the little remaining attention that he can get from his parents, to endure the family crisis without being able to really help, while growing up himself, and not to lose ground during his difficult years. Sara's care for Kate, which takes somewhat extreme forms, is challenged by the other siblings' needs and by her love for all of them. But often she is unable to see these needs at all. At some point she even loses sight of Kate herself as a person, while fighting for her life using all that medicine can offer – against Kate's own struggle and willingness to accept dying, and in this sense, against her family as a whole.

2.3 Entangled Temporalities

The film ends on a sentimental chord. Anna, again resuming her role as main narrator, explains that she does not know why Kate had to die while she, Anna, could live. After Kate is gone, the memories of her are vivid and, as Anna says, "our relationship continues" (Min. 98).

It is noteworthy to see how the film is cut and composed to tell its story and how the multiple narrative layers are intertwined. The film has been criticized for having too many flashbacks that follow emotions and lose sight of reality (Bradshaw 2009). We, however, can see some good sense in this formal choice. There is not a single chronological line that leads through the film. The only part of the story told in chronological order is the court procedure. It extends from the beginning, when the audience hears (from Anna herself as narrator) that Anna is about to sue her parents, to the last minutes of the movie, when Campbell Alexander visits Anna to bring her the documents about the success they finally had in court. The court scenes, the scenes in the lawyer's office, in the office of Judge de Salvo, the judge's visit to Kate in the hospital, and the court sessions themselves are spread throughout the movie – in a straightforward chronological order.

However, the medical procedures, as well as the family stories and the story about Anna and Jesse, are organized by showing flashbacks and by visualising a memory. The family story, and also Kate's story as the patient, are composed of singular stories from different times, partly in the present and partly in the past, filling that present with meanings and depth. They assemble as a *Gestalt* that is temporally construed by moving slowly forward, pulling the characters acting within it, sometimes driving, sometimes being driven by the entangled components of this structure, towards the point of decision about the desperate last attempt of a kidney transplant or palliative care.

How much the memory of earlier viewings of this film can straighten out these temporal curls and wrinkles that make up the screen experience of it! Despite having seen the film at least three or four times, and having used it in academic teaching some years ago, we were both surprised when revisiting the film after a few years for the preparation of this chapter. We remembered the story of Kate and Anna as a much more straight-line story, while the film actually presents it with innumerable temporal folds. This is much closer to how memories are built up while living through difficult situations (Ricoeur 2004).

If this is true, the superposition of temporal layers is also closer to the experiences of the families in our study who have lived through a time of severe illness, care and responsibility. The experience of a slowly but relentlessly forward-moving *Gestalt* of activities and passivities, of decision-making while always remembering and being at the mercy of one's emotions, can be seen as a cinematographic attempt to capture the complex temporal structure of this long-term experience of severe illness and of hope for rescue, of finding the right way forward in a situation that is neither obvious nor morally clear. The film attempts to capture the manifold perspectives that are held by the individual family members. They cannot be interchanged because each person has an existential position based on their particular way of bodily being and their medical, social and familial role within the setting.

2.4 What Can We Learn?

The book and the film have different endings, yet the complexity of the situation remains. In a very convincing way the film gives each person his or her own voice to express concerns or feelings, judgments or values. On a superficial level, we learn that each difficult constellation has more perspectives to it. Since all these different perspectives are uttered in the familial context, the members are challenged to try to understand each other's perspectives. That this is not always easy comes as no surprise. On a deeper level, we can learn that not only is each dimension – the juridical, ethical, familial or medical – controversial, but there may also be tensions between them that cannot be resolved easily.

However, if one aspect is decided in one dimension it will immediately have consequences for another, e.g. allowing children to ask for the help from an attorney can even result in the judge's decision to grant the freedom of decision in medical matters (that children usually do not have). Thus, we may learn that the care for a child's well-being in the medical sphere of difficult decision-making (as we have seen with stem cell transplants) should also include an attorney who juridically consults with the child and who may protect her from the unwarranted demands of parents or doctors.

The film (and the book) grants an insight into a complex moral setting. If we viewed it as just a moral setting, we would reduce it to an unfounded moral dilemma.

However, if such a moral setting is seen as a juridical, ethical, familial, medical and temporal setting, then there may be a chance to deal with this situation in a way that later admits, retrospectively, that the decisions and the actions were undertaken in an appropriate way (Schües and Rehmann-Sutter 2014). A morally difficult situation is always temporally situated and challenged by the power of time. The medical decision often has to be taken "now"; there is no time for deliberation or consultation with each other. The temporal entanglement of the family members does not end with a decision, but provides a framework to prospectively and retrospectively care and carry responsibility for the family and its members – the parents and the children. Nonetheless, a book or a film would not be a piece of fiction mirroring insight into reality without using metaphors, exaggerations, clues and hints to guide the viewer on the path of concern for the ties of a family.

Literature

Bonk, Kiley. 2008. Minors as living organ donors: Protecting minors from martyrdom. *Children's Legal Rights Journal* 28 (1): 45–52.

Bradshaw, Peter. 2009. My Sister's keeper (film review). *The Guardian*. 26 June 2009.

Cassavetes, Nick, dir. 2009. My Sister's keeper. Curmudgeon Films, Gran Via Productions & Mark Johnson Productions, USA.

Elfarra, Ayah. 2018. My Sister's keeper: Compelled donations and a Minor's rights to their own body. *Children's Legal Rights Journal* 38 (2): 160–164.

Faison, Amanda M. 2005. The miracle of Molly. 5280 Denver's High Mile Magazine, 1 August 2005. Retrieved from: https://www.5280.com/2005/08/the-miracle-of-molly/. Accessed 28 July 2020.

Franklin, Sarah, and Celia Roberts. 2006. *Born and made*. An ethnography of preimplantation genetic diagnosis. Princeton: Princeton University Press.

Hendrickson, Molly. 2017. 17 years later, Nash family opens up about controversial decision to safe dying daughter. *The Denver Channel* 14 November 2017. Retrieved from: https://www.thedenverchannel.com/news/local-news/17-years-later-nash-family-opens-up-about-controversial-decision-to-save-dying-daughter. Accessed 28 July 2020.

Kant, Immanuel. 2002. *The critique of practical reason*. Translated by Werner Pluhar. Indianapolis: Hackett Publisher.

Picoult, Jodi. 2004. *My sister's keeper*. New York: Atna Books.

———. 2015. The story behind my Sister's keeper. Audio podcast on https://www.jodipicoult.com/my-sisters-keeper.html. Retrieved 28 July 2020.

Prendergast, Elizabeth. 2008. Book review: *My Sister's keeper* – A view of the genetics debate at a personal level. *Children's Legal Rights Journal* 28 (1): 68–70.

Raz, Aviad, Christina Schües, Nadja Wilhelm, and Christoph Rehmann-Sutter. 2017. Saving or subordinating life? Popular views in Israel and Germany of donor siblings created through PGD. *Journal of Medical Humanities* 38 (2): 191–207.

Rehmann-Sutter, Christoph, and Christina Schües. 2015. Retterkinder. In *Rettung und Erlösung. Politisches und religiöses Heil in der Moderne*, ed. Johannes F. Lehmann and Hubert Thüring, 79–98. München: Fink.

Ricoeur, Paul. 2004. *Memory, history, forgetting*. Translated by Kathleen blamey and David Pellauer. Chicago/London: University of Chicago Press.

Schües, Christina. 2017. The Trans-human paradigm and the meaning of life. In *Future Directions in Feminist Phenomenology*, ed. H. Fielding and D. Olkowski, 218–241. Bloomington: Indiana University Press.

Schües, Christina, and Christoph Rehmann-Sutter. 2014. Retrospektive Zustimmung der Kinder? Ethische Aspekte der Stammzellentransplantation. *Frühe Kindheit* 2: 22–27.

Trifolis, Kristie Lauren. 2014. Savior siblings: The ethical debate. *Law school student scholarship*. 432. Retrieved from: https://scholarship.shu.edu/student_scholarship/432/. Accessed 30 July 2020.

Vandenhouten, Christine L., and Joan Groessl. 2014. My Sister's keeper: An innovative interprofessional ethics teaching and learning strategy for nursing and social work students. Health and Interprofessional. *Practice* 2 (2): eP1055. 1–12.

Open Access   This chapter is licensed under the terms of the Creative Commons Attribution 4.0 International License (http://creativecommons.org/licenses/by/4.0/), which permits use, sharing, adaptation, distribution and reproduction in any medium or format, as long as you give appropriate credit to the original author(s) and the source, provide a link to the Creative Commons license and indicate if changes were made.

The images or other third party material in this chapter are included in the chapter's Creative Commons license, unless indicated otherwise in a credit line to the material. If material is not included in the chapter's Creative Commons license and your intended use is not permitted by statutory regulation or exceeds the permitted use, you will need to obtain permission directly from the copyright holder.

Chapter 3
Dimensions and Tensions of the Child's Well-Being and Stem Cell Transplantation: A Conceptual Analysis

Christina Schües

Abstract The concepts of the child's well-being and the child's best interests are both central to medical practice concerning children. Such concepts become particularly crucial when a healthy child becomes a stem cell donor for her sick sibling. The concept of the child's well-being inheres a tension between her well-being and her will, her present and future well-being, and the child's individual well-being and that of the family as a whole. In this essay, I first unfold some key juridical, ethical and philosophical aspects of the concept of the child's well-being; second, I discuss decision making in the medical realm, asking about the characteristics of the child's will, the tension generated between the child's will and well-being, and the stages of decision-making; and third, I refer to the perspective of temporality, which shifts the tragic problem to an open field that can keep those affected (i.e. the donor child, the recipient, and last but not least the whole family) in communication with one another. The internal relationships of the child's well-being need to be seen in the context of the whole family's well-being.

Keywords Concept of child's well-being · Child's best interest · Stages of decision-making · Rights of the child · UN-declaration on the rights of the child · Law · Temporal structure · Norms · Family · Child's will

In the situation of bone marrow transplantation between children, the aims of medical treatment and of child care are threefold. One aim is to ensure the well-being of the sick child being helped towards recovery; another concerns the well-being of the child whose stem cells are taken in a medically unindicated intervention, for the benefit and well-being of her sick sibling; and a third is directed towards the well-being of the family so that it can remain stable, caring and loving for all its members. In the context of paediatric stem cell transplantation between siblings, two

C. Schües (✉)
Institute for History of Medicine and Science Studies, University of Lübeck, Lübeck, Schleswig-Holstein, Germany
e-mail: c.schuees@uni-luebeck.de

© The Author(s) 2022
C. Schües et al. (eds.), *Stem Cell Transplantations Between Siblings as Social Phenomena*, Philosophy and Medicine 144,
https://doi.org/10.1007/978-3-031-04166-2_3

conceptual tensions are central: the child's well-being and her will on the one hand, and the well-being of the child and the well-being of her family, on the other. This essay focuses on the well-being of the child whose body material has been given to her sibling.

The concept of a child's well-being is rarely used in the language of everyday life. Care for a child is not usually done *because* of the concern for the child's well-being in the juridical and moral sense; in concrete terms, the daily meal is not served with regard to well-being. However, in times of crisis or in situations that endanger a child, the concept of the child's well-being is applied as guidance. When a child suffers or is threatened by injury, violence, mistreatment or injustice, the question of her well-being is posed because of her endangerment (Schües 2016). Thus, the concept of well-being belongs to and is used in situations of crisis. It concerns the vulnerability of the child, her development and her need for protection.

The *United Nations Convention on the Rights of the Child* (1989) considers the will of the child as a central aspect of the child's well-being. While the Convention regards the centrality of the child's well-being in general, this essay concretely focuses on the role of the donor child's will and questions how it can be brought to bear within medical practice and its social and familial context. The question this essay poses is not simply whether or how a child who is unable to consent should participate in the decision-making process. Rather, it is a matter of discussing how the regard and respect for the child's will can be considered in relation to the child's well-being. It is possible that stem cell donation between siblings may prove to be a practice in which both respect and disregard for the child's will lead to a conflictual situation that I would call a tragedy.[1] We generally see that if one member of the family is not well, the other members, or even the family as a whole, are affected.

In this essay, first, I unfold some key juridical, ethical and philosophical aspects of the concept of the child's well-being; second, I discuss decision-making in the medical realm, asking about the characteristics of the child's will, the tragic relationships between the child's will and well-being, and stages of decision-making; and third, I refer to the perspective of temporality, which shifts the *tragic* problem to an open field that may keep those affected (i.e. donor child, recipient, and last but not least the whole family) in communication with one another. The internal relationships of the child's well-being need to be seen in the context of the family's well-being.

The introduction of the concepts of a child's "well-being" and "best interests" in juridical, political and ethical contexts – roughly a hundred years ago – represents a shift from disregard to regard (Invernizzi and Williams 2011; Alderson 2008; German Civil Code 1900). In the early twentieth century, the child's well-being was mostly considered in the context of child abuse, or neglect and violence in the family. Its introduction into medical practice happened later and is widely discussed today (Wiesemann et al. 2003; Wiesemann 2016; Schües and Rehmann-Sutter 2013b).

---

[1] I discuss aspects of the concept of "donation" in this volume, Chap. 15 on intercorporeality.

A stem cell transplant may be recommended if a child is seriously ill, for example with a disease of the haematopoietic system or leukaemia, and if other suitable treatment is not available. A transplant concerns more than one individual, and holds significance for individuals and for the family as a whole, for whom periods of illness (Chap. 8 in this book) are difficult when the children and the parents have different care needs. Having one child be a donor for another is not an everyday idea. For some families, the donation of body material and the necessary medical intervention seem to be taken for granted as a matter of course; for other families or individuals, on the other hand, the donation and its context are difficult and exceptional. In any case, adult consent is legitimating for the medical intervention of serving as a donor. Children who are minors cannot give final consent. Hence, a stem cell transplant between siblings calls the child's well-being (and best interests) into question; the parents have to care for all their children, while in a strictly moral sense they are entering into the conflict of allowing one child (the donor) to be injured in order to help the other (the recipient) (Schües and Rehmann-Sutter 2015). This constellation needs to be discussed with regard to the concept of the child's well-being, decision-making in medical practice, and family relationships.

3.1   The Child's Well-Being: The Juridical Perspective and Its Normative Foundations

In political, social or ethical discussions, both "child's well-being" and "best interests" are used. Compared to best interests, the notion of well-being is a broader concept and is historically primary, whereas the concept of "best interests" is narrower and was introduced later. The child's well-being encompasses all dimensions relevant to a good life of the child and his or her healthy development, the provision of the will of the child, and its basic needs and rights (Schües and Rehmann-Sutter 2015; Dettenborn 2010; Zitelmann 2001).[2] However, the concept of well-being is vague and hypothetical, and depends on concrete interpretations and evaluations, norms and values in society. The observation that it is somewhat vague or hypothetical does not, however, mean that it is an "empty box" (Steindorff 1994), a "sham" (deceptive packaging, Goldstein et al. 1991), or of no use at all for professional decision-making (Figdor 2009). Rather, I argue that the concept of child's well-being *does have* a normative content and, hence, a guiding function for a minimum standard of care, whether with regard to difficulties in daily life, a situation of crisis, or in a specific medical and familial situation, as we discuss in this book. Nevertheless, the concept of a child's well-being needs to be interpreted in its concrete field of tension between theoretical and practical challenges, as well as within its different tensions with the child's will and the well-being of the family. Generally,

---

[2] Contemporary authors agree that children are not "little adults", hence, the question needs to be debated as to how autonomous children can be taken to be (Büchner 2003, 11–27).

the need to interpret the concept arises out of the plurality of styles of life, cultural customs, or social preferences, which might all be very different yet still compatible with the well-being of the children and their families. And concretely, the need for interpretation also arises out of the observation that medical practices include constellations and challenges that cannot be met by compromizses or different styles of care. Injuring a healthy child for the benefit of a sibling is traditionally and intuitively morally debatable; at least not self-evident or something to be taken for granted.

With regard to recent medical possibilities for treatment, we need to ask for a specific *normative perspective* on childhood and children. Recognizing such a normative perspective means claiming that, first, children are persons and have the status of a subject; hence, they have rights, i.e. parents, other humans and society have obligations towards them (Archard 2018; Wiesemann 2016; Brighouse 2002; O'Neill 1988). Children have a full normative status regardless of their age and competence. Therefore, the concept of well-being includes the idea and practice that children deserve respect (Giesinger 2013). Second, they have a "normative status" that is distinct from adults' (Bagattini 2014). Apart from the observation that rights are formulated especially for children and that they are acknowledged by their particular standards of protection, care and support, several aspects must be delineated to fully understand the child's normative perspective with regard to his or her well-being.

3.1.1 The United Nations Convention on the Rights of the Child

In the twentieth century the child's well-being became an issue in juridical, ethical and social debates. In some respects the *United Nations Convention on the Rights of the Child* (UNCRC 1989) formulates what had already been expressed in the *Geneva Declaration of the Rights of the Child*, adopted 26 September 1924 at the League of Nations: "Men and women of all nations, recognizing that mankind owes to the Child the best that it has to give".[3] This sentence was reworded in 1989 by the

---

[3] Geneva Declaration of the Rights of the Child: Men and women of all nations, recognizing that mankind owes to the Child the best that it has to give, declare and accept it as their duty that, beyond and above all considerations of race, nationality or creed:

1. The child must be given the means requisite for its normal development, both materially and spiritually;
2. The child that is hungry must be fed; the child that is sick must be nursed; the child that is backward must be helped; the delinquent child must be reclaimed; and the orphan and the waif must be sheltered and succored;
3. The child must be the first to receive relief in times of distress;
4. The child must be put in a position to earn a livelihood, and must be protected against every form of exploitation;

UNCRC in terms of the idea that the "best interests of the child shall be a primary consideration".[4] It has been ratified by 193 nations (in 1992 by Germany).

The UNCRC proclaims the priority of the child's well-being and describes it with regard to three different clusters of rights: rights of protection, of development, and of participation. The basic standards of the child's well-being are supported by a short definition of who a child is, by the proclamation of the imperative to realize these rights, by the obligation of the state to inform families and children about the convention, and by the obligation of the state to report to the UN on the measurement of and progress towards the implementation of the child's rights. Hence, the well-being of children contains *normative recognition* of the child as someone who has rights and (by way of the right to participate) as someone whose *will* must be respected.[5] Hence, normatively, this expands both the realm of those who are considered subjects of rights, and the framework and range of obligations on the part of parents, society and states. Such expansion is important for legal as well as ethical debates because it sets relationships – in terms of protection, development and participation – between mature and immature persons as the focus of consideration.

These three areas of rights (protection, development, participation) are subordinated under the general Article 3 of the UNCRC:

1. In all actions concerning children, whether undertaken by public or private social welfare institutions, courts of law, administrative authorities or legislative bodies, the best interests of the child shall be a primary consideration.
2. State Parties undertake to ensure the child such protection and care as is necessary for his or her welfare (*Wohlergehen*), taking into account the rights and duties of his or her parents, legal guardians, or other individuals legally responsible for him or her, and, to this end, shall take all appropriate legislative and administrative measures.

Authors often refer to the first part of this article alone. I introduce the whole of Article 3 because this enables me to consider the juridical perspective as well as the underlying philosophical distinction between *well-being* and the *best interests* of

---

5. The child must be brought up in the consciousness that its talents must be devoted to the service of fellow men. (http://www.un-documents.net/gdrc1924.htm)

UN Convention of the Rights of the Child. https://www.ohchr.org/en/professionalinterest/pages/crc.aspx

See for the question of implementation and its consequences for the German practice: Eichholz 2009.

[4] United Nations Convention on the Rights of the Child, Article 3 (1). The UNCRC itself uses the terms "well-being" and "best interests" more or less interchangeably: "best interests" in Art. 3 (1), Art. 9 (1), Art. 9 (3), Art. 18 (1), Art. 20 (1), Art. 21, Art. 37 (c), Art. 40 (2b iii); and "well-being" in the Preamble, Art. 3 (2), Art. 9 (4), Art. 17 and 17 (e), Art. 40 (4). However, in the German translation, in the social context as well as in the family law the notion of "well-being" prevails. In particular, the notion of endangerment of the child's well-being (*Kindeswohlgefährdung*) to be found in German family law suggests the different connotations of the two terms. Taking into account the differences in emphasis, using the larger notion of well-being thus coheres with the German social and juridical context.

[5] In 1946 the World Health Organization (WHO) defined health as an all-encompassing ideal that can rarely be achieved in practice: "Health is a state of complete physical, mental and social well-being and not merely the absence of disease or infirmity".

the child. This leads to the following question: in what sense are they hermeneutically distinct?

Most usages of the notion of best interests (as here in Article 3 of the UNCRC) have been translated into German as *Wohl des Kindes* (which actually means well-being of the child). The UNCRC mentions "well-being" six times and "best interests" eight times. It seems that both notions are important for Art. 3 and that they do not mean exactly the same thing. Best interests and well-being are different not only in emphasis but also in sense; thus, I do not agree with authors who believe that they can be used interchangeably. First, they belong to a different tradition of the history of ideas: the notion of best interests belongs to the Anglo-American tradition of liberalism, which focuses in particular on the rights of an individual, mostly in the sense of protection of rights; well-being, or welfare, on the other hand, comes from the Roman tradition and refers to "the subjective aspects of feeling well and to objective aspects of care, support and protection" (Schües and Rehmann-Sutter 2013a, 198). Furthermore, well-being is associated with paternalism and social care, as given from mature adults to immature children. Contrasting with this trend of paternalism, we could understand the notion of best interests to represent the idea that the child is a subject with his or her own will, opinion and aim of action (Krappmann 2013, 7; Doek 2014). Thus, the fact the Convention contains both notions implies the claim that the child's well-being must include the perspective of the child herself; not just the adults who define and judge a child's rights but the perspective of the child herself and of children as a group should also be considered for the realization of their rights and well-being.

The notion of the child's well-being is the older of the two and goes back to the child protection movement of the late nineteenth century. Its function, at least in Germany, is to reprimand parents who neglect their children and endanger their well-being. This is one of the reasons why German law uses the endangering of well-being of the child instead of other formulations that might define the "good life" of the child. In German social work with children, it is agreed that in case of a conflict, the child's well-being takes precedence over the parents' (Heilmann 2000). But, as I have said, both notions are used in the Convention. I argue, very roughly, that well-being refers to the child who needs care and protection, while best interests brings out the idea that the child is also a subject who has rights and who may participate in decisions that concern her well-being. The underlying intention is that both aspects – best interests and well-being – are needed to support the idea that a child must be provided with conditions in which they can develop and live in relationships based on respect, care, and the responsibility of adults. Children are subjects from the outset, but they rely upon adults to ensure their rights and to provide the support that enables them to enact their right to exercize their will.

The notion of well-being can be used in a very narrow sense, as is the case if the concern is merely for protection against child endangerment, and it can be used in a broader sense that includes religious or ethical conviction. It has certainly often been used to legitimize paternalistic or pedagogical regulations. But the idea of best interests, particularly because of its future directedness, can also be taken as a *forceful notion* for a decision that entails the hypothetical or future autonomy of the child.

In medical practice, for example, the notion of best interests is used by Tom Beauchamp and James F. Childress. For them, respecting autonomy entails the obligation to act in the best interests of the (adult) patient. If there are alternative actions, we are required to choose the one that has the most benefit for the persons involved (Beauchamp and Childress 2001, 102). Thus, in such calculations, something non-well or something bad can also accord with the "highest benefit" for most. The notion of well-being is less suitable for weighing risks and benefits. In discussions about the legitimation of paediatric tissue or organ transplantation, practices that need to use another child's body material to cure a sick child, supporters of these practices can easily calculate the benefit of survival against the risk to the healthy child (Wiesemann 2014; Schües and Rehmann-Sutter 2017). This form of calculation is, however, blind to the donor child's perspective and may easily result in exploitation, abuse or violence.

3.1.2   German National Law

Since our study of the practice of and experiences with stem cell transplantation was conducted in Germany, the context of the national law is important. German law does not clearly define the notion of well-being,[6] which may therefore be taken as a hypothetical concept; yet there is a systematic context that concretizes its normative use depending on an individual case. In Germany, the juridical notion of a child's well-being existing in addition to parental responsibility falls under family law. This is based on Article 6 of the *Basic Law* (*Grundgesetz*, GG), which provides that "the care and upbringing of children is the natural right of parents and a duty primarily incumbent upon them" (Art. 6.2 GG).[7] However, the legislation lacks a definition or explanation of the term "well-being". The law only mentions its counter notion: "endangerment of the child's well-being" (*Gefährdung des Kindeswohls*, my translation). This can be found in the *German Civil Code* (*Bürgerliches Gesetzbuch* BGB, §1666)[8] and in the *German Social Code* (*Sozialgesetzbuch* VIII, *Kinder- und Jugendhilfegesetz*, in § 8a *Schutzauftrag bei Kindeswohlgefährdung*, which was newly introduced in 2005). Hence, the law states that the state has the power to ensure the child's protection. The chosen wording "evaluation of the endangerment" (*Gefährdungseinschätzung*, SGB VIII, §8a) inheres a diagnostic and prognostic

---

[6] This translation is not taken from the official English version of the *Basic Law*: https://www.gesetze-im-internet.de/englisch_gg/englisch_gg.pdf. In the official translation the notion of the child's well-being is mostly generally given as "best interests of the child". This notion, however, follows a different tradition of thought. See also the explanations above.

[7] If not stated otherwise, I follow the official translation: https://www.gesetze-im-internet.de/englisch_gg/englisch_gg.pdf

[8] "The parents must exercise parental custody on their own responsibility and in mutual agreement for the best interests of the child." (Palandt et al. 2009, BGB, §1627).

aspect (Ziegenhain et al. 2007).[9] Thus, with the endangerment of well-being the legislator acknowledges that it is important to assess and evaluate the child's present and past situation as well as her possible future risks. Each case of child endangerment needs a juridical as well as medical, social and ethical interpretation. But if the notion of the child's well-being is to be useful in processes of decision-making and action, it needs an interpretation apart from or beyond its legislative context as well. Hence, I argue that the notion of the child's well-being contains this twofold temporal direction: it refers to the present state of being well (being healthy and content), and to participation in education, daily social and family life, and so on, and also to the child's opportunities to develop towards a good life. Hence, it is always also about the future.

3.1.3   German Law on Transplantation

In order to regulate stem cell transplantation, in May 2007 the German parliament (Deutscher Bundestag) added a new Article § 8a to the *Transplantation Act* (*Transplantationsgesetz*, TPG 1997), intended to amend and supplement the *Medicinal Products Act* (*Arzneimittelgesetz*, AMG), and the other provisions in the *Transplantation Act* (TPG) and the *Transfusion Act* (*Transfusionsgesetz*, TFG).[10] This revision of the law was taken as an opportunity to create governance for tissue donation by minors who belong to the family and who may not legally consent. While the collection of bone marrow from underage donors was not legally regulated until 1997 and had formally been prohibited under a strict interpretation of the Transplantation Act since 1997, it was then explicitly regulated in the added § 8a, which now permits it under certain conditions.[11] Even though a sibling can be considered as a donor, the law provides that there must first be a search for an adult donor. However, the current practice, in Germany and elsewhere, is to test family members first, to see whether they have a matching human leukocyte antigen (HLA) pattern, i.e. compatible tissue characteristics (Busch 2015). When a sibling becomes the (possible) donor child then the question of consent or willingness may arise. But in practice the matching child is already determined as *the* "donor child"; hence, she is already considered to have a (moral) task to donate – just *as if* such duty were evidently, naturally built into the body, as a matter of course.

---

[9] The concept of risk implies empirical scientific measurability and verifiability. In fact, the abuse, neglect and injury of children are generally prohibited. Exceptions are therapeutic treatments for the well-being and in the best interests of a sick child. In practice, however, it is also tolerable to expect underage, healthy donor children to be injured for a bone marrow donation, provided the risk to them is low (Wendler et al. 2005, p. 827; Ross 2002, p. 108; Shah 2011; Kopelman 2004).

[10] Official English version at: http://www.gesetze-im-internet.de/englisch_amg/

[11] In accordance with existing practice, § 8a TPG permits the transfer of bone marrow to close relatives under strict conditions, even for minors and non-competent adults. Deutscher (2007). *Bundesdrucksache.* 543/06, 50.

The following two interview examples illustrate the parents' and physician's attitude towards the family donor.

> The interviewer asks: Your wife and your son were considered as donors: did you think about an unrelated donor or was it clear, that it'll just…? The father responds,
> "of course we DIDN'T at first think about an unrelated donor. No, it was actually clear, one of the two would have to do it." (Kirstein father, 29–30).
> I: And you decided for a sibling donation and against an unrelated donor, because? M: Well that was of course ultimately on the DOCTORS' recommendation, erm (.) they did say that you can't say at this point that the surviv- survival rate is necessarily HIGHER, erm if you take a sibling donation, but the well the SIDE effects erm are often less and it's better tolerated overall in the long run. (Rohde, mother, 82–83).

Before going more deeply into this theme, I shall add two further conceptual layers of the "child's well-being" to our discussion.

3.1.4 Normative Structural Tension of the Child's Well-Being: Will, Time and the Family

So far I have delineated the difference between the child's well-being and best interests, and I have also explained some of the juridical aspects of these notions. It was already implicitly understood that the concept of a child's well-being contains a deeper meaning than that of not endangering the child. It inheres the respect and support of the child's will. Furthermore – and these perspectives will always be open to further discussion – the child's well-being means, among other aspects, welfare, a good life, and living in supportive relationships. In the next step, I shall deepen the analysis of the child's well-being with regard to two *internal* and one *external* dimensions, which are in fact structural tensions. One is between the child's well-being and the child's will (a), the other between the present well-being and the future well-being (b). Both are central to the practice of the donor constellation of stem cell transplantation. Furthermore, and as an *external* tension, the child's well-being may be in tension with the family's well-being (c).

(a) *Will and well-being* – The will of the child as an element of the child's well-being is recognized in the UNCRC, which has the normative status of a declaration of human rights. Article 12 states that the child's will is understood as being a part of the best interests of the child; and indeed, it is an important part of the child's well-being. "The views expressed by children may add relevant perspectives and experience and should be considered in decision-making, policymaking and preparation of laws and/or measures as well as their evaluation" (Committee on the Rights of the Child 2009, Art. 12)[12] Accordingly, it can be argued that the failure to take the child's will into account would constitute an

---

[12] And Art. 13 states the following: "These processes are usually called participation. The exercise of the child's or children's right to be heard is a crucial element of such processes. The concept of participation emphasizes that including children should not only be a momentary act, but the starting point for an intense exchange between children and adults on the development of policies, programmes and measures in all relevant contexts of children's lives."

interference with the child's well-being (United Nations Convention on the Rights of the Child 1989; Moritz 1989, 221; Schües 2013; Dörries 2003). However, some lawyers, psychologists and ethicists see a threat to the child's well-being if the child's will is (substantially) followed contrary to the parents' intentions.[13] The relationship between the child's well-being and will is therefore open to further clarifications and negotiations. Different ideas about what constitutes the child's well-being, and uncertainties about when and how a child's will should be heard or taken into account, are based on different meanings of and attitudes towards the child's well-being.

(b) *Present and future* – The second difficult relationship within the child's well-being lies in its temporal structure of present and future. Every decision or action with or for children radiates into the future. But how should the relationship between present well-being and future well-being be understood? I agree with Christoph Schickhardt, who holds that the "central challenge in dealing with children is to take into account the future well-being of the child" (2012, 176). The child's well-being must be considered in childhood as well as in relation to the future phases of life. But to what extent should the supposed future be taken into account in present discussions? Might the child's well-being in the present be neglected for the sake of well-being in the future? In the context of dental treatment, for example, the answer seems to be obvious: enduring pain and discomfort in the present serves the future well-being of the patient. But subordination of the present to the future in principle would still not be acceptable, especially since the actual occurrence of an imagined future will cannot be guaranteed.

The temporality of the concept of well-being is connected to the debate about the child's will. Oscar Wilde wrote the following insightful piece of text: "In this world there are only two tragedies. One is not getting what one wants, and the other is getting it. The last is much the worst; the last is a real tragedy!" (Wilde, *Lady Windermere's Fan*, Act III n.d.) The relationship between the well-being and the will of the child can be thought of similarly: one tragedy can arise when the will of the child is not taken into account, and the other can be conjured up when it is. In the first case a decision is made against the child's will, and in the second case a decision is made which follows the child's will. In certain circumstances, the second possibility may give rise to the more difficult problem because, for instance, the child may not have foreseen the consequences of the decision, or its outcome may be too much of a burden of responsibility.

The temporality of a child's well-being implies the structural tension between caring for a child in the present and for the future. Successful care for well-being rests between two extremes that parents should avoid: subordinating the present to the future or, with regard to the present, ignoring the future. It may well turn out that

---

[13] Dörries (2003) worries that there is a lack of knowledge about the "determination of the ability of children and adolescents to give consent and the way in which they participate in clinical decision-making processes" (594).

ultimately the question of whether the child's well-being has been adequately taken into account can be judged only in retrospect. But what does it mean to take adequate account of the child's will? In this study, the question is not directed at clear cases endangering the child's well-being (*Kindeswohlgefährdung*) such as severe violence, obvious maltreatment or neglect, where immediate protection of the child would be necessary in the present.[14] The practice of blood stem cell transplantation is established and (usually) takes place within families which care for all their children. Here, families, physicians, or other people involved in the donation practice with children in the context of blood stem cell transplantation do not see, at least as far as empirical studies show, any endangerment of the child's well-being as such (MacLeod et al. 2003; Packman et al. 2004; Wilkins and Woodgate 2007; Wiener et al. 2007). The practice is established, the risks to and the burden on the donor child are not very high and the success rate is quite good.[15] However, there is the illness which leads to a stem cell therapy, the family is in a state of stress and anxiety, and both morally and according common sense a child should not be injured for the benefit of another; as mentioned above, common practice does not follow Germany's legal regulations step by step. In other words, the ethical field of the practice of stem cell donation for siblings is somewhat "grey"; much might depend on how the practice is carried out and how the children and their families are cared for. Injury – not medically indicated – to a healthy child is accepted for the benefit of a sick child. From a purely legal point of view, minors are not able to give consent. Legitimization of the treatment of sick minors is regulated through the proxy consent of the parents (Schmidt-Recla 2009). In the case of a donation of blood stem cells from a healthy child to benefit the sick sibling, the well-being of the healthy child and her right not to be injured conflicts with the well-being of the sick child and her options of recovery. Mature adults may voluntarily suspend their right to physical integrity, and consent to donation. For children, however, there must be another way of justifying the donation. In this rather exceptional situation of illness and therapy by transplantation some of the parents decided, over their children's heads, that the body material should be given to the sick child. But they still find it remarkable, and not simply normal. The emotional level of the conflict and the normative insight is presented in the following sample from a family interview:

> M: I've- I know- I can remember one scene (.), when Kira and I were upstairs (.) standing outside the bathroom and KIRA somehow came out with: (.) "I REALLY DON'T WANT TO DO THIS"-
> D: No, //I didn't want to either//
> M: "I DON'T want to donate any bone marrow" and I was weeping, totally devastated: "and er then then // Klaas will die"//
> D: //[38:31] as bonkers as it looks//
> M: "And is- is that what you want?" and that's how it is with our family. You build up such an insane pressure, (.) you don't want this to happen to one of them [38:39] at all, you

---

[14] With reference to blood stem transplantation, see the cases reported by Lainie Ross, Chap. 12
[15] See Chap. 1 for the parallel between establishing an ethical discourse and the success of the practice.

know you're also (.) basically afraid for both children, but er that's after all the only
chance you can see at that moment, that (..) the sibling can donate (.) to the one who's ill.
F: yes.
M: And (..) no child (.) should have to go through that, (.) no-one (Kunow, family interview,
   304–310)

In some other families it was simply taken for granted, not even questionable or a
matter of decision, that the healthy sibling would undergo the procedure of harvesting stem cells to help her sister or brother. This family interview is an example of
expressing a concern about the medical indication but not considering the therapeutic decisions.

I: Was that a question somehow, I mean (..) whether a a erm a bone marrow transplant
   should be done or not, was evidently no question
F: No. 29 of 66 I: it was simply medically necessary.
M: Yes.
F: Well, we did question it, but we questioned the medical medication, not the therapy itself.
   (Lassen, family interview, 141–145)

According to the present understanding of the importance of exercizing free will, it
seems that the less the child's will is taken into account, the more she appears to be
merely *used* as a convenient remedy for the recovery of another child. It should
therefore be discussed how the child's own will can be included, and how the participation of the donor child can be considered, without falling into the trap described
by Oscar Wilde. A further problem is that the child's will is not really at her disposal, and she does not have the power of decision, because both parents and doctors assume that a child cannot actually refuse. The reason for this lies mainly in the
power of the sibling's life-threatening illness. If the donor child refuses, then – so
the argument presumes – she does so for secondary reasons, such as fear of an injection. Thus, on the one hand, the imminent death of the sick sibling seems to be
enough evidence for rationally and voluntarily giving consent; yet, on the other,
possible reasons for refusal by a donor child do not seem valid and may be taken
even as refusal to help or as an offence against the family, and therefore have to be
ignored.

(c) *Individual and family well-being* – Family is a social institution that comes in
    historically and socially diverse structures. It is "a social group comprized by
    one or more adults and one or more children who are linked together by a spe-
    cial history (for example, as biological kin or adoption) and by sentiments of
    mutual affection." (Macleod, 213 f.; Young 1997, 196) Essential to a family in
    twenty-first-century Western society is a special sort of *affective relationship*
    that may and often does change in quality, kind and even status over the years,
    but is always intergenerational and mostly ongoing by intention (Schües 2012).
    An affective relationship is not necessarily happy or loving, functional or stable.
    The size of a family and the depth of these affective relationships may show
    great variety and distinctiveness. The variety and uniqueness of family brings
    about its ambivalent status, somewhere in between the protected sphere of
    privacy and, generally speaking, vulnerable to possible intrusion by state regu-
    lations or authorities. This sphere of privacy is always also determined by poli-

tics and cultural understandings; it can (and should) be legally and legitimately intervened in where there is psycho-physical abuse, severe neglect of children, or violence.

The threshold of where and when the privacy of family must be breached is a legal, social and cultural question. However, the tension between the family and the state is not one that I will follow up here (Drerup et al. 2016). Rather, I want to indicate the special tension between the child's well-being and the family's well-being. This tension may appear in daily life when, for instance, one family member (whether adult or child) needs disproportionately more attention than other members. In such situations, if some members are exposed to severe injustice or if a child is neglected or abused (regardless of whether she is able to speak about it), then this would endanger the well-being *of* the family and welfare *in* the family. One of the family's tasks is to balance the individual's needs and obligations, care and affection, against whatever keeps the family together as an entity that may endure. In addition, the particular relationship between one child and the family as an entity may become questionable and difficult. This would be the case if one child is faced with a particular task in order to enhance the well-being or ensure the endurance of the family. A child is always vulnerable and dependent by virtue of being a child (e.g. Mullin 2014; Hagger 2009).[16] This is the case because the relationship between a child and her parents is always asymmetrical. Since a child is born into her family, she finds herself in a situation of dependency that may be grounded on love and care but may also be precarious and violent. One function of the family is generally seen as caring for the children and keeping them from harm (Schües and Forth 2019; Lindemann 2014; Betzler and Bleisch 2015). The task of caring for children, however, not only rests upon the parents but also the siblings. The endurance and stability of a family is grounded, among other things, on the efforts and conduct of its members. Nevertheless, questions remain: may one member be subjected to the needs of others in order to preserve the family's stability and enable it to endure? In what sense may the illness and the particular treatment – here, stem cell transplants between siblings – endanger or strengthen the well-being of the family? Should one child sacrifice herself or be sacrificed for the well-being of the whole family? Is a donation actually a sacrifice, or a donation, or something else, in the eyes of a family? Are these questions perhaps wrongly posed? Should we rather consider that *how* a practice and its procedure is communicated, accompanied and acted upon may also determine how individuals feel about it? Illness, therapy or transplant are lived through and experienced very differently. The differences depend on many factors; there is the particular role a person has (for example, being the donor child or the caring father), the quality of the relationship, the general social context of the family, and – certainly – the severity of the illness or the kind of medical practice and personal context.

Families are not entirely stable entities. Families that live through times of illness and difficult therapy may transform, experiencing new, meaningful relationships,

---

[16] See in this book Chaps. 5 and 15.

and new roles for the individual members. The parents become "parents of a sick child"; one parent – often the mother – spends a lot of time at the hospital while the father looks after the remaining child, i.e. the donor, and, perhaps, other children. Often one parent has to give up work or reduce their hours. How the family is structured is no longer constituted by feelings, a particular theme of interests or biographical fact, the parents' professions and so on – but also on the basis of the sickness, the transplant, the recovery of the sick child, the well-being of the other members, and keeping the family together – somehow.

Family members generally have different roles that are not interchangeable. Whatever role they have, they are certainly not supposed to die, unless they are old, perhaps grandparents or great-grandparents. Members of a family are usually concerned for each other in an ongoing way. However, the roles and the concerns may change over the years: parents care for children, who later become adults and may care for their aging parents, as well as for their own young children. Hence, family is about *partiality*, i.e. roles and concerns are filled more or less exclusively in the family, and the *asymmetry of the relations changes* and develops in different ways over the years, yet they remain familial. Most families in our study reported that they wanted to solve the problem within the family, and are glad to have their own recourse to aid the sick child: the "donor child". Once a child is tested for HLA compatibility (blood compatibility), she is announced as the "donor child". With this announcement a transformation of the situation takes place, and roles and constellations seem to be fixed: the ill child becomes medically dependent on the body of the suitable healthy sibling (Rehmann-Sutter et al. 2013). The donor child feels that she must save the life of her ill sibling. Other options, like trying to find an anonymous adult donor from the general register, are no longer in focus.

With regard to the concrete context of illness and transplantation, families function very differently; some fall apart, others display strong resilience. In order to determine the ways in which the family's uniqueness and power can emerge (and be protected), one might ask about the special *goods, meanings and values* that can be realized by the family and within familial relations after learning about the life-threatening disease and going through the transplantation practice. Particularly in times of crisis, dimensions of meaning and value may fall apart, be transformed, weaken or even strengthen. Decision-making in the family may not always be easy; in the medical field decisions have distinctive features, and people may sometimes feel as if they have never *really* decided on the treatment pathway.

3.2 Decision-Making in Medical Conflicts and the Child's Will

Generally, decision-making in medical-ethical conflicts is based on the recognition of the patient's will, her competence of rational insight, and her right to self-determination. But a close look at our study reveals that the issue of decision-making is not very clear. The families and their individual members often felt that they never *really* decided. Even though the parents may have signed an informed consent for the transplantation and, hence, juridically speaking, had taken the steps of being informed, deciding, and providing informed consent. As our study shows, there are families who did not see any conflict of interest or questions of difficult decision making; it was self-evident and a matter of course that the stem cells of the healthy sibling would be taken to treat the sick sibling. Considering decision-making in transplantation and in the paediatric context, I need first to discuss a general view in order to show the general background of principles. They no longer hold when children are involved and are presented as "donors". Then, more concretely, I will turn to the psychology of the child's will and different aspects of her will in decision-making in this medical and familial context.

3.2.1 The Principle of Self-Determination

The established practice of medical ethics focuses on individual informed consent, which requires a person to have the power to make a decision. This requires the clear will of the patient (or affected person) to justify the medical interventions and treatment. The general medical and ethical principles, which have been recognized from ancient times, are non-maleficence, care, benevolence and welfare. Today's establishment of individual basic rights could generate the attribution of the right to refuse or agree to medical interventions, based on the recognition of the will and the legitimate claim to self-determination.

The recognition of the principle of self-determination and the implied demand that people must always be asked and that they may and should decide for themselves, is a result of enlightening and emancipatory movements that started in the eighteenth century. Whereas Immanuel Kant described autonomy as a property of a rational will that enables a person to submit to objective and generally binding moral law, today's discourses in medical ethics are instituted rather on a middle level of "good" decisions between the binding level of laws and the framework of subjective values, individual convictions and personal wishes. Autonomy, non-maleficence, beneficence and justice are presently the most recognized principles in medical ethics (Beauchamp and Childress 2001). With the emphasis on the individual right of decision-making, the concept of will is quite close to the utilitarian tradition of J.S. Mill. A person has more or less free will, often called autonomy, depending on how independent she is of external constraints, other people or influences. Accordingly autonomy, which is based on the idea of free will, is no longer understood in the Kantian sense of a general moral law, but rather as individualistic, gradual and, in recent literature, as relational (Mackenzie and Stoljar 2000).[17]

The will required in clinical practice to legitimize medical interventions and therapeutic treatment concerns personal and significant goals and circumstances of life. A decision by will, made by adults, does not necessarily need to be justified or show "good reason". It is sufficient if the will is expressed as informed consent. Informed consent to a medical intervention must be given voluntarily and on the basis that the person concerned has been informed and has competence to consent. The idea that the medical decision is a consent procedure means that patients do not normally choose between equally important alternatives, but they have certain protective rights that are addressed by the rule that the legitimation of a medical intervention requires a patient's informed consent (Beauchamp 2011). The conclusion that a patient has the necessary decision-making competence is based on the official recognition of her ability to reflect, weigh up a decision, and consider the respective consequences. A person must be informed in such a way that she understands and can judge what is to be decided upon and what she consents to; her decisions should be made without coercion or external influence by other persons. If an adult person is no longer able to make self-determined decisions, then authorised persons, ideally appointed in advance in the form of a patient directive, will make proxy decisions. However, this regulation is only applicable to adults, but not to minors. For children, neither preliminary agreements nor assumptions based on an already lived past can be used as a basis for decision-making.

The informed proxy consent of the guardians (usually the parents) is central to medical ethics in the paediatric field.[18] So far, the focus has been on the final decision that is necessary to determine whether or not an intervention will be carried out. However, this focus does not acknowledge that the final and legal decision is contextualised and is the result of a decision-process that may be well communicated or hidden by routine practice. With older children and adolescents in particular, consideration of and respect for the child's will are seen as important for the decision-making process.[19] This is because exercising her will is understood to be part of the child's well-being. The will in general is realized through the possibility of making a decision. The child's will has to do with the question of the decision as

---

[17] The Kantian concept of autonomy is not of this kind; for Kant, individual autonomy would be an impossible concept. Thus, the child's will cannot be derived from Kant's free will, for "free will" is characterized by abstracting from any feelings and interests, except for wanting to act morally.

Nevertheless, his approach to autonomy in the context of moral duty should not, in my opinion, be excluded from medical ethics, because it is positioned at a higher level of ethical consideration – principle legitimation – which should not be neglected. O'Neill argues for the relevance of Kant's concept of autonomy, since only with it and beyond individual autonomy can one argue for certain moral principles that are inescapable for human relationships. These include the fundamental right to physical integrity, the prohibition of instrumentalization and torture, and the prohibition of slavery. (O'Neill 2002, Ch. 4, 5).

[18] See American Academy of Pediatrics (1995), Informed Consent.

[19] In a conflict over treatment between parents with a duty of care and paediatricians, the "child's well-being" is a term that serves as a legal and ethical yardstick for making decisions. See UNCRC.

well. Phrasing it as a final and legal decision means already differentiating between the decision as the ultimate "informed consent" and a process of co-decision-making, which may take into account the child's opinion, but does not regard it as final and binding. But before discussing this type of decision-making, I shall delineate different psychological aspects of the child's will. This description should help to address how a child's will may be realized in practice.

3.2.2 Psychological Aspects of the Child's Will

The child's will is already present in the child from an early age (Nunner-Winkler 1998, 2016). From a family psychological perspective in the context of divorce and problematic custody constellations, Harry Dettenborn (2010) discusses diagnostics and assessment, dealing with the child's will and its relationship to the child's well-being. Although the will of very young children is not always clearly expressed, children already have the necessary competencies for the formation of a will at the age of three or four. Even at this young age, the will may not be less intense or more prone to disruption than in older children. In order to determine whether a child should be involved in a decision, four characteristics are important: goal orientation, intensity, stability and autonomy (Dettenborn 2010, 70–86).

Goal orientation is achieved when the child is oriented towards the "desired conditions" and is no longer subject to "mood-dependent suffering or undirected change tendencies". *Intensity* means "the insistence and determination with which goals are striven for". *Stability* is assumed when the will is "maintained over a reasonable period of time in relation to different people and under different circumstances". Although the child's formation of the will is a process, the assertiveness of the will in a child may be stronger or weaker. In any case, the *stability* of the will is constitutive for the will because it may transform a purely reactive situational impulse. In this respect it stands for a duration of firmness that extends into the future from the subjective perspective and can be remembered retrospectively. In this approach, the notion of *autonomy*, understood simply as having the ability to understand, judge and make decisions, is taken as the central moment of the will, which has to do with "inner striving and the child's becoming a self" and the feelings of self-efficacy and subjectivity.

Developmental psychology and cognitive insights into the will show that goal orientation, intensity, stability and autonomy do not change significantly over the course of childhood. On the other hand, the ability to formulate, communicate and realize the will does change enormously. Asserting and justifying one's own subjective perspective and interests requires a certain maturity, and reflective and communicative ability. However, parental, medical and simply human sensitivity are also required to hear, understand and comprehend the children's perspectives. Following the UNCRC, and considering the psychological description of the child's will, we can conclude that respecting and believing in the child's will means caring for the child and her well-being. But particularly in difficult situations, this is not the end of the "story": the issue is more complicated.

3.2.3 The Tragedy of Decisions

The importance of the child's well-being and the child's will means that the child's subjective perspective is regarded as being fundamental to her development and life. In light of this, the child's will is considered central to her care, safety or health. In the context of custody arrangements it is therefore often argued that there can be no child's well-being *against* the child's will (Ell 1986). However, in the case of stem cell transplantation (SCT) the path of therapy seems to be taken as so self-evident that the family members feel they have never decided anything. In retrospect, and if the therapy has not led to healing or to the result they expected, the parents or "donor child" may wish they had decided differently. Hence, even if a family acts on the basis of matter of course, ideas about will, decision, and responsibility may creep in through the backdoor.

The problematic constellation of decision-making with regard to the child's will resembles that of a tragedy. A tragedy is based on a fateful conflict or a difficult constellation, from which the hero inevitably emerges "guiltlessly guilty". The colloquial understanding of tragedy is, however, not meant here: the point is not that what happens is miserable or distressing, or that a protagonist is very sad or sorrowful. Even though the concept of tragedy may seem exaggerated in this context at first, it fits in two respects. First, in the sense of Hegel's (1970) concept of "tragic collisions", which implies that two opposing positions both contain something good.[20] Here, I presume an inescapable absoluteness of the positions that leads to a tragic collision. If the child makes a donation (with or against his or her will), the sick sibling will most likely be saved or, at least, get better. If the child does not donate (with or against his or her will), his or her right to integrity and physical integrity remain unharmed. Thus, there seems to be something good about both positions.

Second, the tragedy is not a failure of action; rather, the transfer of an obligation succeeds insofar as someone innocent, the child, becomes burdened with responsibility, since current medical practice requires the whole family to be tested for HLA compatibility if stem cell transplantation is advised. If one sibling's body material is compatible with that of the sick sibling, she is assigned the role of donor. And by becoming a donor, she holds the life and the well-being of the sick sibling "in her hands". The burden of helping is on her, as the other family members are no longer responsible for the stem cell donation itself. In line with the association with tragedy, it is also possible to speak of an inevitable situation of conflict or debt into which a donor child may fall, because the haematological "fit" means the donor child "owes" help to the sick sibling. The conflict seems insoluble, with a child who has innocently found herself in the position of being the only one with the obligation and responsibility to help. Either she decides to help (but then may be

---

[20] Hegel, *Vorlesung über Ästhetik*, p. 522 f.; p. 549 f. In the speculative interpretation of the tragic, Hegel refers to "Antigone", where he sees the collision of two equal powers. Comedy, which Hegel also addresses, is of course not at issue here.

overburdened by feeling responsible if the transplant fails) or she refuses to help (with the result of feeling guilty later in life); or the parents overrule any decision-making on the part of the child and relieve her of this responsibility but in doing so overrule her will, which itself is considered to be contrary to the child's well-being.

3.2.4 The Consideration of the Child's Will in the Process of Decision-Making

Below, I indicate several problems of a *strong* concept of decision and consider arguments for and against including the child's will in the decision. In order to reconcile the two positions and to do justice to both, I suggest a *participatory* concept of decision-making, which is based on a weak notion of the decision.

3.2.4.1 Arguments for Taking the Child's Will into Account

Paediatric stem cell transplantation in which a minor sibling donates involves a difficult constellation of decision-making for the parents, because the values and norms involved are structurally contradictory. Refusal to donate means that the right to physical and emotional integrity has been respected, but the sick child may die, or at least remain seriously ill. If parents consent to stem cell therapy and no adult donor is available, they also consent to injuring the healthy child. Parents and caregivers know that the medical intervention into the body of the healthy donor child[21] is performed without medical indication and only for the clinical benefit of the sick child. The conflict for the parents is that they have the duty to care for both the healthy and the sick child, and they must decide on behalf of both children. In the case of impending therapy using blood stem cells, it is probably a relief for parents if the donor child volunteers, without pressure and perhaps even in quite another context: "I'll do it!" I think this would be important for the parents, and they would be relieved of their responsibility to decide, because they would just follow the child's wish and consent to help. This I call the *argument of responsibility transfer.*

This plea for self-determination can be complemented by an *argument of respect*: taking the child's subjective perspective seriously means acknowledging the will of a child. In this view, the parents or caregivers do not just decide *for* a child, but actually let her decide. Generally, in medical practice we can see a tendency towards giving children more freedom to decide (Ruhe et al. 2015). Involving the child in a decision means recognizing and paying attention to her feelings and interests, listening to her and supporting her in the decision-making process. The dimensions of the child's will described above in terms of the goals of orientation, intensity,

---

[21] Concerning the question of whether the medical intervention concerns *only* the body, see Chap. 15 in this book.

stability and autonomy imply the recognition of and respect for the child's will and the understanding that the will is temporally extended, that it (ideally) has a certain permanence and an effect on the future. One argument for the consideration of the child's will is supported by the presumption that the development of a child into a self-determined, responsible adult can only succeed if the family members, the medical personnel or other persons interact with the child with respect, and thereby promote her self-esteem. Such attention in the encounter with and support of the child is realized by hearing and respecting the child and her opinions. It could therefore be concluded that recognizing the child's will not only ensures that the child behaves in a compliant manner during medical practice, but also promotes self-esteem and thus the child's well-being. Conversely, disregarding the child's will might lead to a lack of willingness to cooperate on the part of the child, but above all it would have to be interpreted as an intervention in the development of the child's personality. This position demands that consideration of the child's will should take priority, even if the child says "no" (for whatever reason) to the donation.

3.2.4.2   Arguments Against Taking the Child's Will into Account

For a blood stem cell donation that is necessary for a sick child, is it appropriate, despite conflicting values and norms, to demand the "donor child" make a decision? It seems downright cynical to ask a child to make a decision when in fact the decision has already been made. This *argument of honesty* claims that a decision, for children or adults alike, should only be required if the result of the decision is really taken as the basis for the subsequent action. Anything else would be dishonest. Of course, it can be said that it is not wrong to ask the children. But it would certainly be wrong to ask for a decision that had been already decided in advance: that would not be an open decision.

This argument is supported by the observation that the question of whether, or when, a child could make a decision rarely arises in the practice of HLA testing. The decision as to whether a healthy child should donate blood stem cells at all is preceded by a test to determine whether the sick child is HLA compatible. Usually, in Germany at least, this test is first performed on all family members for reasons of time and to reduce complexity. The children whose blood characteristics make them ineligible as donors do not need to be considered for further treatment of the sick child. However, if a child fits medically, she is seen as the "donor child" (Rehmann-Sutter et al. 2013). This attribution opens up a treatment path that the testing had already anticipated, and that can now be taken. If a child is seen as the "donor", the scope for decision-making is already channelled towards consent. This practised order leads to the fact that from the child's point of view, the decision is made from the perspective that she is already being approached as a suitable donor child. The decision process has already been decided in that a donation would be the further way to go. The donor child thinks it all depends on her. This argument boils down to the fact that the decisions have already been made anyway, and therefore any request or even admission of a decision by the "donor child" is rather a constructive fake. The *American Academy of Pediatrics* (Ross) has argued for the instalment of a child's attorney, who accompanies the families with regard to the question of whether a child should donate before HLA testing is carried out.[22]

The consideration of the child's will as a *real* decision made by children in a concrete situation might nevertheless leave space for an *orchestration of the child's will*. Parents, doctors or other persons involved want to be sure of the ethical legitimacy of the intervention. They may also feel uncomfortable about the parents' proxy consent. There are different models for imagining or constructing voluntary consent by the donor child: the child's will in the subjunctive (1), the interests of the child (2), and the will in retrospective consent (3) (also Schües and Rehmann-Sutter 2014). These three models are different in structure, but similar in outcome, because they do not provide a role for the involvement of the child in the decision-making process itself.

The model that presents the child's will in the *subjunctive* (1) does not ask the child, but claims that the child would want to donate if she were able to decide. In the assumption that the child does not have the capacity to decide at all, the child's consent is assumed. In this model, the parents transfer their beliefs to the child in accordance with their own values and norms, and assume that the child would have wanted it the same way.

The model that decides in the *interests* of the child (2) offsets the psychosocial benefit of the donation against the inconvenience (American Academy of Pediatrics 2010; Pentz et al. 2004, 2008). This model understands the term "best interests of the child" in the sense of the child's future interests. However, it seems that the consideration of the child's will plays a role only if she comes to the same decision as the adults who have a duty of care. With the argument that the child, if she refuses to donate, would not have her future interests in mind, one would try to change the child's will in the present or, at worst, ignore it. The basic conviction of this position is that the healthy donor child cannot actually have "good reasons" for refusal. The frequently mentioned fear of injections is no reason to refuse a donation, but rather a fear of and aversion to injections. However, the harder question is what "good reasons" could be found to prohibit an HLA-compatible sibling, who is perfectly willing to donate, from participating in the donation.

The search for reasons to consent or even to refuse donation, against a child's expressed will (but in the case of legal incapacity to consent) leads to the decision *model of retrospective consent* (3). This approach does not leave the decision for or against a donation to the child herself either. However, proponents of retrospective consent try to decide in such a way that they can hope the child may later understand

---

[22] In the US there has been vigorous debate about the implementation of child advocacy. Led by L. F. Ross, the *American Academy of Pediatrics* (2010) formulated recommendations on how a donor child can be supported when confronted by the issue of a stem cell transplant. One of the recommendations is the implementation of a donor advocate who should be trained in child development, have verbal and non-verbal communication skills, and have some medical knowledge. This idea and practice provoked a pro/contra debate. In Germany, most hospitals provide some social-pedagogical support for the children.

with hindsight, and share and approve the decision made. Certainly, remembering the circumstances of the donation may also contribute to how the past that had been present and the decision taken at that time is seen, understood and judged in retrospect. Ideally, the older or grown-up child will give retrospective consent, or at least understand the parents' reasons and motives at the time when the therapy of transplantation was under discussion. For this model of retrospective consent, I would like to distinguish more precisely between retrospective consent concerning the concrete decision made at the time, and that with regard to the difficulty of the situation, the general care and respect shown by the parents, and their motives and reasons for the decision, particularly if the grown-up child ultimately does not agree with the decision. If the transplant has been unsuccessful, in particular, retrospective consent may become more difficult. Questions may be posed, such as: Is the recipient child alive? How is she or he? Are there any difficult health problems, such as graft-versus-host disease? However, in our empirical study we found no examples of regret expressed by those who had donated. All three models stage and construct the child's will at the time of the actual decision. The hope that the decision will be confirmed at least in retrospect is expressed by the third model of retrospective consent.

A strong argument *against* considering the child's will is based on the possible consequences of the decision and the question of responsibility. This *consequentialist argument of responsibility* can be explained as follows: Suppose the practice of bone marrow transplantation is such that the child can decide before testing, and that both consent and refusal would be taken into account when deciding which way to go. Whoever decides is also responsible for the consequences of that decision. The feeling of being responsible is important for how the consequences or outcomes of a decision or action are dealt with. Thus, the extent to which a child's will should be taken into account depends not only on the child's ascribed capacity to consent, but also on the type of treatment, the situation, the conflicting norms and values inherent in the decision itself, and on the possible long-term consequences that medical therapy such as stem cell transplantation may have.

The experiences after a transplant may be very different: the sick child may be healthy and continue to live well. This is the positive case. It may be that in retrospect the family, and the donor child, do not even talk in terms of a decision because helping was such an obvious thing to do. Another consequence of the donor child's decision to donate could be that she may later on put pressure on the sibling who has recovered because of the help given. She can blame her sister or brother for putting her, the donor, in the situation of being injured for her body material. The formerly sick child may also feel indebted, although not to be blamed, because her disease has made her force her sister or brother feel indebted towards her. So the formerly sick child remains in the (guiltless) debt of the healthy, generous donor child, who has willingly done their part. However, it is also possible that the child treated with blood stem cells dies, and thus the therapy with stem cells from the healthy child was unsuccessful. It is possible that the child survives but needs another donation or suffers from severe complications, such as graft-versus-host disease (GvHD), a strong immune reaction of the donor immune system against the recipient, and that the immunosuppressive drugs do not work. All this means severe stress not only for the recipient sick child, but also for the donor child and the whole family.

Does the donor child feel responsible, obligated, even guilty, because she agreed to the donation, which was not curative? Along with mourning for the possible loss of the sibling, part of the tragedy of the constellation of stem cell transplantation between siblings is the self-transference of guilt for an unsuccessful donation and for the death of the sick child.

The responsibility argument of the transfer of feeling guilty is also applicable if the intended donor child refuses to donate, and if this refusal were accepted. If the sick sibling dies, the intended donor child may be seen as responsible for the death of her brother or sister based on her decision (Klitzing 2015). Having chosen to be a donor seems to overrule the judgement that the sick child ultimately died because of her illness.

We are confronted with the difficulty that, on the one hand, the well-being of both children should have priority and consideration of the child's will is part of the child's well-being and, on the other, that following the child's will (here, the donor child's will) may be problematic. The different lines of thinking showed that arguments on both sides, in favour of allowing or disallowing the child to exercise her will through a decision, are numerous. If the will of the child is not taken into account, her decision will be disregarded along the lines of the argumentation of the principle of self-determination and the right to integrity. Not being asked, not being heard, not having a voice means, from the adults' perspective, a violation of personal integrity and the right to self-determination, which is perhaps even more tragic than the violation of physical integrity for the benefit of the sibling. Why should it be different from the child's perspective?

In order to discuss how a child, who may have been already tested as HLA compatible with the sick sibling, can participate in decision-making processes that affect her existentially now and for the future, I have already presented the psychological characterizations of the child's will in terms of goal orientation, intensity, stability and autonomy. These aspects are important for seeing where a child stands with regard to her abilities, but they also show that even young children of under 4 years old may have a will that should be taken seriously. The insight that a will, and its content and temporal structure, may have different qualities gives rise to the idea that, first, children should participate in decision-making processes, and second, they may do so without taking all the responsibility.

3.2.5 Communication and Stages of Decision-Making: Children Should Participate

The child's will is expressed and realized according to the scope of decision granted to a child. In the context of medical practice, the child's will can be expressed in different stages and as a participatory decision. But a child should not take the final decision, for which responsibility must be taken retrospectively or with regard to the consequences.

As a consequence of this paper and in order to reconcile the concerns described, I would like to sketch out a way that the will of the child can be considered and taken into account, in the case of a medically beneficial intervention, for a sibling donation. It is important to consider a decision as a process with different steps or stages of communication.

It is not just a question of the fundamental legitimacy of transplantation practices, but of how children can make participatory decisions in the paediatric context of stem cell transplantation. I would like to suggest that a weaker concept of decision, which is open to participation in different dimensions, may be more suitable for the family context, and can be understood in terms of a *co-decision* without having to bear responsibility. Participatory decision-making should take the will into account appropriately, without expecting a final decision or assumption of responsibility. There may still be tragic moments and a certain inevitable feeling of obligation, for example when the result of the HLA test becomes known. Any *real* decision-making process contains a lot of information that has to be absorbed, processed and weighed up; emotional components of fear, worry, perhaps courage, trust, hope or pessimism; and rational approaches that try to understand the practice, the information and suggestions and to objectify the state of emergency.

A decision-making process involves different stages and can be accompanied by professionals in different ways: at each stage, different dimensions of the child's will can be addressed and discussed. Based on an approach developed by the psychologist Priscilla Alderson (Alderson 2008, 36; Schües and Rehmann-Sutter 2014, 26) we can distinguish five stages. Each stage claims a dimension in the decision-making process that is important for respecting the child's will, which can and should be considered independently and in conjunction with the others.

1. *Listening* – This first stage is about equality with regard to listening to the feelings, concerns and perspectives of all family members. It is not just the sick child's medical situation that is important here, but also the sentiments and feelings, fears and concerns of all individual family members. This space for conversation is fundamental for the formation of the child's will, because it is here that she can express herself and be heard.

2. *Information* – At the second stage, all family members, including non-donor siblings, are informed of the medical details and the chances and risks, such as the possible death of the recipient child, or any long-term consequences. Young children can also be talked to or played with in order to give them an idea of what might happen.

3. *Expressing an opinion* – This third stage relates to the dimension of communication by exchanging personal views. Everyone – the donor child, parents and other children – is allowed to express their opinions, feelings and concerns. Fears have their place here, as well as questions, perhaps even very odd questions. Donor children sometimes deal with questions based on very unexpected ideas. For example, one girl worried whether her brother would also have her allergies

after the transplant. Another boy wondered whether his sister would like to play with cars after receiving his stem cells (Di Gallo 2015; Lux 2016). Although a family may be overburdened with a child who is life-threateningly ill, and the psychosocial service sometimes has little time for extra conversations, these discussions are important in the long run. Fears can be taken away, and those affected can support each other. But there are limits: such difficult situations and their possible explanations remain within the framework of the existing family structure and family relationships between parents and their children. Regardless of a sensibly staged decision-making process, a family in which a rough and cold tone prevails will be unlikely to find a loving and open relationship in such a situation. Therefore, institutions can only provide the best protected space and supportive framework that they can.

4. *Weighing opinions* – The fourth stage takes the opinions and weighs their influence on the final decision. A child must also be heard here. It is important that she *feels* involved, and that she actually *is*, and that – at least, if she is old enough at the time of the donation – she can later remember that she was listened to and that her opinion had been heard. At this stage it must be made clear to the child that she actually will not formally decide. She can strongly express her opinions and wishes, and if she is heard and understood, deeply and empathetically, then the child is also taken seriously in her perspective. The child's self-esteem has its place here.

5. *The final decision* – At the fifth stage, final decisions are made, and made on behalf of the child. At this level only the parents (or other caregivers), with their assumption of responsibility, play a role. The child is not expected to take any final decision or responsibility.

These five steps of a decision-making process allow the child's appropriate participation in a process of communication. Although, ethically and socio-psychologically, the inclusion and participation of children in consent processes is promoted, this does not mean that children should ultimately decide; their participation is based on their opinions and wishes. They must be heard, and must be given a space to express themselves. Children and young people benefit legally, psychologically, medically and ethically from participatory decision-making, at the centre of which their concerns and needs, their opinions, and also their rights are positively addressed and received. Thus, the donor child's well-being, as formulated in the *UN Convention on the Rights of the Child*, is realized by receiving appropriate information about the diagnosis, the illness, the course of treatment of the sick sibling as well as about the medical intervention itself, and the difficulties and risks involved for both siblings. Furthermore, the communication that leads through these different stages of decision-making should not stop with the final decision. Each individual aspect of the different steps from one to four should be given room in the future and after the action – whether a transplant or a decision against it – that follows the final decision. Being excluded after participating in a "yes, I want to do the transplant" decision might feel like a betrayal. The continuation of communication is thus very important.

The participation of children and young people in such important areas as medicine and health means that the social and familial practices are regarded as not just a legal matter between a doctor and a legal representative. Rather, family relationships touch on dimensions that cannot or should not (only) be regulated by law (Honneth 2000). From the context of separation and divorce in families, it is known that children and adolescents are not primarily concerned with the right of sole decision. It is important to them that they are informed and heard, that they experience care and empathy from the people close to them.

3.3   Temporality of the Child's Well-Being and the Family

The relationship between the well-being of children and the will of the child has so far been the explicit focus of our study in Lübeck. No less important, however, is addressing and clarifying possible tensions between the present and future well-being, as well as between the child and the family.

May or should the child's well-being in the present be subordinated to (presumed) well-being in the future? How should we understand the temporal dimensions of the child's well-being, which is always embedded in complex relationships, special situations and narrative structures? How much does the well-being of the family count against the well-being of a child?

A decision for or against a donation is based on the family's previous history, often hours of silence and worry, open and unasked questions – overall, a complex narrative dimension of meaning destined to be remembered. The decision therefore has a prospective, future-oriented dimension, which has inscribed itself as a dimension of meaning in the child's life; on the other hand, this narrative dimension of meaning can also be hermeneutically reinterpreted retrospectively. Such a retrospective reinterpretation may change the meaning or validity, colouring and weighting of some aspects. This narrative perspective in retrospect is different to an attempt to reconstruct past events objectively.

With this distinction, I would like to draw attention to four aspects of the relationship between the well-being of the child and the will of the child in a temporal consideration and familial context:

1. How a sister or a brother, a daughter or a son was seen at the time before the donation, the relationships a potential donor had with the other family members, in what way she was able to participate in the upcoming decisions, whether her worries or fears were heard or questions were discussed, whether she was able to express her opinion or wishes, whether she was able to express her opinion emphatically, how the decision was ultimately made by the parents and whether this decision was really understood and felt as a decision in the long term at all, and last but not least, how the family relationships are shaped – all this and more influences the biographical meaning of the transplantation practice and the dimensions of the stories that emerge.

2. Within the question of the child's well-being, the aspect of the child's will is just one of many. Here, the problem of participation in the decision to donate may not be the most important[23]: What is really important is being involved in the stories, in the emotional situation, in the worries, being perceived, being informed, knowing what is coming ... above all, the overall stability of the relationships between the family members. The child's well-being has to do with appreciation and consideration of the child's will, but also with relationships of trust, security and general care. Such relationships are not realized if parents try to trick their children into believing that the world is "ideal", even though the children have known for a long time that they are very worried and possibly desperate. Or, for instance, parents can overburden their children with the demands of decision-making or frighten them with their emotions and worries. Here, we can touch upon certain general standards or ideas, but each family is different. It is there-fore impossible to state precisely and in detail *how* the participation of children in the overall process can best succeed. At best, this article can provide some valuable structural information on paediatric decision constellations and their temporal and familial embedding. Biographical retrospectives, as collected in our study, show that the children's participation is important for their well-being and later family life.

3. Depending on how the time of the donation was experienced and how it was talked about, what happened and to what extent the donation was successful, the positive integration of these events into a donor's biography will be more or less successful. There is an interpretative permeability between past, present and future. Depending on the form of the past future, which is now the present, the past will be shown. A past is not simply closed; essential events remain, but their meaning for a person's further life can change; equally, a dramatic past can influ-ence the present and the future for a long time to come.

4. Depending on the familial structures, its ways of communicating and its resil-ience, a family may hold together more or less. There is no one criterion for how to answer the question of what characterizes the well-being of the family. But we can possibly say that a child is only well if she lives in good relationships. Hence, the child's well-being may also be a kind of mirror for how the family could care for its members. However, having said this, I should not absolutize the entangle-ment in the familial concept either. Individuals – children or adults – can cer-tainly become unwell, despite a functioning family.

The question posed at the beginning, of whether the child's well-being can exist even without consideration of the child's will, can now be answered more clearly. The child's will, in the sense of opinions, feelings or wishes, must be taken into account. This position corresponds to the *UN Convention on the Rights of the Child*

---

[23] See Tiesmeyer 2012; also Weisz, Robbenolt (1996). Our book project includes an interview study. A narrative has the task of bridging the disruption between the linear sequence of what has happened, what was experienced, and what is remembered. It gives existence its sense and it enables the emergence of intergenerational life contexts.

and a positive definition of the well-being of the child. However, I do not consider it to be supportive of the child's well-being and the subjective development of the child in the future if the legally incompetent child also bears responsibility for the decision to donate (or not to donate) blood stem cells to her sibling. If the consequences of a decision to donate and, accordingly, to have a transplant are tragic, if the sick child dies or suffers from other difficult diseases due to the sibling blood stem cells, the donor child may feel responsible for her decision in the long run and be exposed to severe psychological stress. Therefore, the child – here perhaps a preschool child – should be given the certainty that she has expressed *only* an opinion and that this opinion has been heard and taken into account. The final decisions must be made by the parents, who are responsible and – ideally – accompany the child with the whole family history into the future, both biographically and narratively.

An imposed decision or attributed responsibility does not necessarily strengthen the child's will or her development to maturity. In everyday situations, it is often right to take the will of a child into account, let her decide, and also to follow her decision. But in exceptional situations, such as those that occur in the field of transplantation medicine, it may be more likely to strengthen the child's will in the long term if one listens to the child but then gives her the sense that she does not have to bear the decision herself. Prioritizing the child's will can, in the worst case, lead to weakening it and thus to unstable self-esteem in the future. The responsibility must remain with the adults, with the parents. Both the strong concept of decision, i.e. compliance with the child's will in the final decision, and alternatively disregarding the child's will, takes a donor child into a tragic system of unfounded obligation and disregard.

Overall, it would be welcoming for research to succeed in finding healing methods that do not need transplantation therapy and its familial intercorporeal or interpersonal entanglement. Whether the well-being of the child was protected and supported in times of crisis might influence how events are remembered in retrospect. Is one's own person remembered as having been valued and respected? Did the parents, the doctors or others turn to the child who is to donate? Did they listen to her? Was his or her opinion understood? Can she retrospectively agree with her parents' decision? Is there a trusting relationship within the family? Many more questions can be asked and are relevant. It is not simply a question of whether the decision to donate was right or wrong. A number of other criteria mentioned above determine whether the well-being of a child has been taken care of – in the present, and for the present and the future. The question of whether the child's well-being – and actually the child as a person – has been well cared for in childhood is always evaluated in the actual present, which once was the future.

Literature

Alderson, Priscilla. 2008. *Young Children's rights*. London and Philadelphia: Jessica Kingsley.

American Academy of Pediatrics. 1995. Informed consent, parental permission, and assent in pediatrics practice. *Pediatrics* 95: 314–317.

American Academy of Pediatrics Committee on Bioethics. 2010. Policy statement – Children as hematopoietic stem cell donors. *American Journal of Pediatrics* 125 (2): 392–404. http://pediatrics.aappublications.org/content/125/2/392. Accessed 14 October 2020.

Archard, David. 2018. Children's rights. In *Stanford encyclopedia of philosophy*, ed. Edward N. Zalta. https://plato.stanford.edu/entries/rights-children/. Accessed 14 October 2020.

Bagattini, Alexander. 2014. Child well-being: A philosophical perspective. In *Handbook of child well-being, Vol. 1*, ed. Asher Ben Arieh et al., 163–186. Switzerland: Springer.

Beauchamp, Tom L. 2011. Informed consent: Its history, meaning, and present challenges. *Cambridge Quarterly of Healthcare Ethics* 20 (4): 515–523. https://doi.org/10.1017/S0963180111000259.

Beauchamp, Tom L., and James F. Childress. 2001. *Principles of biomedical ethics*. 5th ed. Oxford: Oxford University Press.

Betzler, M., and Barbara Bleisch (eds.). 2015. *Familiäre Pflichten*. Frankfurt/M: Suhrkamp.

Brighouse, Harry. 2002. What rights (if any) do children have? In *The moral and political status of children*, ed. David Archard and Colin M. Macleod, 31–52. Oxford: Oxford University Press.

Büchner, Peter. 2003. Kinder und Kindheit in der Erwachsenengesellschaft – ein Blick in die Stellung des Kindes aus kindheitssoziologischer Sicht. In *Das Kind als Patient*, ed. C. Wiesemann, A. Dörries, G. Wolfslast, and A. Simon, 11–27. Frankfurt/New York: Ethische Konflikte zwischen Kindeswohl und Kindeswille.

Busch, Lina. 2015. Geschwisterspender oder Fremdspender: Wer zuerst? – Diskrepanzen zwischen Gewebegesetz und klinischer Praxis hinsichtlich der Knochenmarkspende nichteinwilligungsfähiger Minderjähriger. In *Rettende Geschwister. Ethische Aspekte der Einwilligung in der pädiatrischen Stammzelltransplantation*, ed. Christina Schües and Christoph Rehmann-Sutter, 149–166. Münster: mentis.

Committee on the Rights of the Child. 2009. Fifty-first session Geneva, 25 May–12 June 2009. https://www2.ohchr.org/english/bodies/crc/docs/AdvanceVersions/CRC-C-GC-12.pdf. Accessed 14 October 2020.

Dettenborn, Harry. 2010. *Kindeswohl und Kinderwille. Psychologische und rechtliche Aspekte*. 3rd ed. Munich: Reinhardt.

Deutscher, Bundestag. 2007. *Bundesdrucksache*. 543/06, DIP21 Extrakt. Accessed 14 October 2020.

Di Gallo, Alain. 2015. Mit Kindern sprechen. In *Rettende Geschwister. Ethische Aspekte der Einwilligung in der pädiatrischen Stammzelltransplantation*, ed. Christina Schües and Christoph Rehmann-Sutter, 91–100. Münster: mentis.

Doek, Jaap E. 2014. Child well-being: Children's rights perspective. In *Handbook of child well-being*, ed. Asher Ben Arieh et al., 187–217. Dordrecht: Springer.

Drerup, Suhrkamp, Gunter Graf Johannes, Christoph Schickhardt, and Gottfried Schweiger, eds. 2016. *Justice*. Education and the Politics of Childhood, Berlin: Springer.

Dörries, Andrea. 2003. Ethische Entscheidungsfindung in der Pädiatrie. *Pädiatrische Praxis: Zeitschrift für Kinder- und Jugendmedizin in Klinik und Praxis* 63: 589–595.

Eichholz, Reinald. 2009. Der Vorrang des Kindeswohls nach Art. 3 UN-Kinderrechtskonvention. Konsequenzen für die bundesdeutsche Praxis. IzKK-Nachrichten 2009-1: UN-Kinderrechtskonvention – Impulse für den Kinderschutz: 12–20.

Ell, Ernst. 1986. *Psychologische Kriterien bei der Sorgerechtsregelung und die Diagnostik der emotionalen Beziehung*. Weinheim Deutscher Studien Verlag.

Figdor, Helmut. 2009. Im Namen des Kindes. Zur Kritik herkömmlicher Sachverständigen-Praxis aus psychoanalytisch-pädagogischer Sicht. In *Jahrbuch für Psychoanalytische Pädagogik*

16, ed. Wilfried Datler, Urte Finger-Trescher, Johannes Gstach, et al., 61–84. Giessen: Psychosozial-Verlag.

German Civil Code. 1900. German Civil Code BGB. Accessed 20 September 2020.

Giesinger, Johannes. 2013. Kindeswohl und Respekt. *Ethik Journal* 1 (2): 1–15.

Goldstein, Joseph, Anna Freud, and Albert J. Solnit. 1991[1974]. *Jenseits des Kindeswohls. Mit einem Nachwort (zur Ausgabe 1991): Weitere Bemerkungen zur Anwendung des Standards der am wenigsten schädlichen Alternative*. Frankfurt a. M.

Hagger, Lynn. 2009. *The child as vulnerable patient: Protection and empowerment*. Surrey: Ashgate.

Hegel, Georg W. F. 1970. Vorlesung über Ästhetik III. In *Werke in 20 Bdn., vol. 15*, ed. Eva Moldenhauer and Karl M. Michel. Frankfurt/M.: Suhrkamp.

Heilmann, Stefan. 2000. Hilfe oder Eingriff? *Zentralblatt für Jugendrecht* 87: 41–80.

Honneth, Axel. 2000. Zwischen Gerechtigkeit und affektiver Bindung. Die Familie im Brennpunkt moralischer Kontroversen. In *Das Andere der Gerechtigkeit*, 193–215. Frankfurt/M: Suhrkamp.

Invernizzi, Antonella, and Jane Williams. 2011. *The human right of children. From visions to implementation*. London/New York: Routledge.

Klitzing, Kai von. 2015. Die Knochenmarkspende zwischen Geschwisterkindern aus entwicklungspsychologischer und kinderpsychiatrischer Sicht. In *Rettende Geschwister. Ethische Aspekte der Einwilligung in der pädiatrischen Stammzelltransplantation*, ed. Christina Schües and Christoph Rehmann-Sutter, 77–90. Münster: Mentis.

Kopelman, Loretta M. 2004. What conditions justify risky nontherapeutic or "no benefit" pediatric studies: A sliding scale analysis. International risky and comparative health law and ethics: A 25-year retrospective. *The Journal of Law, Medicine & Ethics* 32: 749–753.

Krappmann, Lothar. 2013. Das Kindeswohl im Spiegel der UN-Kinderrechtskonvention. *Ethik Journal* 1 (2): 1–17.

Lindemann, Hilde. 2014. Why families matter. *Pediatrics* 134 (2): 97–103.

Lux, Sebastian. 2016. Kiwi-Allergie nach Stammzellspende. *Allergo J* 25 (3): 8. https://doi.org/10.1007/s15007-016-1063-4.

Mackenzie, Catriona, and Natalie Stoljar. 2000. *Relational autonomy: Feminist perspectives on autonomy, agency, and the social self*. Oxford: Oxford University Press.

MacLeod, Kendra, et al. 2003. Pediatric sibling donors of successful and unsuccessful hemapoietic stem cell transpants (HSCT): A qualitative study of their psychological experience. *Journal of Pediatric Psychology* 28 (4): 223–231.

Moritz, Heinz P. 1989. *Die (zivil-)rechtliche Stellung der Minderjährigen und Heranwachsenden innerhalb und außerhalb der Familie*. Berlin: Duncker & Humblot.

Mullin, Amy. 2014. Children, vulnerability and emotional harm. In *Vulnerability. New essays in ethics and feminist philosophy*, ed. Catriona Mackenzie, Wendy Rogers, and Susan Dodds, 266–287. Oxford: Oxford University Press.

Nunner-Winkler, Gertrud. 1998. Zum Verständnis von Moral – Entwicklungen in der Kindheit. In *Entwicklung im Kindesalter*, ed. Franz E. Weinert, 133–152. Weinheim: Beltz.

———. 2016. Wissen und Wollen beim Kind und in der Nähe des Todes. In *Randzonen des Willens. Anthropologische und ethische Probleme von Entscheidungen in Grenzsituation*, ed. Thorsten Moos, Christoph Rehmann-Sutter, and Christina Schües, 63–90. Frankfurt/M: Peter Lang.

O'Neill, Onora. 1988. Children's rights and Children's lives. *Ethics*: 445–463.

———. 2002. *Autonomy and Trust in Bioethics*. Cambridge: Cambridge University Press.

Packman, Wendy, et al. 2004. Psychosocial adjustment of adolescent siblings of hemapoietic stem cell transplant patients. *Journal of Pediatric Oncology Nursing* 21 (4): 233–248.

Palandt, Otto, Peter Bassenge, et al., eds. 2009. *Bürgerliches Gesetzbuch (BGB)*. 68th ed. Munich: Beck.

Pentz, Rebecca D., Ka W. Chan, Joyce L. Neumann, Richard E. Champlin, and Martin Korbling. 2004. Designing an ethical policy for bone marrow donation by minors and others lacking capacity. *Quarterly of Healthcare Ethics* 13: 149–155.

Pentz, Rebecca D., Ann E. Haight, Robert B. Noll, Raymond Barfield, Wendy Pelletier, Stella Davies, Melissa A. Alderfer, and Pamela S. Hinds. 2008. The ethical justification for minor sibling bone marrow donation: A case study. *The Oncologist* 13 (2): 148–151.

Rehmann-Sutter, Christoph, Sarah Daubitz, and Christina Schües. 2013. "Spender gefunden, alles klar!" Ethische Aspekte des HLA-Tests bei Kindern im Kontext der Stammzelltransplantation. *Bioethica Forum* 6 (3): 89–96.

Ross, Lainie F. 2002. Do healthy children deserve greater protection in medical research? The Department of Paediatrics. Mclean Centre for Clinical Medical Ethics, University of Chicago, Illinois.

Ruhe, Katharina M., Tenzin Wangmo, Domnita O. Badarau, Bernice S. Elger, and Felix Niggli. 2015. Decision-making capacity of children and adolescents – Suggestions for advancing the concept's implementation in pediatric healthcare. *European Journal of Pediatrics* 174: 775–782.

Schickhardt, Christoph. 2012. *Kinderethik: Der moralische Status und die Rechte der Kinder*. Münster: Mentis.

Schmidt-Recla, Adrian. 2009. Kontraindikation und Kindeswohl. Die "zulässige" Knochenmarkspende durch Kinder. *GesR* 11: 565–572.

Schües, Christina. 2012. Was gibt der Generativität Sinn? Über Geburt, Zeit und Narrativität. In *Statu nascendi. Geborensein und intergenerative Dimension des menschlichen Miteinanderseins*, ed. Tatiana Shchyttsova, 89–107. Nordhausen: Bautz.

———. 2013. Kindeswohl. In *Wörterbuch der Würde*, ed. Rolf Gröschner, Antje Kapust, and Oliver W. Lembcke, 354–355. Munich: Fink.

———. 2016. Epistemic injustice and the children's well-being. In *Justice, education and the politics of childhood*, ed. J. Drerup, G. Graf, C. Schickhardt, and G. Schweiger, 155–170. Berlin: Springer.

Schües, Christina, and Hannes Forth. 2019. Elternschaft. In *Handbuch Philosophie der Kindheit*, ed. Gotthard Schweiger and Johannes Drerup, 90–98. Stuttgart: J.B. Metzler Verlag.

Schües, Christina, and Christoph Rehmann-Sutter. 2017. Has a child a duty to donate hematopoietic stem cells to a sibling? (with Christoph Rehmann-Sutter). In *New issues in ethics and oncology*, ed. Monika Bobbert, Beate Herrmann, and Wolfgang U. Eckart, 81–100. Freiburg/Munich: Alber.

———. 2013a. The well- and unwell-being of a child. *Topoi* 32 (2): 197–205.

———. 2013b. Hat ein Kind eine Pflicht, Blutstammzellen für ein krankes Geschwisterkind zu spenden? *Ethik Med.* 25: 89–102. https://doi.org/10.1007/s00481-012-0202-z.

———. 2014. Retrospektive Zustimmung der Kinder? Ethische Aspekte der Stammzelltransplantation. *Frühe Kindheit* 2: 22–27.

———. 2015. *Rettende Geschwister. Ethische Aspekte der Einwilligung in der pädiatrischen Stammzelltransplantation*. Münster: mentis.

Shah, Seema. 2011. The dangers of using a relative risk standard for minimal risk. *The American Journal of Bioethics* 11 (6): 22–23. National Institutes of Health.

Steindorff, Caroline. 1994. Zur Einstimmung in das Thema. In *Vom Kindeswohl zu den indesrechten*, ed. Ders., 1–6. Neuwied, Kriftel u. Berlin.

Tiesmeyer, Karin. 2012. *Familien mit einem krebskranken kind*. Bern: Huber.

United Nations: Convention on the Rights of the Child. 1989. http://www.ohchr.org/en/professionalinterest/pages/crc.aspx. Accessed 7 June 2020.

Weisz, Victoria, and Jennifer K. Robbenolt. 1996. Risks and benefits of pediatric bone marrow donation: A critical need for research. *Behavioral Sciences & the Law* 14: 375–391.

Wendler, David, Leah Belsky, Ezekiel J. Emanuel, and Kimberly M. Thompson. 2005. Quantifying the federal minimal risk standard. *JAMA* 204 (7): 826–832.

Wiener, Lori, et al. 2007. Hematopoietic stem cell donation in children: A review of the sibling donor experience. *Journal of Psychosocial Oncology* 25 (1): 45–66.

Wiesemann, Claudia. 2014. Der moralische Status des Kindes in der Medizin. In *Wissen. leben. ethik –Themen und Positionen der Bioethik*, ed. Johann D. Ach, Beate Lüttenberg, and Michael Quante, 155–168. Münster: mentis.

———. 2016. *Moral, equality, bioethics, and the child*. Switzerland: Springer.

Wiesemann, Claudia, Andrea Dörries, Gabriele Wolfslast, and Alfred Simon, eds. 2003. *Das Kind als Patient*. Frankfurt: Campus.

Wilde, Oscar. n.d. Lady Windermere's fan, Act III: Mr. Dumby.

Wilkins, Krista L., and Roberta L. Woodgate. 2007. An interruption in family life: Siblings' lived experience as they transition through the pediatric bone marrow transplant trajectory. *Oncology Nursing Forum 2007*. 34 (2): E28–E34.

Young, Iris M. 1997. *Intersecting voices. Dilemmas of gender, political philosophy, and policy*. Princeton: Princeton University Press.

Ziegenhain, Ute, Jörg M. Fegert, Teresa Ostler, and Anna Buchheim. 2007. Risikoeinschätzung bei Vernachlässigung und Kindeswohlgefährdung im Säuglings und Kleinkindalter – Chancen früher beziehungsorientierter Diagnostik. *Praxis der Kinderpsychologie und Kinderpsychiatrie* 56 (5): 410–428.

Zitelmann, Maude. 2001. *Kindeswohl und Kindeswille: Im Spannungsfeld von Pädagogik und Recht*. Weinheim: Beitz.

Open Access This chapter is licensed under the terms of the Creative Commons Attribution 4.0 International License (http://creativecommons.org/licenses/by/4.0/), which permits use, sharing, adaptation, distribution and reproduction in any medium or format, as long as you give appropriate credit to the original author(s) and the source, provide a link to the Creative Commons license and indicate if changes were made.

The images or other third party material in this chapter are included in the chapter's Creative Commons license, unless indicated otherwise in a credit line to the material. If material is not included in the chapter's Creative Commons license and your intended use is not permitted by statutory regulation or exceeds the permitted use, you will need to obtain permission directly from the copyright holder.

Part II
Mapping Responsibilities

Chapter 4
Mapping Responsibilities: Report from the Qualitative Interview Study

Martina Jürgensen and Madeleine Herzog

Abstract One of the main themes emerging from the interviews with 17 families about their long-term experiences of bone marrow transplantation was the perception and distribution of responsibilities among the members of the family. Families reported that they felt it was a shared responsibility to help the sick child, and therefore considered donation a matter of course, even a family duty, which contributed to a dynamic differentiation of responsibilities among family members. Donors, for instance, acknowledged a responsibility for the success or failure of the transplant, and some said that their duty extended over time and included more transplants later in life. In retrospect, most donors valued their donation positively.

Keywords Transplantation medicine · Family duty · Family responsibility · Sibling donation

One group of questions especially important for family members were those connected to responsibility. How are responsibilities distributed within the family and how do they change due to the events of the illness? How do they guide the decision-making about donation and the transplantation? We have analysed the interviews with this guiding question: How are responsibilities allocated, negotiated and understood in the complex relational network of patient, donor, other siblings, parents, physicians, and caregivers in the social environment?

All families in our study experienced the time of the illness and of its treatment as a major rupture. During this time, they had to (newly) allocate and negotiate responsibilities within the nuclear family as well as with their external network. What unifies the families in the sample of this study is that they had the possibility of using an intrafamilial donor for a bone marrow transplant (BMT) and that they ended up doing so. All families in this study took the option of genetic HLA typing

M. Jürgensen (✉) · M. Herzog
Institute for History of Medicine and Science Studies, University of Lübeck, Lübeck, Schleswig-Holstein, Germany
e-mail: martina.juergensen@uni-luebeck.de

© The Author(s) 2022
C. Schües et al. (eds.), *Stem Cell Transplantations Between Siblings as Social Phenomena*, Philosophy and Medicine 144,
https://doi.org/10.1007/978-3-031-04166-2_4

within the family, in order to find a suitable donor, as a matter of course. They did not struggle much with that idea. However, they chose different ways of making it happen. The approaches they took following the result of genetic typing, after learning that there was a suitable donor among the siblings, varied greatly between the families.

One unexpected finding of our study is that most families did not actually consider searching for an unrelated donor to be an option, as soon as they found out that one of their children was suitable as donor. The reasons for this vary. In their narratives the families often told us that finding an unrelated donor is doubtful and uncertain; having one in the immediate family is like winning the lottery. In some other cases, time played a significant role and the need to find a donor as soon as possible put a great deal of pressure on the families. In these cases, intrafamilial donation was chosen because it seemed the fastest option. Yet another, more profound motive might have been that many felt a need to find the solution to the crisis within their own family. Being able to heal the disease with family-internal resources seemed to be a way to reclaim power over the life-threatening disease and the experience of helplessness connected to it.

4.1 Donation as a Family Responsibility: A Matter of Course ("Selbstverständlichkeit")?

The family is regarded as the primary place for solving the "illness"/ "transplantation" problem.

Members of several families unanimously reported that they felt it is a shared responsibility of the family to solve "the problem" and do all they could to save the ill children's life. Getting tested as well as deciding to donate the blood stem cells was a matter of course, not to be questioned or discussed. In the interviews it becomes clear that the mere thought that a family member would think about not being tested for compatibility, or reject a donation if one were possible, is something most study participants considered unthinkable – both parents and children.

> Interviewer: But you say there was no question for you that you would like to do this and
> Non-donor brother: NO, of course not. Well I think don't remember at all now, well I'd be surprised if someone said: nah, I don't want – can't get myself typed, I would never (laughs) donate bone marrow to my sister. (Minz)

In several families of our study, the intrafamilial donation was taken for granted by all members. To be able to provide a donor is seen as a gift and a special strength and ability of the family and a means of regaining control and power in their difficult situation after the rupture caused by the disease.

Even if the donation was seen as a matter of course by the families, many of them emphasized that the donor children had made a voluntary decision. They did not feel any contradiction between these two interpretations of the situation: on the one hand, there was no question, no decision to be taken, in the sense of a choice between yes or no as options, but on the other, it was a decision that the donor *had* to take.

4.2 Donation as a Family Duty?

In some families, the blood stem cell donation by the suitable sibling was viewed – mainly by the parents – as a familial duty. This view did not have much of an impact on families in which the potential donor agreed to the transplantation. By contrast, it led to situations of conflict in those families where the potential donor refused to donate the bone marrow cells in the first place.

The main reason for potential donors not wanting to donate was fear of the expected stay in hospital and of the potential for harm to their own bodies.

In some families the duty to donate as a familial duty was perceived to be so powerful that it could override all concerns about acting against the will of the donor child. Since the child is part of the family, the child must submit to family duty, even if they personally made a different decision about donation. Since donors in our study were underage children, the will of the parents was ultimately decisive – they were responsible for deciding what seemed best for the family as a whole. The parents weighed up the pros and cons and came to the conclusion that the possible negative effects of a donation on the donor child were negligible compared to the advantages of sibling donation for the family.

One mother did ask the donor whether she agreed to donate but said the demands of the situation were so strong and so obvious that there was no real chance to refuse, even by the donor child herself. She was aware that she had put the donor child under massive pressure and that the child had no real possibility of refusing to make the donation. Therefore, asking was in fact a charade:

> Mother: As she says, I knew, I had to do it, I she sensed the PRESSURE, she HAD TO- she didn't have a choice. We asked her and explained it to her, said to her, ARE you going to do this, do you want to do this, but actually everything was really obvious, she's got to do this, even if we ask her, it was a charade, you see. It was clear to all of us and SHE sensed the pressure, yeah great, I am terribly scared. No way could I dare say- I can't say no. (Bahr)

The donor child mentions a series of elements that build up this perceived situational moral demand, most importantly: (i) the parents putting pressure on her, telling her that she just had to do it, (ii) because it is "your brother after all"; (iii) that she would not forgive herself later in life if she did not, and (iv) that she didn't want to take responsibility afterwards vis-à-vis other people for not having donated.

4.3 Differentiated Responsibilities and Obligations

Parental duties in the situation of bone marrow transplantation between siblings were manifold and contradictory in part. They included caring adequately and acting responsibly for all their children in a conflict that emerges in relation to the donation and transplantation. In reading the interviews we were guided by these questions. Do they feel guilty when recounting how they handled the situation? Do they or other family members identify any dilemma?

Many parents felt they were at the mercy of the system, or of the doctors; they experienced a lack of control and associated great insecurity. Together with this experience came a sense of no longer being able to fulfil their "proper" role as parents, i.e. protecting their children and providing them with security.

Several parents described a *dilemma* in relation to caring for their sick and their healthy children equally. The sick child needed more resources and the parents faced a conflict between responding to the sick child's needs while still fulfilling their parental role for the other healthy child(ren). This dilemma became especially significant when a decision needed to be made on the donation: a medical intervention into the donor's healthy body was necessary, in order to provide a potential treatment for the recipient child. With this medical intervention, the parents accepted that the healthy child's body is temporarily "made sick" to provide treatment for the benefit of their other child.

In our interviews, the dilemma was described in particularly clear ways. Parents reported various strategies for dealing with it. Some just pushed their conflicting thoughts away and decided to do what they (supposedly) "had to do". Others point out that the donation was no big deal for the donor – a safe and barely stressful procedure (analogous to nail trimming) with immense positive effects.

Most donors shared this view with their parents and could, at least in retrospect, understand the dilemma in which the parents found themselves. In their opinion, too, the parents had no other option, even if they themselves as a child had found it difficult to donate.

4.4 Donors' Responsibilities Before Donation: The Chance for a "Rescue Attempt"

Several families reported that the donor has, to a certain degree, the responsibility to stay healthy and secure in order not to risk the donation not taking place successfully. Being the potential donor changed views of the body of the donor child. It became something that needed to be particularly protected and kept healthy, as it now had a different role to fulfil, that of a source of the potential medical treatment for the sick child. From this perspective, the body no longer belonged only to the child itself, but became an important resource for the survival of the sick sibling and thus the well-being of the entire family. The resulting restrictions – for example, some said they had to limit their social life in the run-up to the transplant in order not to get sick themselves – had to be accepted by the future donor. In the interviews it became clear that they were willing to do this and to accept this role.

> Donor: Yes like I said, you really have a great responsibility and erm (..) I really tried to like keep myself away from people who were ill, so that nothing happened to me so that I'd like get ill, some kind of cold or something. I mean I really tried, erm to be fit and you really have, 'cos you've always got it in the back of your mind: what'll happen if you're ill, then (.) if the operation actually has to be postponed for such a small thing, because you didn't want it at all and yeah, [the] responsibility was great, but you were actually

pleased about it too, being erm able to do it, being a match and well like I said, you did try not to come into contact with pathogens like that, so that you don't really meet people who are ill, because I thought myself, that something like that really doesn't need to be part of the situation, because you just wanted the operation to take place when it was supposed to, yeah. (Kötter)

4.5   Responsibility for the "Success" or "Failure" of the Transplant?

In many families we interviewed for this study, the connection between a successful or unsuccessful transplant and the donor's sense of responsibility or blame was discussed. Several donors reported that they experienced a feeling of responsibility for their sibling's health and for the outcome of the BMT.

The reaction of the parents or physicians to this notion of responsibility, however, was always the same in all families in this study: that the donor child was *not responsible* for the outcome. Yet the feelings of responsibility remained for many donors, and were something they struggled with. This sense of responsibility was related not only to the survival of the sick child but also to potential aftereffects of the transplant, such as Graft-versus-Host Disease.

After a failure occurs there is a real challenge to clarify responsibilities, and the child might have difficulty accepting the release offered by the parents.

4.6   Long-Term or Life-Long Duty for Further Donations?

In some families, the donation of blood stem cells and other body material (in one case a lacrimal gland) was necessary more than once. In other families, the possibility of needing further body material from the donor remained present. The responsibility of the donor child to provide body materials in the longer term was discussed in several families. The donor children also faced questions of how long they wanted and needed to keep themselves ready for further donations; some had the sense of being a "depot of spare parts", as the donor sibling in the Wahl family put it:

> Donor: that THEN for the first time ever this thought CAME to me, that now I- if I now was a, like at some point I expressed it really badly, whether I was now a SPARE PARTS DEPOT for him. (Wahl)

The prospect of more possible transplants in the future was clearly present in two families. For example, one donor of blood stem cells was asked, years after the BMT, when her brother suffered from a GvHD-related pulmonary dysfunction, why she would not donate a lung to her sick brother. This question showed her that having served once as a donor to her brother was interpreted by others as a lifelong obligation to donate. Although she was quite ready to donate part of her lungs to her brother (which was not possible for medical reasons), this transfer of responsibility to her (or rather her body) was a significant burden for this girl. For her, the material physical composition of her body and the resulting potential to serve her brother as a donor created the impression of a responsibility that exists independently of her own will.

Another donor sibling said in the family interview that he considered joining the official donor registry in order to be able to donate blood stem cells to sick people outside the family. His mother pointed out to him that his sibling might yet need another donation and that this could be endangered if he had just donated to a stranger. He should therefore please refrain from official registration in order to remain available as a donor for his sibling at any time. This argument made sense to the donor - he accepted the long-term responsibility of "rescuing" the sibling in an emergency.

4.7   Does the Recipient Owe Something to the Donor?

In contrast to the case of a stem cell transplant from an unrelated donor, the recipient of an intrafamilial donation knows whose body material has been used for her treatment. To this knowledge are connected several ideas and feelings: of responsibility, to gratitude for this donation, the "gift", and notions of debt towards the donor.

Many participants reported that this image of responsibility or gratitude has never been thought of or discussed in their families. But other interviewees reported expectations on different levels to value the donation, the "gift of life", in an appropriate way or, for the recipients, to show their gratitude.

Some brought up the donation jokingly when there were disagreements, others expected the recipient child to live a life according to the donor's or the family's ideas about what is right and wrong. In these cases, the donation of body material was transformed into a tool of control; and the recipient was expected to show gratitude for the donation by living up to the family's expectations, as the following quotation shows.

> Father: I mean Karsten always has something of an attitude (groans) like: she could be a bit thankful to me for doing all that, couldn't she? (Kirstein)

In one family, gratitude to the donor took a dramatic turn when the recipient became depressed, drug addicted and suicidal. Her brother, the donor, interpreted this as an affront and accused her of throwing away the life he had given her and so not appreciating this gift sufficiently.

4.8   In Retrospect

In the families' stories, it became obvious that in retrospect most donors felt positively about the donation. They were proud to have helped their siblings – even in families where the sick child had severe side effects or died. Taking responsibility for the well-being of the sibling and the entire family and being able to help had short-term and long-term advantages for the donors. In the short-term it became clear that the donation makes the donor the focus of attention of the parents, other siblings, medical stuff and the social environment. This sounds profane, but in a situation in which all attention is usually directed to the sick child, it is immensely important for a sibling. In addition, the donation and the associated medical procedure gives the donor sibling access to the world of the hospital – a world into which the parents often disappeared together with the sick child over long periods of time and from which the siblings were otherwise largely excluded. Getting to know this world was described by several donor siblings as a positive experience.

It is impressive that even those donors who said that as children they had found the perceived obligation to donate burdensome were able, in retrospect, to sympathise with their parents' plight and dilemma and to understand their decisions. None of the donors in our interviews accused the parents of abusing them for the benefit of the sick sibling.

Open Access   This chapter is licensed under the terms of the Creative Commons Attribution 4.0 International License (http://creativecommons.org/licenses/by/4.0/), which permits use, sharing, adaptation, distribution and reproduction in any medium or format, as long as you give appropriate credit to the original author(s) and the source, provide a link to the Creative Commons license and indicate if changes were made.

The images or other third party material in this chapter are included in the chapter's Creative Commons license, unless indicated otherwise in a credit line to the material. If material is not included in the chapter's Creative Commons license and your intended use is not permitted by statutory regulation or exceeds the permitted use, you will need to obtain permission directly from the copyright holder.

Chapter 5
Mediating the Risks of Mutual Care: Families and the Ethical Challenges of Sibling Bone Marrow Donation

Claudia Wiesemann

Abstract Bone marrow transplants from one sibling to another are a challenge for medical ethics. How can the decision to donate be made freely and without coercion if the life of a child depends on it? I examine how sibling bone marrow donation can be reconciled with the moral ideal of family, specifying the meaning of care, and focusing particularly on the role of minors. I also take the example of intrafamily bone marrow transplantation as a test case to identify the dangers of care and ask how to best mediate them.

Keywords Medical ethics · Child · Family · Parents · Care ethics · Care · Autonomy · Trust · Bone marrow transplantation

5.1 The Ethical Challenges of Sibling Bone Marrow Donation

Bone marrow transplants from one sibling to another are a serious challenge for medical ethics. An informed consent, essential prerequisite for any medical intervention and especially one without benefit to the donor, is highly questionable. How can the decision be made freely and without coercion if the life of a sibling depends on it? Saying no to donation would threaten the life of the brother or sister. The reactions of other family members – accusations, rejection, isolation – would be dire. Being aware of these consequences would create a particularly severe form of implicit coercion and is undoubtedly capable of undermining self-determination to such an extent that consent might be considered invalid.

C. Wiesemann (✉)
Institute of Medical Ethics and History of Medicine, Goettingen University Medical Centre, Goettingen, Germany
e-mail: cwiesem@gwdg.de

© The Author(s) 2022
C. Schües et al. (eds.), *Stem Cell Transplantations Between Siblings as Social Phenomena*, Philosophy and Medicine 144, https://doi.org/10.1007/978-3-031-04166-2_5

To complicate matters, donors are minors and often at an age when full informed consent may not yet be possible. Even though bone marrow transplantation is an intervention whose nature, significance, and scope is comparatively easy to understand, it cannot be taken for granted that children under the age of 12–14 years will be competent to consent. Parents as their legal representatives must give consent on behalf of the child. However, the parents' consent has to be based on what is in the donor's best interests. An intervention without benefit to the donor child, such as a bone marrow donation, can hardly be justified by the commonly used concept of the donor's best interests.[1] Interventions in minors without potential personal benefit may be justified if they are associated with only minimal risks and burden. However, although it is disputed what exactly counts as minimal (Radenbach and Wiesemann 2009), a surgical intervention under anaesthesia in bone marrow donation certainly involves more than minimal risks and burden. Not surprisingly, and for all these reasons, medical ethicists have called into question the ethical justification of bone marrow donation by a minor sibling.[2]

The parents in the Lübeck study on intrafamily bone marrow transplantation,[3] too, express such fundamental concerns:

> Father: This this exact issue (.) has cropped up in several places. Is it actually somehow permissible, erm, to use this- a child as a construction site for the other? (Wahl)

The answer to this obviously rhetorical question can only be no. Or does it? In what follows, I will examine how bone marrow donation can be reconciled with the moral ideal of family. To that purpose, I will specify the meaning of care, focusing particularly on the role of minors. Moreover, I will take the example of intrafamily bone marrow transplantation as a test case to identify the dangers of care and ask how to best mediate them.

5.2   What Are Families For?

The intuition of many of the family members interviewed in the Lübeck study – and the general public, as well – seems to point in a different direction. Shouldn't everyone in a family be prepared to stand by the other family members? Isn't that exactly what families are there for? Many answers from parents, all of whom are undoubtedly people with a high sense of responsibility and parental love for their children, and also from siblings suggest this view:

---

[1] For a critical analysis see Schües 2015.

[2] Schickhardt 2015. Schües and Rehmann-Sutter 2013a, b rightly point to the fact that there are no justifications of minor sibling bone marrow donation based on the argument of life as a higher good.

[3] The Lübeck study is a qualitative empirical study on bone marrow transplantation between siblings, conducted from 2016 to 2019 by Madeleine Herzog, Martina Jürgensen, Christoph Rehmann-Sutter and Christina Schües of the Institute of History of Medicine and Science Studies, University of Lübeck.

Mother: Well, it became evident relatively quickly that erm (.) Greta was a match, that that would work and then it was actually a matter of course for us. We didn't have any other (..) thoughts on the matter, did we". (Grohmann)

Father: I don't know, he always took it for granted. There wasn't anyone else who put him (.) under pressure or anything, there (.) there WAS no discussion at all. 'I'll do that for my brother'. (Kötter)

Non-donor sister: that she has to have bone marrow and that we all need to get ourselves tested, (.) or whether we wanted to get ourselves tested and I think, that's actually not something to question. (Kirstein)

These responses from a mother, a father, and a non-donor sister do not suggest that bone marrow transplantation is an exceptional act of altruism. These so-called supererogatory acts would be praiseworthy, but not morally required. In an ethics of rights and duties, they go beyond what can be demanded of someone (Heinrichs 2015). If someone registers in a database as stem cell donor and is willing to donate bone marrow to a stranger in case of a match, this is indeed considered a heroic act, a special act of selfless charity. For example, a German advertising campaign for tissue typing expresses this view by inviting potential candidates: "Do you want to be a hero?"[4] In contrast, bone marrow donation in the families studied here is not celebrated like heroic behaviour. The families see it as a "matter of course", the testing for suitability as a stem cell donor as something that simply cannot be called into question. As if this particular caring act was not an extra, not a special "on-top", but simply a moral given. It is somehow foundational to the moral identity of the families involved.

In families, many things are different in a way that is unusual – and sometimes even irritating – for ethics. The family maintains a special role which to some ethicists is dubious and even worrisome. A major problem associated with the special role of the family in ethics dates from a time when men and women did not enjoy equal rights in marriage and partnership, when the husband was still considered the head of the family and the wife and children his subordinates (Okin 1989; Fineman 1999). Women in the countries of the global North have largely freed themselves from this form of legal, political, and social dependence. But the problem remains that children are still largely subject to parental authority (Archard 2003). Legal regulations, such as the parents' duty to promote the well-being of the child, are intended to limit this power of authority (Schües and Rehmann-Sutter 2013a, b). The child rights movement also seeks to strengthen the rights of children as morally relevant individuals. However, any form of political and legal emancipation of children reaches its limits because of their invariable need for protection (Schickhardt 2012; Wiesemann 2015).

And yet most of us will not classify the reactions of the families studied here as unusual. The self-evident nature of help in families, their willingness to stand up for each other, is not surprising. Just because it seems so self-evident it has often not been given further consideration in academic ethics (Beier et al. 2016). As a

---

[4] „Willst Du ein Held sein?", Deutsche Knochenmarkspenderdatei (DKMS) https://www.dkms.de/de/anzeige-willst-du-ein-held-sein. Schaper et al. (2019) analyse the implicit messages of similar health campaigns from an ethical point of view.

consequence of a methodological as well as normative individualism, traditional ethics has ignored the special moral connection in families and thus implicitly treated it as irrelevant (Blustein 1982; Schoeman 1980; Lindemann Nelson and Lindemann Nelson 1995). This should indeed worry us because, after all, this way of life has relevance for almost everyone. Most of us grew up in families and are currently living in one. And many ethical questions, at least in health care, relate to persons in family relationships (Lindemann Nelson and Lindemann Nelson 1995; Verkerk et al. 2014).

The difficulty of understanding the family from an ethical perspective is also due to the fact that a multitude of life styles are common today. Some types of family have only recently been legally recognised. For the sake of simplicity, the term family I will use here shall be understood to mean all social groups of at least two persons who live together or manage the major part of their day-to-day life together, and comprise at least one child and one caretaker, regardless of whether the caretakers are married or unmarried, or genetically or socially related to the child. The stories told here are about families with at least two children: one who is ill and one who is to donate bone marrow. In what follows, I will focus on groups of people who include underage children because this way of life is prototypical for the moral image of the family: it assumes that the members take care of each other. But, of course, two adult persons living together can also see themselves as a family and strive to live up to the same ideal.

5.3   The Moral Ideal of Family

How does this moral ideal look like? Simply put, families are places of care for each other. Iris Marion Young understands family to be

> people who live together and/or share resources necessary to the means of life and comfort; who are committed to taking care of one another's physical and emotional needs to the best of their ability; who conceive themselves in a relatively long-term, if not permanent relationship; and who recognize themselves as family. (Young 1997, 196)

Young's idea of the reciprocity of care, however, creates a philosophical problem. Isn't the care for children rather unidirectional? Parents take care of their children, but children do not take care of their parents in the same way, at least not when they are young. And whether and to which degree children as adults have a duty to care for their old parents is philosophically controversial.[5] So, what might reciprocity of care mean? In order to understand this concept, one has to consider that, for one thing, families are not short-lived groups. They are conceived as groups that are

---

[5] Hugh LaFollette (1996) states that because of the lack of reciprocity (in the conventional sense) children and parents cannot have a truly personal relationship. To the contrary, Magdalena Hoffmann (2014, 204f) advocates a special form of "basal reciprocity" in the interpersonal relationship. See also Schües and Foth 2019, 96.

meant to last for a long time, even indefinitely. As a consequence, the identity of families is not bound to certain persons. It can be maintained even if individual members leave the family or die. Care is often not returned to the original caring person, but is passed on to the children of the next generation. Reciprocity is created by the children as adults taking over the role of parents and passing on the love, warmth and care they received to their own children. Thus, reciprocity relates to roles rather than to persons. Moreover, if reciprocity between persons is achieved, it is usually not an exchange of the same type of care. Children do take care of their parents, but rather in ways they can master. Their care is not material by nature. But they do perceive the needs of their parents and, if necessary, may try to comfort and support them. When such gestures are made by young children, who themselves are in considerable need of help, this can be particularly touching.

In order to maintain family relationships in the long run, all persons involved must somehow practice caring. Receiving care and taking care becomes part of everyday routines. This applies to adults and children alike. Even small children imitate the parent-child relationship by, for example, playing with their dolls and thus practicing caring behaviour. When, in the absence of parental control, older children have to care for their younger siblings this can also be an exercise in this practice.

The meaning of family care is not easy to grasp from an ethical perspective. Essential aspects of parental responsibility are, in the words of Samantha Brennan and Robert Noggle, "care, advocacy and protection" (Brennan and Noggle 1997, 12). In everyday life, care often boils down to acts of advocacy or protection. However, in the course of the child rights movement it has become clear that the child should not only be an object of advocacy and protection, but also be treated like a real subject of human relationships. Care does not only aim at satisfying needs and representing interests, but at paying respect to the person cared for. From the perspective of liberal ethics, it is unclear how this can be realised in the context of family relationships and, in particular, when children are concerned. Respecting a person is usually understood as respecting the autonomy of the person which in families is compromised in various ways. I have argued elsewhere that young children can nevertheless be acknowledged as morally relevant persons if their carings are respected, carings being complex emotional attitudes with which a person identifies and which form part of their identity (Wiesemann 2016, 97). Carings are internal in the sense that they are our own; they represent our self. We cannot easily distance ourselves from them or feel that they are just imposed on us by our nature. The concept of caring allows us to distinguish the merely sensual desires of a person from those attitudes the person identifies with and can reflect on with some subtlety. In the context of bone marrow donation, a young child may particularly care for his/her sick brother or sister, and although donating bone marrow may not yet be the result of an autonomous decision, it may nevertheless arise from of a deep caring emotion that should be respected. The intuitive responses of siblings to the request for donation reflect the fact that they considered the caring act as something deeply ingrained in their family identity.

Non-donor brother: NO, of course not. Well I think (.) don't remember at all now, well I'd
  be surprised if someone said: 'nah, I don't want – can't get myself typed, I would never
  (laughs) donate bone marrow to my sister'. (Minz)
Non-donor sister: that she has to have bone marrow and that we all need to get ourselves
  tested, (.) or whether we wanted to get ourselves tested and I think, that's actually not
  something to question. (Kirstein)
Father: I don't know, he always took it for granted. There wasn't anyone else who put him
  (.) under pressure or anything, there (.) there WAS no discussion at all. 'I'll do that for
  my brother'. (Kötter)

5.4   The Dangers of Care

It is obvious that family is not solely based on the autonomous decisions of the
persons involved. Parents may have agreed together to start a family, but their children did not decide to belong to that family. Annette Baier has argued that it is precisely such unchosen relationships, and especially care relationships, that acquire a
special moral significance, if only because they are so common in human life (Baier
1987). Yet, care relationships can be morally challenging in that they construct the
person being cared for as passive and tend to have a paternalistic patronizing effect,
thus threatening to undermine the idea of the moral equality of all human beings
(Held 2006). There is no doubt that such a demanding and complex practice is in
many ways in danger of degenerating into something negative. Some of these concerns are also evident in the family interviews:

Mother: And because of that it was clear to me, without us having a massive discussion with
  Zorro, that Zorro WILL donate whether he wants to or not. (Zucker)
Non-donor sister: because if you believe you're losing a child then it's- then this child has
  a different status in the family. (Minz)
Mother: [During the time of illness, the other children] actually needed me TOO, but it just
  didn't happen, you know. (Kirstein)

As we can see from these answers, danger always looms large when care is
requested (Hoagland 1991, 252f; Feder Kittay 1999, 34). Care can be misunder-
stood as a duty of sacrifice and self-abandonment, it can be imposed on individual
members like a servitude, it can be granted arbitrarily, favouring only a few or, in
these cases, just one child over the other children, it may even be hypocritical and
disguise selfish motives. Clearly, the conditions under which intrafamily bone marrow transplantation takes place are a major challenge to the ideal of family care.
Typically, the following questions arise: How is it still possible to treat each child as
an individual and a person if one of them requires so much attention that the others
must be neglected? How is it possible to maintain a common identity when the pressure on a single person is so intense? How can the ideal of reciprocity be maintained
when someone receives a gift so special that it cannot be returned?

In a father's comment, the serious danger of the donor being instrumentalized
and treated only as an object resounds:

Father: This this exact issue (.) has cropped up in several places. Is it actually somehow permissible, erm, to use this- a child as a construction site for the other? (Wahl)

The father points out the ultimate danger of objectification which is looming with this kind of therapy. Quite interestingly, it would seem that objectification is threatening not only the care recipient but also the caring donor. Carers often feel like being objectified. Especially in long and demanding care relationships, they may perform their tasks merely mechanically and they may no longer feel that they are regarded as a person with a life and interests of their own. An important question, therefore, is whether and how families succeed in confirming both donor and carer as subjects and morally relevant persons, despite this impending danger.

The donors tried to achieve a more active role by adopting the role of the caring person and the responsibility associated with it out of their own accord.

Donor: Yes like I said, you really have a great responsibility and erm (..) I really tried to like keep myself away from people who were ill, so that nothing happened to me so that I'd like get ill, some kind of cold or something. (Kötter)

Another donor compares donation to pregnancy.

Donor: I have to (..) erm because for that I- because I'm not just responsible for MY body but also for another body, erm like and act like that. (..) I mean I feel like that now I'm pregnant as well (laughs). (Wahl)

This is a very telling interpretation. Even more so than in the case of bone marrow donation, the body of the pregnant woman is instrumentalised for the growth of the foetus. The comparison is particularly interesting because pregnancy is not only a very good example for the ethical issues involved in instrumentalising the body of a person and, thus, the person herself (Wiesemann 2018). It is also a prerequisite for the very existence of donor and recipient. Instrumentalizing the body of someone is not alien to the idea of family, but rather constitutes it. A positive concept of family can emerge when pregnancy, or comparable types of instrumentalization, are successfully interpreted as a beneficial and constructive care relationship. The ability to accept and constructively interpret such ambivalences is an essential achievement of the good family (Jansen 2004).

That is why it is so important that the donors playfully assume a position of power - as a deliberate contrast to the feeling of impotence necessarily associated with the instrumentalisation of their bodies.

Mother: Melissa was also TOTALLY cool, yeah? and Mighel had just been um discharged from the BMT and the two fought again for the first time (.). 'oh', Melissa says to me, (loudly), 'YEAH YOU KNOW WHAT AND NEXT TIME YOU WON'T GET ANY MORE BONE MARROW FROM ME' (laughs), I thought that was so cool. I had to LAUGH so much, because it was so cool, so childish, so normal you know, yeah. (Molle)

By playfully threatening not to donate next time, Melissa resumes authorship of her life. Her mother sees this as her way of restoring normality. Normality in this context means: the relationship is reciprocal again – dependencies are again shared equally between donor and recipient.

The powerful position of the donor also manifested itself in another, rather dramatic, family story. Some time after donation, the recipient girl from the Kirstein family got depressed and attempted suicide. Her sibling donor severely reproaches her for that:

> Recipient: well [I was] also very depressed and then I tried to kill myself and um my brother could never approve of that like, because he said: 'I SAVED your life and now you just want to throw it away!' (Kirstein)

Obviously, the game of power has become serious. The balance of mutual care – which is also a balance of power – is threatened once again.

> Recipient: what worried me a bit for quite some time, was that I felt I OWED him something, on the principle of: 'Yes, you saved my life and I owe you something'. But erm for one thing I can't owe him erm my whole life long erm- I mean that he like, I mean that I have a DEBT towards him or something. That can't be the case, can it, and it can't be the case either that erm he makes some kind of statements and I just HAVE TO listen to them and be sad. That can't be the case either, you know? Because he doesn't have a RIGHT either to say, no way: you don't have the right to KILL YOURSELF, because um I donated bone marrow to you or whatever, yeah? So he got in a huff and when I say: why don't you just ask me WHY I tried to kill myself anyway, you know? (Kirstein)

Reacting to this shift in power, the sister emphasizes that her brother, even though having *saved* her life, has no *right over* her life. She no longer wants to be just the person who received a bone marrow donation. She demands her brother to face up to the reasons for her suicide, to consider the life she led after transplantation. She will not be forever trapped in the role of the grateful recipient, but is moving forward in her development, even if her life takes an adverse turn.

Care relationships must be negotiated again and again. They have to be dynamic and continue to evolve as long as they exist.

5.5   Conclusion

The statements of the various family members examined here clearly demonstrate the moral complexity of family relationships. From a moral point of view it is important, on one hand, to recognize each family member as a person and as morally significant and, on the other, to maintain the identity of the family as a whole. In the family, each member is responsible for the well-being of all. Such reciprocal care can only be realized over time, depending on the abilities of each individual. Persons who as childrens were the recipients of parental care will later in life do their share of care by raising future generations. Such a dynamic realization of reciprocity secures the existence of the family over long periods of time. To accomplish this goal, every member of the family has to exercise her- or himself in the practice of care. Even young children are not exempted from this task, although they may often realize it in a more playful manner. Relationships of care can thus acquire a high degree of complexity.

Under these circumstances, the danger of turning care relationships into abusive ones also looms large. In particular, there is the serious risk of family members being instrumentalised for the welfare of others. However, one has to keep in mind that care work is always threatened by this kind of danger. It is decisive for the moral ideal of family whether it is possible to mediate this risk, i.e., to constructively reinterpret forms of instrumentalization as particularly laudable examples of personal commitment and responsibility.

The families that present themselves here try in various ways to mediate the danger of the misuse of care. Bone marrow transplantation among siblings is a special challenge because persons who are still minors have to provide care for their siblings. The resulting imbalance of power must be redressed not only between siblings, but also between parents and children. It helps that the moral ideal of family is not static, but dynamically realized over time. The stories the family members tell illustrate that, if everything goes well, it is even possible to affirm the family's moral identity in a particularly felicitous way.

Literature

Archard, David W. 2003. *Children, family, and the state*. Aldershot: Ashgate.

Baier, Anette C. 1987. The need for more than justice. *Canadian Journal of Philosophy* 13: 41–56.

Beier, Katharina, Isabella Jordan, Claudia Wiesemann, and Silke Schicktanz. 2016. Understanding collective agency in bioethics. *Medicine, Health Care and Philosophy* 19: 411–422.

Blustein, Jeffrey. 1982. *Parents and children: The ethics of the family*. 1st ed. New York: Oxford University Press.

Brennan, Samantha, and Robert Noggle. 1997. The moral status of children. Children's rights, Parents' rights, and family justice. *Social Theory and Practice* 23: 1–26.

Feder Kittay, Eva. 1999. *Love's labor. Essays on women, equality, and dependency*. New York/London: Routledge.

Fineman, Martha A. 1999. What place for family privacy? *George Washington Law Review* 67: 1207–1224.

Heinrichs, Bert. 2015. Die normative Bewertung der Pädiatrischen Stammzelltransplantation. In *Rettende Geschwister. Ethische Aspekte der Einwilligung in der pädiatrischen Stammzelltransplantation*, ed. Christina Schües and Christoph Rehmann-Sutter, 121–131. Münster: Mentis.

Held, Virginia. 2006. *The ethics of care: Personal, political, and global*. Oxford: Oxford University Press.

Hoagland, Sarah Lucia. 1991. Some thoughts about "caring". In *Claudia Card*, ed. Feminist Ethics, 247–263. Lawrence: University Press of Kansas.

Hoffmann, Magdalena. 2014. What relationship structure tells us about love. In *Love and its objects. What can we care for?* ed. Christian Maurer, Tony Milligan, and Kamila Pacovská, 192–208. Basingstoke: Palgrave Macmillan.

Jansen, Lynn A. 2004. Child organ donation, family autonomy, and intimate attachments. *Cambridge Quarterly of Healthcare Ethics* 13: 133–142.

LaFollette, Hugh. 1996. *Personal relationships: Love, identity, and morality*. Oxford, Cambridge: Blackwell.

Lindemann Nelson, Hilde, and James Lindemann Nelson. 1995. *The patient in the family. An ethics of medicine and families*. New York: Routledge.

Okin, Susan M. 1989. *Justice, gender and the family*. New York: Basic Books.

Radenbach, Katrin, and Claudia Wiesemann. 2009. Risiko und Belastung als Kriterien der Zulässigkeit von Forschung mit Kindern und Jugendlichen. In *Ethische Aspekte der pädiatrischen Forschung*, ed. Georg Marckmann and Dietrich Niethammer, 37–49. Köln: Deutscher Ärzte-Verlag.

Schaper, Manuel, Solveig L. Hansen, and Silke Schicktanz. 2019. Überreden für die gute Sache! Techniken öffentlicher Gesundheitskommunikation und ihre ethischen Implikationen. *Ethik in der Medizin* 31: 23–44.

Schickhardt, Christoph. 2012. *Kinderethik. Der moralische Status und die Rechte der Kinder.* Münster: Mentis.

———. 2015. Bedeutung und Wert von Einwilligung unter besonderer Berücksichtigung der Gewebespende zwischen Geschwisterkindern. In *Rettende Geschwister. Ethische Aspekte der Einwilligung in der pädiatrischen Stammzelltransplantation*, ed. Christina Schües and Christoph Rehmann-Sutter, 101–119. Münster: Mentis.

Schoeman, Ferdinand. 1980. Rights of children, rights of parents, and the moral basis of the family. *Ethics* 91: 6–19.

Schües, Christina. 2015. Dem Willen des Kindes folgen? Das Kindeswohl zwischen Gegenwart und Zukunft. In *Rettende Geschwister. Ethische Aspekte der Einwilligung in der pädiatrischen Stammzelltransplantation*, ed. Christina Schües and Christoph Rehmann-Sutter, 215–239. Münster: Mentis.

Schües, Christina, and Hannes Foth. 2019. Elternschaft. In *Handbuch Philosophie der Kindheit*, ed. Johannes Drerup and Gottfried Schweiger, 90–98. Berlin: J. B. Metzler.

Schües, Christina, and Christoph Rehmann-Sutter. 2013a. Hat ein Kind eine Pflicht, Blutstammzellen für ein krankes Geschwisterkind zu spenden? *Ethik in der Medizin* 25: 89–102.

———. 2013b. The well- and the unwell-being of a child. *Topoi* 32: 197–205.

Verkerk, M.A., Hilde Lindemann, Janice McLaughlin, Jackie L. Scully, Ulrik Kihlbom, Jamie Nelson, et al. 2014. Where families and healthcare meet. *Journal of Medical Ethics* 41: 183–185.

Wiesemann, Claudia. 2015. Ethik in der Kinderheilkunde und Jugendmedizin. In *Praxisbuch Ethik in der Medizin*, ed. Georg Marckmann, 313–325. Berlin: MWV Medizinisch Wissenschaftliche Verlagsgesellschaft.

———. 2016. *Moral equality, bioethics, and the child.* Cham: Springer.

———. 2018. Which ethics for the fetus as a patient? In *The fetus as a patient. A contested concept and its normative implications*, ed. Dagmar Schmitz, Angus Clarke, and Wybo Dondorp, 28–39. London/New York: Routledge.

Young, Iris M. 1997. *Intersecting voices. Dilemmas of gender, political philosophy, and policy.* Princeton: Princeton University Press.

Open Access This chapter is licensed under the terms of the Creative Commons Attribution 4.0 International License (http://creativecommons.org/licenses/by/4.0/), which permits use, sharing, adaptation, distribution and reproduction in any medium or format, as long as you give appropriate credit to the original author(s) and the source, provide a link to the Creative Commons license and indicate if changes were made.

The images or other third party material in this chapter are included in the chapter's Creative Commons license, unless indicated otherwise in a credit line to the material. If material is not included in the chapter's Creative Commons license and your intended use is not permitted by statutory regulation or exceeds the permitted use, you will need to obtain permission directly from the copyright holder.

Chapter 6
Responsibility, Care and Illness in Family Relationships

Jutta Ecarius

Abstract Family as a relationship of cooperation and solidarity refers to responsibility and education between generations. Often, the intermingling of mutual responsibility of all family members and upbringing within a specific parent-child relationship is not at all obvious. But it is set in motion when a child falls ill with leukaemia and the sibling becomes a donor, because care of the sick child changes the family structure, and thus what parents understand by responsible action and the significance that education has. In the first section, I deal with education, responsible parenthood and family issues. The second part discusses family and illness. This is followed by an analysis of the Kirstein family from the Lübeck project on bone marrow donation between siblings, in which a child has been diagnosed with leukaemia. Finally, I work through the different dimensions of responsibility in education and family interaction in the family structure.

Keywords Responsibility · Illness · Family · Education · Bringing up · Siblings · Responsible parenthood

Family, as a relationship of cooperation and solidarity, refers to responsibility and education between older and younger generations. The family is a relationship based on cooperation and solidarity. The birth of a child or children turns two adults into a father and mother, and as such they have responsibilities. Ideas of responsible parenthood exist (Hünersdorf, 2014), but they overlook the fact that parents usually have two or more children, and their responsibility is to each child as well as to the sibling relationships – and siblings in turn develop their own responsibilities. It is often not obvious that the mutual responsibility of all family members is mixed in with the specific parent-child relationship of bringing up children. But such responsibilities are set in motion if a child becomes critically ill with leukaemia and a sibling becomes a bone marrow donor. The proximity of death, and fear and

J. Ecarius (✉)
Faculty of Human Sciences, University of Cologne, Cologne, Germany
e-mail: jecarius@uni-koeln.de

© The Author(s) 2022
C. Schües et al. (eds.), *Stem Cell Transplantations Between Siblings as Social Phenomena*, Philosophy and Medicine 144,
https://doi.org/10.1007/978-3-031-04166-2_6

solicitude for the child, all change the family structure, this community of the family, with its patterns of behaviour and thus what parents understand to be responsible action, how siblings relate to each other, and what significance their upbringing has.

The first section of this chapter deals with *Erziehung*,[1] – the bringing up of children – responsible parenthood and related family issues. In the second part I look at family and illness. This is followed by an analysis of the Kirstein family, which has a child diagnosed with leukaemia, from the Schües and Rehmann-Sutter project on bone marrow donation between siblings (Herzog et al. 2019). I conclude by teasing out the different dimensions of responsibility in *Erziehung* and family interaction within the family structure.

6.1 Family: Parents, Children and Siblings

The family is a complex private way of living (Böllert 2010), combining different generations and thus varying biographical time structures (Ecarius 2013). Intimacy is considerably more embedded in this relationship network than in other social systems. The family comprises a specific "relationship of cooperation and solidarity" (Wonneberger, Stelzig-Willutzki 2018, p. 506); it is a "family of relationship and upbringing" (Honig 1999, p. 492), to address two dimensions. Supportive activities and acknowledgement of the other(s) are characteristic for maintaining structures of interaction and communication (Ecarius, 2013).

This can also be understood as a claim about a successful family life. Jurczyk (2014) emphasises that the family in late-modern societies is no longer self-evident, that it can no longer simply fall back on traditional standards of a shared life (marriage, children, gender and generation-specific norms), but must be established consciously and responsibly. This entitlement to producing a deliberate and mutually recognising family has itself become a norm, although it is not always expressed in the real-life interactions between parents, children and siblings. They may act responsibly towards one another, but envy, blame and competitiveness can also dominate – whether or not illness is present.

Family practices are generated in a "space of conjunctive experience" (Mannheim 1928) over generations, as communicative knowledge about one's own family gradually unfolds, even though this knowledge is coloured by individual members' viewpoints. Embedded in this space are family themes (Ecarius 2003), some adopted by new generations, but also transformed and sometimes discarded. Themes such as "being ambitious" or "taking on responsibility" weave themselves into the family's space of conjunctive experience, often with very little communicative knowledge

---

[1] The German concept of *Erziehung* encompasses personal, social and moral pedagogy, as well as what English-speakers would understand as bringing up or raising children. Nor is it equivalent to "education", a more formal concept of teaching provided by schools, universities and other institutions of learning. We have therefore decided to leave *Erziehung* or *Erzieher* (the person providing the *Erziehung*) as the German term where there is no proper English translation.

about them. When illness becomes the dominant theme, family interaction is reconfigured or new interactions are added. Family issues can become virulent if, for example, personal responsibility can no longer be practised in familiar ways. But how children are brought up can also change.

Interactions of *Erziehung* take place between two subjects of different generations. This bisubjectivity comprises teaching or imparting on the one side, and learning or acquisition on the other, as the two activities of *Erziehung* (Sünkel 2016, p. 23). And yet there is often a third element as well, the activity of demonstration (Prange 2012, p. 67). *Erziehung* thus has a reciprocal, practical structure in the context of teaching and learning, with the action of indicating something, whether an object, a behaviour, a moral choice or a requirement (Ecarius 2018). There are responsibilities on both sides: the older generation has the responsibility to teach, and the younger one to learn and to grasp relationships with themselves and with the world, for that generation to become independent. This also includes the fact that *Erziehung* is always open, and both the child and the *Erzieher* can refuse or reinterpret their roles. Contingency (Luhmann, Schorr 2015) is immanently embedded in education.

Illness and bone marrow donation can bring about fundamental change to sedimented family and sibling interactions, as *Erziehung* is no longer foremost, but has been replaced by nursing and medical treatment (Peter, Neubert 2016), and a deep-seated fear for the child's life can predominate. How do such fears and the complex challenge of the child's illness influence family members' interactions and responsibilities to one another? The question also arises as to how parents shape the family through their "duty" to raise the children, and what part siblings play. Looked at in this way, the family becomes an interdependent structure (Elias 1976).

How we handle illness is shaped by cultural and socio-historical factors (Foucault 1979) and is thus subject to normative expectations that "interpellate" the family (Reckwitz 2018). The high degree of self-regulation that late-modern societies demand – in other words, self-responsibility (Ecarius et al. 2017) – interpellates both the sick child and the donor. Each family designs its own ways of dealing with the situation, based on its historical biographical experiences, specific family themes, and unique sibling interactions. If one child has leukaemia and a sibling is a bone marrow donor, the demands on the family are enormous: there can be a crisis of generativity and a loss of responsibility. Equally, families are often called upon to provide lay support to the medical and healthcare system (Morris 2000). What has previously been everyday is not only in flux but also under pressure.

6.2 Illness as a Continuum

A disease such as leukaemia should not be understood solely biomedically, as symptoms deriving from an identifiable cause. Illness requires the person concerned, and their whole family, to adopt a particular way of life (Gerhardt 1976): the diagnosis of leukaemia should be distinguished from the subjective feelings and ways of dealing with it. If the family is understood as an interactive structure, the illness of one child and a sibling's donation of bone marrow encompasses the entire family (Herzog et al. 2019). As well as causing damage and frailty, illness is also significant in changing the generational structure of the family.

This way of looking at it differs from the approach of resilience research, which seeks resources and practices "that contribute to being resilient and adaptable in the face of crisis situations" (Sonnenmoser 2016, p. 170). Managing highly risky life situations better than expected is understood to be resilience (Opp & Fingerle 2008), which thus becomes competence (Rönnau-Böse & Fröhlich-Gildhoff 2015) in coping with leukaemia and bone marrow donation. A kind of normativity of good and bad thus creeps into the underlying assumptions.

From this perspective the focus is not just on symptoms and medication, and how to handle them correctly and resiliently, but also on illness as a continuum between being healthy and being ill (Antonovsky 1997), and this continuum of sickness and health affects family interactions. Thus, despite experiencing illness, the sick person always benefits in some way as well: a mother cares more for a sick child, and the sick child receives more attention and becomes the centre of the family, even while suffering, while the siblings who are not sick miss out on maternal care.

At this point the question arises of the extent to which *Erziehung* and illness such as leukaemia can be two opposing phenomena. The child at risk of dying is unable to meet the requirement to become independent in the world, and needs comprehensive support and care from others such that life-threatening situations make *Erziehung* towards a self-responsible life recede into the background. Illness can thus lead to the parents suspending their activities as *Erzieher*, and modifying their responsible parenthood for the other children as well. The case below comes from the BMBF-funded project "Stem cell transplants between siblings", in which 17 families were interviewed (16 family interviews and 66 individual interviews) using qualitative research methods (Jürgensen, Herzog 2019; Herzog et al. 2019), under the direction of Prof. Christina Schües and Prof. Christoph Rehmann-Sutter. Written materials relevant to the Kirstein family were kindly made available to me for my research.

For my analysis of the Kirstein family, I used Grounded Theory (Strauss 1991) and the Documentary Method (Bohnsack 2010). The key categories were "*Erziehung*", "responsibility", "family structure; parents, children, siblings", and "illness as a process". The two steps of analysis involved formulating and reflecting interpretation (Nohl 2016), with qualitative analysis focusing on this one case. The abstractions of reflecting interpretation cannot be generalized, but they provide information about possible courses of action and problems concerning illness, responsibility and upbringing in the family structure.

6.3 The Kirstein Family: "We Gave Everything, You Made Nothing of It"

The Kirstein parents are living with their three children and grandmother on a farm when the youngest, at 9½, falls ill with leukaemia. To keep the farm going, the father works full-time as a lorry driver; the mother is a trained seamstress, but also works full-time on or for the farm. The farm is the centre of the family's life, and everyone is involved in animal care and agriculture. The interviewees (father, mother, donor, recipient, sister) describe a family theme of care and responsibility for the well-being of the animals and the farm: it has positive connotations, and everyone participates. For example, the sister of the child with leukaemia says: "I never felt I had to, I always enjoyed doing it." The son also helps as a matter of course and enjoys doing so.

At the age of 9½ Karolin falls ill with leukaemia. She receives chemotherapy at a hospital 120 km away, where her mother stays with her day and night. The mother takes up the family theme of gladly taking responsibility for the farm and the animals, and thus for others, and extends it to include the illness: "This had to work" – meaning her taking care of the child with leukaemia, and the two other children and their grandmother taking over responsibility for the farm. The recipient Karolin says, "we were a great team." When Karolin comes home after her first stay in hospital, the farm environment is supposed to be as sterile as possible. Karolin's health deteriorates after three quarters of a year. She has a relapse and there is a search for a donor; her brother donates his bone marrow. Her mother is also considered as a potential donor, but the doctors recommend using the son. The son is happy to donate and says: "Fortunately, two donors were suitable. (.) Well, um (...), YES (sighs), let's say, in the end it was clear to me from the beginning, if the day comes and they ask (.), do you want to donate, that uh, it was out of the question for me to say no, (.) not from the very beginning." Karsten connects this with his upbringing: "You can DO something and um, (.) let's say (.), I was never brought up like that, if I could do something (.) POSITIVE that I shouldn't do it, (.) well, that's how my parents brought me up." For him it is a positive experience: "You are put on a little pedestal and you are (.) a LITTLE hero, if you like, yeah? You can DO something." Karsten is about 18 years old at this time, and the middle sister Kerstin is 16 years old.

The process of change as family members take over responsibilities is not accompanied by conversation: Karolin's sister Kerstin, in particular, misses emotional support, comfort and praise. She milks the cows early in the morning while also taking a training course; she feels very overworked and eventually breaks down, but manages to finish her apprenticeship. The grandmother supports her a little. Her brother appropriates the family theme as responsibility for other people (donation), other things (the farm), and also himself, by deciding not to spend a year abroad. As donor, assuming responsibility for the farm and for his own work becomes a life strategy, because if he works a lot, he "forgets everything", and understands donating bone marrow as resulting from the *Erziehung* his parents have provided. The father is often away earning money as a lorry driver and only rarely present, but even when there he is helpless. When he cries, Kerstin consoles him despite being in need of comfort herself, while the mother looks after the seriously ill Karolin round the clock. Karolin receives the family's whole attention because of her illness. The mother's activities of care and *Erziehung* are "subtracted" from the two "healthy" children and her husband, and diverted towards the sick daughter. The division of labour between family members for the upkeep of the farm becomes a responsibility for Karolin, and subsequently into a responsibility for each individual, characterised by self-discipline and doing without.

After recovering, Karolin returns to school, where she experiences bullying. She also has several operations as a result of her illness. When Karolin is between 13 and 15 years old, arguments break out between her parents and her brother, in which he accuses them of having neglected his *Erziehung* because they "let Karolin get away with everything". There is a fight "between me and my parents, because I said this is not acceptable, you can't just let her get away with it." Their mother also says, "she caught up on her adolescent phase in an extreme form at 15, she didn't know her limits." They also refer to indulging Karolin. The bone marrow recipient Karolin puts it differently: "My siblings are a little bit older, aren't they, and I'm Daddy's little girl, aren't I, and on top of it also a sick little girl (laughs), well, he always wants to help me." The son, in reminding his parents of their responsibility to raise their children, emphasizes that this has been transformed by Karolin's illness into perpetual support and indulgence. This contradicts the family theme of taking responsibility, as he reminds his parents. But Karolin's patterns also change: leukae-mia, bullying, her drug and alcohol addiction make her blame the illness and disre-spect from others for her situation. The responsibility to fight for her own life turns into helplessness and surrender – finally, she has a drunk-driving accident and aban-dons her vocational training. When she becomes addicted to alcohol and drugs, her brother, who has been running the farm during and after the acute phase of illness, and is the bone marrow donor, tells her: "Get your life under control so that others can have a life again."

The quarrel is fed by the bone marrow donation and thus Karolin's and Karsten's relationship, which had already been tense. Karolin says: "My brother and I// really NEVER HAD the best relationship." Karolin experiences her brother's donation to her as a burden, and when she tries to commit suicide, her brother reacts reproach-fully: she says, "I tried to kill myself and, um, my brother could never approve of that because he said: I SAVED your life and now you want to throw it away!" Their father broaches the subject from his point of view: "Well, Karsten's attitude is always (.) um (groans) like (.) a little bit like (.) well: she could well be a bit grateful to me for doing all this, couldn't she?" For Karsten this results in a difficult relation-ship: he was happy to donate, but Karolin did not recover, and so there were "strange expressions like from my mother that I am um (.). ... yes and I (.) have ALWAYS been very strong-willed. ... and then there are sayings like 'you could have put a bit of your willpower into Karolin' and that's the thing where I say (.) you can't TRANSPORT that, (.) can you?"

Kerstin also recognises the family problem: "because, like I said, because she always SHOWS us, um, what she's making of her life, i.e. nothing at all. And um with alcohol and drugs that somehow destroy everything ... And then I always think (takes a deep breath), YES (sighs), I think that's very stressful for him, because he thinks it's a pity, because he would like his sister to be healthy and (.) HAPPY." But she also realises that Karsten has special significance in the family because of donat-ing bone marrow, and that he has changed roles as well: according to Kerstin, Karsten "gladly took on a fatherly role, beside my father actually. I mean he was even stricter than my actual fa-- my real father (laughs). We always did have our shortcomings, and afterwards even a bit more, because um (.), yes, well I had, as I said, I also had depression in my adolescence."

The family theme of taking on responsibility for a collective thing (the farm) in order to live well as a farming family has changed over the years. Karolin's two siblings, who could or wanted to avoid the guilt of a possible death by taking responsibility for the farm, and by the brother's donation, now demand that their sister take responsibility for becoming independent. The brother takes on the role of an *Erzieher* and demands that Karolin take responsibility for her own life. The mother wants the bone marrow transplant to "transform" Karolin's character traits so that she gains willpower. For both mother and father, the responsibility for *Erziehung* has become concern for Karolin's life, which also meant the other two siblings have to take on more responsibility at an early age. At the same time, their daughter's illness has meant her *Erziehung* has been neglected, and she has become used to receiving constant attention without the setting of boundaries; she rejects her brother's attempts to be an *Erzieher* and feels he compromises her. What was initially taking on responsibility has turned into mutual accusation.

6.4 Perseverance Persistence

The family perseveres, at cross-purposes but – so far – without breaking apart. However, even at the time of the interview – i.e. after more than 20 years – there is no space for talking about taking responsibility, self-responsibility, blame/accusations, helplessness or concern, or for finding solutions. Communication like that seems possible only when Karolin actively hears the appeal to shape her life independently. She rejects the responsibility, using the excuse of depression, although she recognises that her father does support her. Her mother has repeatedly distanced herself from her daughter, which causes Karolin distress. Her brother currently lives with his wife and two children in one part of a semi-detached house, bought by their parents after selling the farm. The middle daughter lives in the same village. Karolin, who is ill, lives 30 kilometres away. Here, too, the spatial distance signifies the state of family communication.

The family theme of responsibility for something shared has changed over the years. At first it mutated into self-discipline of the "healthy" children, using a strategy of perseverance without communication and with little support from the parents; commitment to the life of the sick daughter; and the brother's donation. While for the "healthy" siblings responsibility for the farm turned into self-discipline, Karolin did not respond to this interpellation as her health improved. *Erziehung* – the older generation's responsibility to instruct and the younger one's to become independent – has been pushed into the background by the illness and, coupled with the donation, has changed the generation gap: the father and the sick daughter become the needy ones, while the brother becomes the head of the family and *Erzieher* by taking on responsibility and donating bone marrow, and the sister Kerstin grows up before her time. The siblings demand that their sick sister Karolin take responsibility for herself; they have paid off their "debt" by the donation and by taking over responsibility for the farm. The mother initially merges with her daughter to form a kind of support team for her. The parents are more entangled in their daughter's neediness: she remains her father's little girl, and her mother seems to try to escape the role of perpetual carer by distancing herself from Karolin. The family remains in this constellation, with internal injuries caused by open neediness.

6.5 Levels of Responsibility in the Family

The illness has increased ambivalences and experiences of difference enormously. The relationship of cooperation and solidarity (Wonneberger, Stelzig-Willutzki 2018) as *one* characteristic of family is affected, and the topic of illness saturates it. The whole family structure swings to and fro on a continuum between health and illness (Antonovsky 1997). It is difficult to see who is resilient and who is not, and who the dominant person in the family is, whether the bone marrow donor or Karolin, the sick child. The family interactions and relationships would probably change "positively" if the sick daughter were to start work and thus come into line with the family theme of self-responsibility, although this would also correspond to late-modern requirements for self-regulation and taking responsibility for one's own life plan (Bröckling 2007).

Karolin seems to have had very little *Erziehung* as such. Her brother appeals to their parents to set boundaries, to involve Karolin bisubjectively in the kind of interactions that enable her to learn self-responsibility (as a third person). *Erziehung* requires an interplay of parents and child, but is at the same time contingent, and refusal or failure are possible (Ecarius 2020). The sister, Kerstin, stresses that there are "two" fathers, or that donating bone marrow turned her brother into an *Erzieher*, the person who takes responsibility and who thus has the right to raise others. The generational relationship as a bisubjective interaction between older and younger people (Sünkel 2016), between father/mother and child, is thus changing. In the sibling relationship, despite Karolin's opposition the brother lays claim to act as *Erzieher*, something which can only happen because the father does not take this role himself, thus creating a "void". A sibling can, by all means, become an *Erzieher*, but this interaction is not based on generativity, since Karsten is not the father but remains Karolin's physical brother.

The moment *Erziehung* is evaluated as successful or unsuccessful, benchmarks of alignment with responsible parenthood, in the sense of the best possible upbringing (Landhäusser 2020), creep in. These benchmarks are also used as a basis for scientific analyses and evaluation. Responsible parenthood is a model (Diabaté et al. 2015) presented in statutory regulations that are relevant for social workers (Athanassiadou et al. 2015): parents' responsibility and thus also their possibility of bringing up their children, where *Erziehung* must be in the best interests of the child. The child also has a responsibility to want to learn and to become independent as he or she grows up. This standard of responsible parenthood, which involves the eager learner child, suggests that the family should be established as an educational sphere (Müller, Krinninger 2016), that every child should be recognised in its development, needs and abilities and always (variously) supported and prepared for the demands of society (Winkler 2015) in the best possible way, taking into account sibling relationships.

The illness brings about changes in the generational structure of the Kirstein family: Karolin does not acknowledge her brother as her *Erzieher*, while Kerstin views him as a "second" father. *Erziehung* may be sidelined if parents have increased caring activities for sick children – and thus also try (one-sidedly) to satisfy the demands of responsible parenthood. Parents in such situations are confronted with a degree of incompatibility between *Erziehung* and care for the sick child, especially when the child might die and the parents themselves be in need of help. The persistent illness may then cause the positioning of individuals in the family structure to change inter- and intrageneratively.

Successful family life, the creation of family (Jurzcyk 2014), follows standards of mutual recognition and consideration of different needs in the context of late-modern interpellations of singularization (Reckwitz 2018) and optimization (Bröckling 2007). In the Kirstein family, however, family interactions take a completely different form, and uncertainty and ambivalence (Lüscher, Liegle 2003) as well as guilt become the dominant themes of family responsibility. Social expectations require the family to cope with illness, meet the challenges, and develop intergenerational solidarity.

Trying to cope with taking on responsibility for a critically ill child and having a donor brother in the family is quite different from "normal" family life. Illness influences family behaviour over many years (Ohlbrecht, Peter 2016). The wish to return to "normality" in the sense of a "healthy" family, appeals to take responsibility and associated blaming, produce ambivalences and cause the health-disease continuum (Antonovsky 1997) in the spectrum of leukaemia and bone marrow donation to be constantly in flux.

The indefinite duration of leukaemia and the confrontation with death require affective coping and equally a specific solidarity between parents and siblings (Hildenbrand 2009), which cannot be tackled using previous family behaviour patterns. *Erziehung* and parental care (in the form of the child's welfare) are joined by medical treatment and the accompanying semi-professional care (Jellen et al. 2018). Here it is the women who take on the tasks, as in the Kirstein family. The brother and sister – Kerstin and Karsten – are also sucked in by having to take on tasks, such as Karsten's donation and Kerstin's self-discipline. However, the individual persons are not "neutral helpers" (Steffen 2015, p. 43). The needs of the carers, both parents and siblings, become less important when a family member is seriously ill (Ohlbrecht, Schönberger 2010). The responsibility for the carer's own well-being becomes secondary when the sick child's well-being is primary, when the struggle for life is foremost. But the siblings have their own needs (Wihstutz, Schiwarov, 2018), and the parents also need time for themselves. They have gainful employment to attend to, while children have to go to school, finish their education and enter the workforce; they are all embedded in further normative expectations for living in society (Morris 2000).

Illness and bone marrow donation as a long-term family figuration transform behaviour, which affects the biography of the family as a whole as well as the biographies of individual family members (Bury 2009). Work has to be done on identities, positioning has to be redeveloped, and mother, father and siblings have to reposition the responsibility of self-care for their own lives, and reshape their relationships with each other. Siblings develop their own relationship configurations (75% of children in Germany grow up with siblings, Federal Statistical Office 2018), each with subjective interpretations and feelings in family and social contexts, establishing their own patterns of action and attributions, directly exchanging feelings such as joy and disappointment (Punch 2008).

In this example all the sick child's family members neglect or change their own caring activities, becoming stronger (the brother) or weaker (the sister Kerstin and the father). Different levels of responsibility interlace in the family. The illness switches responsibility for *Erziehung* (1) from the parents to the brother through the dominance of the responsibility to care (2) for the sick child, while neglecting the other siblings through the family theme of taking responsibility (3). Responsibility for *Erziehung* and responsibility to care for the life of each child (Schües 2016) are knotted together with the family theme in a peculiar way, and result in mutual recriminations between the siblings and with their parents. Things the family takes for granted in terms of daily life, *Erziehung*, self-care and caring become questionable, as the self-evident is lost. Family biography changes into the biography of a "sick" family, in which each individual responds differently to responsibility for caring and self-care, as well as for *Erziehung*, thereby repositioning him- or herself within the family topic of responsibility and at the same time transforming it.

Finally, it can be said that although family life in the everyday does contain harmonious elements, the generational structure has to process different forms of responsibility, in responses which can lead to conflict among siblings, as well as excessive demands and repositioning such that they (can) also become *Erzieher*. But even parents who attempt to parent responsibly can find the task of caring for and bringing up children produces excessive demands, fear and helplessness. Family life is not purely harmonious: it is also characterized by tensions and ambivalences due to the generational difference between older and younger family members, and between siblings, as well as the different needs of all the family members and their varying perceptions of family issues and social demands such as learning, caring and responsible parenthood, all of which are challenged by illness.

Literature

Antonovsky, Aaron. 1997. *Salutogenese. Zur Entmystifizierung der Gesundheit.* Tübingen: dgvt.

Athanassiadou, Zoi, Matthias Euteneuer, Frank Mücher, and Uwe Uhlendorff. 2015. Familienkonzepte – ein sozialpädagogischer Blick auf die Gestaltung familialer Lebenswelten. In *Neue Aufmerksamkeiten für Familien (12. Sonderheft Neue Praxis. Zeitschrift für Sozialarbeit, Sozialpädagogik und Sozialpolitik)*, ed. Susann Fegter, Catrin Heite, Johanna Mierendorff, and Martina Richter, 12–25. Lahnstein: Neue Praxis.

Bohnsack, Ralf. 2010. Die Mehrdimensionalität der Typenbildung und ihre Aspekthaftigkeit. In *Typenbildung und Theoriengenerierung: Methoden und Methodologien qualitativer Bildungs- und Biographieforschung*, ed. Jutta Ecarius and Burkhard Schäffer, 47–72. Opladen: Barbara Budrich.

Böllert, Katrin. 2010. Familienformen im sozialen Wandel – Pluralität von Familienleitbildern in der Kinder- und Jugendhilfe? *Soziale Passagen* 7 (12): 191–204.

Bröckling, Ulrich. 2007. *Das unternehmerische Selbst*. Frankfurt/M: Suhrkamp.

Bury, Michael. 2009. Chronische Krankheit als biografischer Bruch. In *Bewältigung chronischer Krankheit im Lebenslauf*, ed. Doris Schaeffer, 75–90. Bern: Huber.

Diabaté, Sabine, Detlev Lück, and Norbert F. Schneider. 2015. Leitbilder der Elternschaft: Zwischen Kindeswohl und fairer Aufgabenteilung. In *Familienleitbilder in Deutschland*, ed. Norbert F. Schneider, Sabine Diabaté, and Kerstin Ruckdeschel, 247–268. Opladen/Berlin/Toronto: Barbara Budrich.

Ecarius, Jutta. 2003. Biografie, Lernen und Familienthemen in Generationsbeziehungen. *Zeitschrift für Pädagogik* 48 (4): 534–549.

———. 2013. Familie – Identität – Kultur. In *Familientraditionen und Familienkulturen: theoretische Konzeptionen, historische und aktuelle Analysen*, ed. Meike Baader, Petra Götte, and Carola Groppe, 53–70. Wiesbaden: Springer Fachmedien.

———. 2018. Vom Verhandlungs- zum Beratungshaushalt: Familie in der Spätmoderne und verantwortete Elternschaft. In *Familie – Bildung – Migration*, ed. Olaf Kapella, Norbert F. Schneider, and Harald Rost, 139–153. Opladen-Berlin-Toronto: Verlag Barbara Budrich.

———. 2020. Erziehung in Familie. In *Handbuch Familie. Erziehung, Bildung und pädagogische Arbeitsfelder*, ed. Jutta Ecarius and Anja Schierbaum. Wiesbaden: Springer VS. (in the appear).

Ecarius, Jutta, Alena Berg, Katja Serry, and Ronnie Oliveras. 2017. *Spätmoderne Jugend – Erziehung des Beratens – Wohlbefinden*. Wiesbaden: Springer VS.

Elias, Norbert. 1976. *Über den Prozeß der Zivilisation*. Frankfurt/M: Suhrkamp.

Foucault, Michel. 1979. *Die Geburt der Klinik*. Frankfurt/M: Fischer.

Gerhardt, Uta. 1976. Krankenkarriere und Existenzbelastung. *Zeitschrift für Soziologie* 5 (3): 215–236.

Herzog, Madeleine, Martina Jürgensen, Christoph Rehmann-Sutter, and Christina Schües. 2019. Interviewers as intruders? Ethical explorations of joint family interviews. *Journal of Empirical Research on Human Research Ethics. Special Issue: Research Ethics in Empirical Ethics Studies* 14 (5): 458–461. https://doi.org/10.1177/1556264619857856.

Hildenbrand, Bruno. 2009. Die Bewältigung chronischer Krankheit in der Familie – Resilienz und professionelles Handeln. In *Bewältigung chronischer Krankheit im Lebenslauf*, ed. Doris Schaeffer, 133–155. Bern: Huber.

Honig, Michael-Sebastian. 1999. *Entwurf einer Theorie der Kindheit*. Frankfurt/M: Suhrkamp.

Hünersdorf, Bettina. 2014. Verantwortete Elternschaft. In *Das Bildungssystem und seine strukturellen Kopplungen*, ed. Elmar Drieschner and Detlef Gaus, 147–165. Wiesbaden: Springer.

Jellen, Josephine, Heike Ohlbrecht, and Torsten Winkler. 2018. Strategien im Umgang mit Krankheit. In *Medizinische Soziologie trifft Medizinische Pädagogik*, ed. Heike Ohlbrecht and Astrid Seltrecht, 173–193. Wiesbaden: Springer VS.

Jurczyk, Karin. 2014. Familie als Herstellungsleistung. In *Doing family*, ed. Karin Jurczyk, Andreas Lange, and Barbara Thiessen, 50–71. Weinheim/Basel: Beltz Juventa.

Jürgensen, Martina, and Madeleine Herzog. 2019. *Studie über die Erfahrungen von Familien mit Blutstammzelltransplantationen zwischen Geschwisterkindern*. Lübeck: Informationen für Studienteilnehmerinnen und Studienteilnehmer.

Landhäusser, Sandra. 2020. Familie und verantwortete Elternschaft. In *Handbuch Familie. Erziehung, Bildung und pädagogische Arbeitsfelder*, ed. Jutta Ecarius and Anja Schierbaum. Wiesbaden: Springer VS. (in the appear).

Luhmann, Niklas, and Karl E. Schorr. 2015. *Reflexionsprobleme im Erziehungssystem*. Suhrkamp: Frankfurt/M.

Lüscher, Kurt, and Ludwig Liegle. 2003. *Generationenbeziehungen in Familie und Gesellschaft*. Konstanz: Universitätsverlag Konstanz.

Mannheim, Karl. 1928. Das Problem der Generationen. *KZfSS* 7 2: 157–185. 3, 309–330.

Morris, David B. 2000. *Krankheit und Kultur*. Munich: Kunstmann.

Müller, Hans-Rüdiger, and Dominik Krinninger. 2016. *Familienstile*. Weinheim: Beltz Juventa.

Nohl, Arnd-Michael. 2016. Grundbegriffe und empirische Analysen als wechselseitige Spiegel. In *Theorien in der qualitativen Bildungsforschung – qualitative Bildungsforschung als Theoriegenerierung*, ed. Robert Kreitz, Ingrid Miethe, and Anja Tervooren, 105–122. Berlin, Toronto: Verlag Barbara Budrich: Opladen.

Office, German Federal Statistical. 2018. *Datenreport 2018*. Bonn: Ein Sozialbericht für die Bundesrepublik Deutschland.

Ohlbrecht, Heike, and Claudia Peter. 2016. Gesundheit und Krankheit bei Kindern und Jugendlichen. In *Handbuch Kindheits- und Jugendsoziologie*, ed. Andreas Lange, Herwig Reiter, Sabina Schutter, and Christine Steiner, 569–592. Wiesbaden: Springer VS.

Ohlbrecht, Heike, and Christine Schönberger. 2010. *Gesundheit als Familienaufgabe*. Weinheim, Munich: Juventa.

Opp, Günther, and Michael Fingerle, eds. 2008. *Was Kinder stärkt*. 3rd ed. Reinhardt: Munich.

Peter, Claudia, and Carolin Neubert. 2016. Medikalisierung sozialer Prozesse. In *Soziologie von Gesundheit und Krankheit*, ed. Klaus Hurrelmann and Matthias Richter, 273–285. Wiesbaden: Springer VS.

Prange, Klaus. 2012. *Die Zeigestruktur der Erziehung 2nd corrected and expanded edition*. Paderborn: Ferdinand Schöningh.

Punch, Samantha. 2008. "You can do Nasty Things to your Brothers and Sisters without a Reason": Siblings' Backstage Behaviour. *Children & Society* 22 (5): 333–344.

Reckwitz, Andreas. 2018. *Die Gesellschaft der Singularitäten. Zum Strukturwandel der Moderne*. Suhrkamp: Berlin.

Rönnau-Böse, Maike, and Klaus Fröhlich-Gildhoff. 2015. *Resilienz und Resilienzförderung über die Lebensspanne*. Stuttgart: Kohlhammer.

Schües, Christina. 2016. *Philosophie des Geborenseins*. 2nd ed. Freiburg: Alber.

Sonnenmoser, Marion. 2016. *Resilienz in Familien*. Dt. Ärzteblatt.

Steffen, Hermann-T. 2015. *Epilepsie und Familie. Familialer Umgang mit chronischer Krankheit und Krankenrolle*. Bielefeld: Universität Bielefeld.

Strauss, Anselm L. 1991. *Grundlagen qualitativer Sozialforschung*. Munich: UTB.

Sünkel, Wolfgang. 2016. *Erziehungsbegriff und Erziehungsverhältnis*. Weinheim: Beltz Juventa.

Wihstutz, Anne, and Juliana Schiwarov. 2018. Kinder als Sorgende – Anmerkungen aus Kindheitssoziologischer Perspektive. In *Handbuch Kindheits- und Jugendsoziologie*, ed. Andreas Lange, Herwig Reiter, Sabina Schutter, and Christine Steiner, 315–330. Wiesbaden: Springer VS.

Winkler, Michael. 2015. Familie – Verwüstung doch nicht ganz ausgeschlossen. In *Das neue Misstrauen gegenüber der Familie*, ed. Steffen Grosskopf and Michael Winkler, 55–93. Würzburg: Ergon.

Wonneberger, Astrid, and Sabina Stelzig-Willutzki. 2018. Familie. In *Familienwissenschaft. Grundlagen und Überblick*, ed. Astrid Wonnberger, Katja Weidtmann, and Sabina Stelzig-Willutzki. Springer VS: Wiesbaden.

Open Access This chapter is licensed under the terms of the Creative Commons Attribution 4.0 International License (http://creativecommons.org/licenses/by/4.0/), which permits use, sharing, adaptation, distribution and reproduction in any medium or format, as long as you give appropriate credit to the original author(s) and the source, provide a link to the Creative Commons license and indicate if changes were made.

The images or other third party material in this chapter are included in the chapter's Creative Commons license, unless indicated otherwise in a credit line to the material. If material is not included in the chapter's Creative Commons license and your intended use is not permitted by statutory regulation or exceeds the permitted use, you will need to obtain permission directly from the copyright holder.

Part III
Dealing with Illness

Chapter 7
Experiences in Times of Illness: Report from the Qualitative Interview Study

Martina Jürgensen and Madeleine Herzog

Abstract How did the families we interviewed after a bone marrow transplant experience the illness for which the donation from a sibling child was a cure? Some families first responded by denial of the fatal diagnosis, hoping that it was a mistake. Many families suffered from the severe loss of control in several areas of their lives. The illness changed family roles and also raised the question of how long a child should be seen as "ill". We found four different patterns of coping: toughening up, resignation, ignoring, and acceptance. Families also found different things helpful in dealing with the situation and in making sense of the events around the illness: keeping or regaining control, maintaining routines, hoping that it will be all right, or making the best of bad things. In hindsight, many families felt that the experience of the disease also had a positive impact on the family as a whole, and that individual family members could learn from it.

Keywords Meanings of illness · Dealing with illness

This chapter focuses on how families experience the illness of a child and how they make sense of it. How are different family members affected by the severe disease of a child? How do they describe and narrate it? How do they interpret what it means to be ill? If the transplant is successful, when does illness end? Parents, children (donors and recipients and third siblings) and healthcare professionals understand illness differently. The interviews that we conducted with 17 families about their long-term experiences with a bone marrow transplant provide ample material.

First of all, it was evident that for all families in our study, the onset of the disease and the diagnosis represented a comprehensive and overwhelming crisis that hit the family without warning. The approaches then chosen by families to handle this situation were quite different and influenced by many factors. They sometimes already

M. Jürgensen (✉) · M. Herzog
Institute for History of Medicine and Science Studies, University of Lübeck,
Lübeck, Schleswig-Holstein, Germany
e-mail: martina.juergensen@uni-luebeck.de

© The Author(s) 2022
C. Schües et al. (eds.), *Stem Cell Transplantations Between Siblings as Social Phenomena*, Philosophy and Medicine 144,
https://doi.org/10.1007/978-3-031-04166-2_7

had different crisis coping strategies. Other factors included the existence and use of resources, as well as family belief systems, and their way of making sense of the diagnosis. Furthermore, structural aspects such as the parents' work situation, the infrastructure in the home, proximity to the treating clinic, etc. are all important factors that can make dealing with the situation either easier or more difficult.

7.1 What Does It Mean to Be Ill?

All families in this study were confronted with their child's diagnosis without any warning. Most families talked about the diagnosis as a "shock", a significant moment that completely changed their whole life, at least temporarily.

No matter how long ago the period of illness, in the interviews we could always feel the dismay families had undergone when they found out about the diagnosis. Especially when the child had leukaemia, a disease that is well known in society and has a lot of connotations, the fear that the child might die became very present. In other cases, when the children were suffering from rarer diseases, a research process would set in, where families tried to understand the extent of the crisis and what they would have to face in the time to come.

The handling of this new situation was influenced by many factors. Previous experiences of the family were central – especially experiences of illnesses and other critical life events, which led to specific family coping strategies. Further factors included the existence and the use of resources as well as family belief systems, their way of making sense of the diagnosis.

7.2 Denial: "We Don't Belong Here!"

Many families described very evocatively the moment when they got the diagnosis and found themselves in an oncological unit. They reported feeling that they were in a "wrong movie", a place that up to then they only knew from TV or the media. They saw sick children, bloated from cortisone treatment or hairless due to chemotherapy. They saw tiny rooms in which children and parents lived together for months.

A typical first reaction of families was the attempt to deny the diagnosis in the hope that it was a mistake. From the narratives of several families it was clear how unimaginable it was for them (at the beginning of the illness) to accept that they now belonged to the medical system of "oncology" – to a kind of "parallel world" that they only knew from TV or the newspapers. A world they refused to be a part of – while (secretly) suspected that this would be their reality for their near future.

Mother: They are really (laughs) like as though they were set in a film like that [...] and always think, hey I don't belong here, this is all wrong. I know, I once said to a doctor, this is- this is a mistake (laughs), this is a mistake too, there's been a mix-up and I still remember how pityingly that doctor looked at me, he thought, oh God that poor woman. I said, THIS must be a MISTAKE, just look (laughs) at the name, you know (Bahr)

7.3 Loss of Control, Being At the Mercy of Something

Many families facing a life-threatening disease in a child perceived a loss of control over several areas of life. Treatment of the children was mostly determined by standardized medical protocols with few if any possibilities for parents to influence it. They also felt that they were losing control of their everyday family life, which was now largely determined by hospital visits and the health status of the ill child. Parents who accompanied their child to the clinic found themselves in a completely new world that had its own unfamiliar rules. In particular, the parental role, which involves protecting one's own children and providing them with security, was challenged since parents themselves felt insecure and could not judge or really influence what would happen next. Given that "perceived control is a powerful resource when dealing with stressful life events" (Skinner and Zimmer-Gembeck 2011), the effects of losing control should not be underestimated.

How strongly this loss of control was perceived depended on the family's character (active, reactive?) and resources and additional structural circumstances.

In our sample there were families who said that they had a distance of six driving hours between their home and the hospital, while others had an oncology clinic in their neighbourhood so that parents were able to sleep at home if they wanted, and siblings could visit the sick child regularly. In some families cooperation between the parents worked very well and the workload of taking care of the children, earning money, and spending time at the hospital was evenly distributed. In other families one of the parents took on significantly more work to deal with the situation. All these and many more factors determined how the whole family and individual family members experienced the loss of control.

Furthermore, families differed fundamentally in how they dealt with challenges in general. Families who usually take their lives very actively into their own hands and trust (only) their own strengths found it more difficult to lose control than those families who are generally more reactive and trust in institutions and authorities. These families sometimes felt that what others perceived as "loss of control" was a "relief".

7.4 Who Is Ill? And for How Long?

The question of who should be considered and treated as (still) ill was mentioned in several interviews. While the starting point of the disease for all families in our sample was very clear, the end was not clearly defined and remained open to interpretation. Leaving the hospital after transplantation was not the end of the disease. Children were medicated and needed special treatment, special hygienic measures, special food and so on. But even after this recovery time there were often physical disabilities, and the fear they might relapse remained.

Regarding the question about who is seen as ill and for how long, very different topics were addressed: Family roles, expectations and commitments, parental care and the child's privacy, anxiety, shame, jealousy, and anger.

In our interviews it became very clear that the question of whether the sick child was still considered sick was often answered differently by those involved. Parents tended to regard the "affected" children as ill long after the actual illness. The (formerly) sick children often resisted this view – they wanted to be seen as healthy and "normal again".

Children considered to be (still) ill were at the centre of the family, playing a special role. On the one hand, they benefited from this special treatment: they were treated with consideration, and parents tried to satisfy all their wishes and needs and were less strict towards them, or "showered" them with presents. On the other hand, being considered ill often meant being exposed to constant and comprehensive parental control. This made it difficult for children and adolescents to develop in an age-appropriate manner and to return to "normality" beyond the disease. In the interviews, the "affected" children/adolescents emphasized that it was very important for them to be viewed as a "normal" person with strengths and weaknesses, and not reduced to the disease.

The healthy siblings of the children considered to be ill were often willing to subordinate their own needs during the time of illness – even if they felt neglected and were jealous of the sibling. After a certain time, however, many sibling children (and parents) began to feel that the "exceptional situation of illness" should have ended and that the special treatment of the (formerly) ill child was no longer justified.

Different assessments by family members of whether the child could and should still be regarded as ill could lead to serious intrafamilial disagreements, as one mother recalls:

Mother: then over time Karolin harped on a bit- a bit on this (takes a deep breath) well, "I was sick and you all have to love me" (laughs) (..), yeah? And then as parents, you're betw-between three stools, if I can put it like that (laughs) (..) and you always have to arbitrate, kind of "you're not sick any more", yeah" (imitates her daughter – moaning) "OH, I don't feel at all well today". Then hm (..) yes. (..) She did thrash it a bit, that she was ill. (Kirstein)

7.5 Dealing with Illness (Coping Strategies)

Families described different ways of coping with the child's illness. Their different attitudes reflected both their previous experiences and their basic attitude toward the world (whether they were hopeful, catastrophizing, resigned ...). The interviews showed that most families went through a process of learning how to deal with the child's illness. There was a development over time of several coping strategies, used depending on particular situations and aspects of the disease and also on changing individual moods and frame conditions (e.g. current state of health of the child, current occupational requirements).

7.6   Toughening Up

Toughening up was a frequently described coping strategy. Families pointed out that they had no other choice than to toughen up and just deal with the situation as it came. The disease of the child did not leave much space for sentimentality and forced many family members to put on their "strong suit". In the interviews, this was often revalued as a point at which no one had time for individual needs as all energy was put into the functioning of the family. Here is one example:

Mother: No, you have to, let me say, if you, (..) all of that, that you're experiencing, it's not just your own child, the- your whole environment, what you're experiencing, you DO become tough, you HAVE to become tough. If you don't get tough you go under with all that. (Jaschke)

7.7   Resignation

In other moments, when family members were feeling overwhelmed with the situation, resignation or giving up became some sort of an exit strategy in their minds. Parents reported several ways in which they had wanted to give up. Drowning in own's misery was named, as well as thoughts about committing suicide. Yet parents felt the need to stay strong for their (other) children and to keep the whole family going. Their sense of responsibility did not allow them to give up and leave the situation.

Father: You'd prefer to drown in your misery. What kept me above water was my children (..) I'd rather... (Bahr)

7.8   Ignoring/ Having Done with It

Another coping strategy was to ignore the subject as a whole. In our sample, one father did not even want to participate in the interview and talk about his experiences. His wife and the donor daughter (the sick daughter died) told us that he had refused to talk about the disease, the BMT or the death of his daughter since everything had happened seven years previously. That is a very extreme case of avoiding the memory of it. But other families (or single family members) also reported that they chose not to think or talk about the illness and the transplant too much as they experienced that recalling it generated a bad mood or feelings that were hard to cope with, or that talking about it (frequently) was not helpful.

Recipient: but otherwise I really do try to avoid the subject, as far as I can. Because it's a subject, I think, that for one thing generates a very bad mood. Somehow that's always immediately a depressive, "everything's stupid" mood, if you even just mention the word cancer, erm, yeah and simply because I try myself to have done with it. Or, I'd very much like to have done with it, the subject, but I know that won't work, I mean it's- it's just, you CAN'T have done with it, it's always a part of me or of all of us, erm, but I do try to have done with it as far as possible. Really to leave it behind me, not necessarily to suppress it, but through, by trying to have done with it, you suppress it, let's say, a bit, like, like along those lines. (Speidel)

7.9   Acceptance

No family in this study did not report that after some time they reached a state of acceptance. Acceptance however could also mean giving in, a moment of subordination to the situation. Mostly, the acceptance of the new life situation only arose after a certain period of adjustment in which families rebelled against the new situation and questioned the truth of the diagnosis. But after this phase, families said they felt that they could not change the situation anyway and there seemed no other possibility than accepting the circumstances.

Acceptance made it possible for the families to focus on coping with various challenges and not to waste their energies and strength in a futile fight against the situation. In this context, one mother described the disease as a fate that she simply had to accept – and she did:

Mother: then I really had a couple of days like, that I (..) really did want to dissolve into SELF-pity and somehow I think after five days I thought, how DUMB are you actually. This is fate, what you're having to tackle right now and it was, I can remember that precisely. We've got a Lidl [name of a supermarket chain] nearby and I'd been shopping and I was thinking, who knows how many people are in the shop right now who have also suffered a harsh fate and strangely, right there in the supermarket it was, I said to myself, no, now just stop this, you've got this situation after all, you have to see how you manage it, and from then on I really did tackle it. Then (..) you deal with it bit by bit. (Preuss)

7.10   What Is Helpful in Dealing with the Situation?

Families reported that they found different things helpful in managing the challenges, conflicts and difficulties which they experienced. Four main patterns emerged from a comparative analysis of the interviews in our 17 families.

7.11   Keeping in Control/ Regaining Control

The perceived loss of control was a very important experience for many parents. As they described, they were entering a new world with new actors and new terminology, and needed to learn how to navigate this new environment. Family members had to react without being able to take control of the situation. Often, they were unable to continue their work, had to move to another city for the clinic and so on. Furthermore, parents had to give consent to medical treatments with effects they could not judge and which were mostly determined by standardized medical protocols with few if any possibilities of parental influence. Some parents felt that the fate of their child was now in the hands of the medical system and that they had no control over it.

A frequently described way of maintaining or regaining control was to collect as much knowledge as possible about the disease, therapeutic possibilities and potential outcomes. In most families, one of the parents had taken on the role of familiarizing themselves with the medical aspects of the disease and transplantation and of communicating with doctors and other professionals.

Mother: otherwise I really have to say, for myself, to feel good, to have everything under CONTROL all the time, to keep a grasp on it all, I had to know everything, all the blood test results, everything (Bahr)

7.12   Maintaining Everyday Life/ Structure & Functioning

As mentioned, the illness of the child meant that the normal everyday life of the family was largely no longer available. In order to maintain security and stability for all involved, many families in our sample tried either to retain as many aspects of their everyday life as possible or to establish a new everyday framework.

Another aspect was that many family members needed a place to "get away" from the situation – even if it was just for a short time. Healthy siblings stated that it was good for them to go to school and meet "normally" with friends or in a sports club – to have a place that was not about the illness or anything like that. For the parents, it seemed to be harder than for the children to find their own place of distraction or respite. Few parents said that they were able to find and use such a space.

The strategy of many families was to switch to a "functional mode" and try to get through each day as well as possible – in order to be able to look forward to the next. It was helpful for them when the disease and the transplant were interpreted as temporary and they were able to focus on "the time afterwards".

It was precisely the overwhelming challenges that the families faced that apparently drove this switch to a functional mode that was perceived as helpful – the situation simply did not allow looking to the right or left. This favoured a focus on the now primary tasks and made it possible to ignore the things that would normally have seemed important in everyday life.

> Mother: It's not life any more, it's just really, you're functioning, yeah. That is, you try to think about it- about it as little as possible, simply really just do what needs to be done, what you have to do and everything else actually doesn't matter. Yes, and that's how the days go. (Jaschke)

7.13 Hope/ Belief That Everything Will Be All Right

Another important resource for many families was the strong hope that everything would be fine. Many families stressed that they never believed that their child could die or that the transplant could not succeed. This unshakeable belief in a good outcome, which left no room for doubt, gave them the strength to get through this difficult time – always keeping an eye on the light at the end of the tunnel.

Where this belief comes from differed, and most families could not specifically name the origin. Only a few study participants were religious and derived this hope from their faith. For the majority, however, it seemed to be more a firm conviction in the sense of a positive worldview and a general trust that what *should* not happen *would* not happen. Like the father in the following quote, several other family members also emphasized their trust in medical skills and doctors in this context.

> Father: yes sure, of course I knew: this is now something that's life-threatening, you know, but WHAT that really means right now, it wasn't clear at that time either, is it leukaemia, cancer or whatever, what the er, thing- (.) what it's about, but for me somehow it was already, from the first minute, no, actually actually at the moment I drove off in the hospital park and then even more that evening back in the hospital, one thing: it will it will be all right, you know? It will (.). From- from the start I had this trust, erm the doctors will know what they're doing and it will er (..), we will get through this together and Marlena will survive this. Yes, later on I kept occasionally having these thoughts: what will happen if your child dies? But er this- this positive trust, this was what I held onto actually for the whole year until the end, you know. (Minz)

7.14 Making the Best of It

This hope and trust gave the families the power to make the best of the situation and to look forward positively, focusing on the good things they had rather than the bad. For example, compared with other forms of leukaemia, the type of leukaemia the child had appeared to be a stroke of luck because it is relatively curable:

> Mother: with everything that we drew out it, that you say, well yes, we have a potful of shit or whatever, we picked the piece out that still looked the best (laughs). YES, that's how it is, you've just got to go for the positive (laughs), like, that's how it is, exactly how it is (Speidel)

In the interviews, several families described occasions in which they managed to experience joyful and even happy moments despite all the fears, sadness, burdens and insecurities. They talked about afternoons of fun together with other sick children in the clinic, about closeness and imaginative activities even within the limited possibilities of the isolation ward, and about friendships with nurses and therapists.

Some of these scenes dealt with the hairloss associated with chemotherapy. While the loss of hair was perceived by many families as drastic and traumatizing, some – like the one in the following quote – managed to create a happy shared event out of it:

> Mother: when Mighel's hair started to fall out it was so (laughs) COMICAL, 'cos Melissa was at school (swallows) and then Mighel said, hm: Mummy look, you know, I said, oh now it's starting, what do you want to do? Do you want to lose a few each day or should I shave it off for you or what and then he said: "I can PLUCK it out!" I said, "yes, you can." And then he had the idea he wanted to wait until Melissa was there and then he wanted him and her to pull all of it out over the bath. And when Melissa came home from school both of them went to the bathroom, so we told her, then both of them went into the bathroom and PLUCKED his entire HEAD over the bathtub and had hellish fun (laughs) (Molle)

7.15   Sense-Making of the Illness

All individuals who participated in the study made it clear that the onset of life-threatening illness was a major crisis for the entire family. In many families it was not just everyday life that was threatened, but basic certainties or taken for granted facts (for example, that both parents work, that the family has several children, that the children will grow up, finish school, build their own families) were shaken. We all know that sense-making can help people to handle trouble by making a situation of crisis understandable and meaningful. Getting a feeling of sense helped the individuals in our families, and the family as a whole, to organize the perceived chaos of their lived experiences.

The participating families associated the disease with different meanings. Some of them referred to spiritual or religious beliefs, but most saw the disease as a stroke of fate. Interestingly, it was only for a few families in our study that the "why us?" question seems to have been important.

> Mother: on the first day there was this mother who had also found out on that day that her child had cancer and she was just crying and saying to me: oh oh WHY? You don't ask yourself why of all people your child? And I looked at this mother and said no […] I NEVER asked myself, why of all people MY child, NEVER, like because firstly that would, I think, I'd thought about it and I said to the mother, no, that would also mean that (.) that it would be more OK for another child or something and I, er er I also asked myself where he got it from or something like that, because my husband and I we're both smokers, so I could have just gone and topped myself. And the psychologist also told us not to go poking around there right now because we also knew that everything here was about children of smokers, there's no point right now, you know, yes. Yes, we didn't pile that on ourselves at that time. (Molle)

In the last quote, another perspective on "sense-making" is apparent: the question of individual guilt appears in the explanations of why the disease developed. Another strategy of sense-making was to place the disease in a temporal context and to conceptualize it as a phase of life that passes (there is a "before" and an "after").

One mother described her understanding of the situation using a very evocative image. For her it was as if she had boarded a train at the beginning of the illness and did not know where it was going. There was only the choice between getting on that train or standing on the platform without knowing when the next train was coming. This image also depicts how the parents find themselves in a situation in which they have to make decisions without really being able to assess what they imply (loss of control).

7.16   Guilt/Punishment

The sense of guilt or of being punished for something can also be understood as a form of sense-making and meaning-provision. In some interviews, the parents wondered how they could have deserved this fate and raised the idea that the child's illness could be a punishment for their own wrongdoing.

Mother: I was also, at the time when he WAS an alcoholic, I kept asking him "have you had a drink"? I smelled it, you know, and he said to me oh, that's also a stronger reason, he swore to me on the children's lives that he hadn't drunk anything. Then he went dry and when we later got the diagnosis for Mighel (.) he, so that was the business with the phone call, after that he said, everything's my fault. I said (quietly) "how so?" "Because at the time I swore on my children's lives even though I REALLY had had a drink" (Molle)

7.17   In Retrospect

In hindsight, several years after the events, family members described them as something that has become an integral part of their lives, or even that it had proved beneficial to the family.

7.18   "It Is a part of My life"

In retrospective, all interviewees identified the disease (and in some cases also the BMT) as a central theme of their lives. They had however handled the disease very differently. Some families tried to conceal the (earlier illness as much as possible and to eliminate it from their lives and thoughts. Teenagers and young adults in particular reacted in this way, pointing out that for them the illness was associated with feelings of shame. They underlined that they wanted to be "normal" and not be identified or labelled as "ill", "formerly ill" or "sibling of a sick child". Apart from the worry that they might be considered "not normal", young people feared social exclusion because their peers often had little health knowledge and were therefore afraid of being infected by them.

> Recipient: I don't actually want to know anything about this disease. I just want to be normal (Preuss)

Other families emphasized that the (earlier) illness was a central life experience for them, which they can neither forget and they would not have wanted to miss.

7.19 "Like a Gift Actually"

A large proportion of the families surveyed said that the experience of the disease had a positive impact on the family as a whole and on individual family members. They spoke of a new quality of deep feelings, both joy and intimacy as well as sadness, fear and pain. They told of important experiences which had brought them closer together, and that they had learned to set new priorities in life.

> Mother: it's a pity that you have to learn something like that, but I think I can say that, since that first day of being ill, we as a family really have lived every day as if it were our last, every day. It IS like that. And they say it so lightly, but EVERY day we go as a family, we do lots and lots of things, we are conscious every day that we are together as a family, that Sven is here, that the world is beautiful. Money is money, well okay. COMPLETELY unimportant! There are so many things that are important, erm, and we live like THAT, and that, well it's a pity, but as I said, the illness also brings a lot that is good. Like Sebastian said, it, we also see a lot of positives in it, that your viewpoint is set differently, yes it really is like that. (Speidel)

Learning so much that is new and important through these incisive experiences led some participants to consider the disease and the transplantation, in retrospect, as a gift.

> Mother: it's in that respect actually despite everything still (..), well, I dunno, like a gift actually, you have to look at it positively, even if it's a TERRIBLE and BAD and stupid thing, but in the end it actually worked out perfectly for us, yeah. (Grohmann)

Literature

Skinner, Ellen A., and Melanie J. Zimmer-Gembeck. 2011. Perceived control and the development of coping. In *The Oxford handbook of stress, health, and coping*, ed. Susan Folkman, 35–59. New York: Oxford University Press.

Open Access This chapter is licensed under the terms of the Creative Commons Attribution 4.0 International License (http://creativecommons.org/licenses/by/4.0/), which permits use, sharing, adaptation, distribution and reproduction in any medium or format, as long as you give appropriate credit to the original author(s) and the source, provide a link to the Creative Commons license and indicate if changes were made.

The images or other third party material in this chapter are included in the chapter's Creative Commons license, unless indicated otherwise in a credit line to the material. If material is not included in the chapter's Creative Commons license and your intended use is not permitted by statutory regulation or exceeds the permitted use, you will need to obtain permission directly from the copyright holder.

Chapter 8
Illness and Family Decision-Making

Amy Mullin

Abstract This chapter discusses how philosophy can help us understand family responses and decision-making when one child serves as a donor of bodily tissue to a seriously ill sibling. Drawing on interviews conducted with families in which one child served as the donor, I explore how a relational understanding of autonomy might help map initial decision-making, how an ethics of care can contribute to understanding the balancing of personal needs against what is wanted for a seriously ill child, and how gratitude, rather than indebtedness, is the appropriate response to sacrifices aimed at saving a sibling.

Keywords Children · Families · Illness · Health care decision-making · Relational autonomy · Donation · Gratitude · Decision-making

When a young child's serious illness is diagnosed, the child's entire family is drastically affected. In addition to coping with worry, fear, and the child's pain and suffering, the family must learn to navigate a complicated health care bureaucracy, and make decisions, often with little time for thought, that have the impact to change all their lives. Clearly the family requires more than just medical care for their child, and can benefit from a variety of supports. It may seem that philosophers have little to contribute, and yet they and other theorists can help understand what is happening to the family, and what help they might need, beyond medical treatment for their child. This is particularly true when one minor child in the family is a bone marrow match for the ill child, and has the potential to have bone marrow extracted and inserted into the sibling. If successful, the implanted bone marrow can generate blood and other bodily material on an ongoing basis and therefore help heal the previously ill sibling.

In this chapter, I begin with a discussion of the complex nature of family responses and decision making in these circumstances. Parents can experience

A. Mullin (✉)
Department of Philosophy, University of Toronto, Toronto, ON, Canada
e-mail: amy.mullin@utoronto.ca

© The Author(s) 2022
C. Schües et al. (eds.), *Stem Cell Transplantations Between Siblings as Social Phenomena*, Philosophy and Medicine 144,
https://doi.org/10.1007/978-3-031-04166-2_8

significant pressure, both because of the urgency of the decisions that face them, and because their circumstances involve healthy children making sacrifices for an ill sibling. Their children, in turn, may face pressure both because of parental expectations and because of concern for their sibling. Then I explore three interrelated sets of questions that arise at three different time periods – when making the initial decision to use one child's bone marrow to help save another, when the families are living with uncertainty and what they hope will be a period of recovery, and after the ill child has received medical treatment and the resolution is largely known.

At the time of diagnosis, does pressure to respond quickly about a vitally important concern, along with complex family dynamics involved when both bone marrow donor and recipient are children, make it difficult to make informed medical decisions? How might a relational understanding of the nature of autonomy help us think about this decision making? Next, once a decision has been made, and while family members are dealing with a child's ongoing serious illness, how do they balance their personal needs against what they want for their ill family member? What can an ethics of care contribute to theorizing the situation? Finally, after the medical treatment has occurred, how might the family think about what, if anything, is owed in return for the donation? Here I distinguish between gratitude and indebtedness and argue that making this distinction clearer could be helpful for some families.

My remarks are inspired by material from interviews conducted with seventeen families in which one minor child served as a donor to another, as to what they experienced following their seriously ill child's diagnosis (Jürgensen and Herzog 2018). These interviews were part of a qualitative multidisciplinary study carried out at the Institute of History of Medicine and Science Studies, University of Lübeck, on bone marrow donation between sibling minor children. In the records of the interviews, each family is anonymized. All those family members willing to speak were recorded, with the recordings later transcribed and translated into English. Most but not all of the ill children survived, as discussed in the Introduction to this volume.

8.1   Expectations, Ethics, Pressure, and Family Decision Making

When a child was diagnosed as seriously ill and in need of bone marrow, the families typically encountered this as a crisis, demanding almost immediate decisions about treatment options. One image they used is striking: several families spoke of feeling like they were suddenly living "in the wrong movie." (### reference to intro II ###) Not only does this metaphor convey the idea of radical and inexplicable change but also the suggestion that one's actions post diagnosis feel scripted. The illness strikes and changes the lives of everyone in the family and now doctors, rather than film directors, mandate what needs to happen next. Clearly the parents in these families felt themselves to be under incredible pressure.

In addition to suddenly finding themselves in a high pressure medical drama, the ill child, parents and siblings, can feel as if they have no real options and that there is no need to discuss decisions, whether within the family or with outside sources of support, because there is no decision to be made. According to the script, everyone in the family should be tested to see if they are a good match for bone marrow donation; if someone is a good match, or the best match, they must have some bone marrow removed, and then everyone waits to see if the ill child can use this bone marrow to heal.

Speaking about her donor daughter, the mother in the Bahr family says[1]: "she (.) sensed the PRESSURE, she HAD TO- she didn't have a choice. We asked her (.) and explained it to her, said to her, ARE you going to do this, do you want to do this, but actually everything was really obvious (.), she's got to do this, even if we ask her, it was a charade, (.) you see. (.) It was clear to all of us (.) and SHE sensed the pressure, yeah." In the Bahr family, the donor was asked, but in the Grohmann family, this never happened. The Grohmann mother says: "I was asked by friends years later, er: 'did you actually ask Greta if that was what she wanted?' and I said: 'it never, it never occurred to us, for us it was actually ALWAYS going to be (.) the case, like, if Greta was a match then that's what would happen (swallows), you know?'" Similarly, the father in the Preuss family says: "Of course we (laughs) asked Pascal (.), you know, but he also (.), well, saying no was never an op- OPTION for him. So (.) none of us thought about NOT doing it, (.) you know (..) that was absolutely never an option for us."

As the quotes above suggest, often there were different reasons why family members felt they had real choices. In some cases the ill child's siblings refused to consider an alternative to attempting to save their sibling's life. For instance, a non-donor sibling in the Kirstein family, who was not a match, describes herself thinking: "she has to have bone marrow and that we all need to get ourselves tested, (.) or whether we wanted to get ourselves tested and I think, that's actually not something to question." Similarly the daughter in the Preuss family wanted to donate, even though she wasn't sure what that involved: "I didn't know at that time what I was supposed to donate or what a transplant was. I didn't know what bone marrow was etc. etc. (.). All I knew was that (.) if they ask me if I'd like to donate and I say yes (.), that I would be saving my sister's life."

In other families there was no discussion about whether anyone would be tested to see if they were potential matches, and no discussion about whether potential donors would donate. Another non-donor sibling, says: "I can't now remember the moment when my parents asked me, Manuel, would you like to get typed? It was a sort of thing, that you, like it SHOULD be like this in the family." The members of this family assumed that what they thought ethically best is what would be done.

Even when parents asked their children if they were willing to donate, they knew they would almost certainly override any refusal. The costs of donation for the donor child, including the need to keep free of infection before the donation, some

---

[1] Interview quotes refer to the excerpts in the appendix of this book.

fear, pain, risk of medical complications, and worry about whether or not the donation will help, paled in comparison to the risk of death to the ill child without the
sibling's donation. Nonetheless the parents were aware of the costs to the donor
child. For example, the mother in the Kelling family speaks about her donor child:
"And they hadn't prepared her for it, not properly I felt, that now she- and that was
really bad for her, so she was afraid of falling asleep and it hurt and actually there
was nothing in there but she's a child and there was still that feeling there was a
needle in her."

All of the families interviewed had a child who provided bone marrow for a sibling. Although I describe them as 'donors', following the practice of the interviewers, it is unclear if all should be seen as donating, if that is taken to involve making
an unconstrained choice. Parents either simply expected their children to donate, or
applied emotional pressure. This is because medical professionals often suggested,
or at least were interpreted as saying, that having a sibling serve as a donor was
ideal. The mother in the Zucker family describes a doctor they consulted: "he ALSO
can't understand how, like, anyone can go searching for an unrelated donor when
you have SUCH A MATCHING donor f- like Zorro." Despite what the families felt,
one matched donor is actually as good as another in terms of survival rates. However,
there are justified worries that, should the family go looking for an alternative donor
rather than one of their children, suitable bone marrow might not be found, the price
expected for the bone marrow and associated expenses might be high, and/or the
search for another donor could lead to a delay that would compromise the health of
the ill child.

While the parents were typically not prepared to accept a refusal from any of
their children, the donor siblings usually cited a combination of concern for their
sibling, feelings about what, morally speaking, they should do as a result, and considerable emotional pressure from their parents as their motivation to accede to
parental expectations. The children agreed despite confusion and fear about what
serving as a donor might involve. The donor daughter in the Kunow family says:
"because then I got so much PRESSURE from (.) my parents: come on, and you
have to do this, he's your brother after all and erm (.), if you don't do this, then erm
(..), yes, then- you you won't forgive yourself for the rest of your LIFE and come
on, just do it. And then at some point I'd been put under such emotional pressure
that I just said: OK, you know what, (.) you're not going to give up anyway and I
don't want afterwards to have to take responsibility." This donor describes a complex mixture of bowing to parental pressure and acknowledging her ethical obligations, with her references to not forgiving herself and not wanting to take
responsibility for a bad outcome.

The fact that bone marrow donation involves incorporating bodily tissue from
another person into one's own body, and having that tissue function on an ongoing
basis, complicates how family members think about both unrelated and familial
donors. Some families may find it more reassuring, apart from largely unjustified
beliefs about the greater efficacy of familial donations when it comes to avoiding
tissue rejection, to accept bodily assistance from someone in the family. Nonetheless,
several donors, recipients, and other family members consider it to be uncanny for

a child to receive bodily tissue from another family member. For instance, a non-donor sister in the Rohde family says: "that was kind of funny, to (.) know that the cells are taken out of one of them and PLANTED into the other one, let's say. It was (.) a bit spooky."

People found this particularly challenging when the bone marrow was supplied by a sibling whose biological sex did not match that of the recipient child. The donor daughter in the Wahl family says: "I'm a GIRL and I've donated my stem cells to him, you sometimes say [turns towards her mother; MJ] you know, that erm (.) (swallows) that he now has female (laughs) stem cells or something, and now because of that some ways of behaving are eh erm DIFFERENT." The mother in that same family says: "that something like something soft, female, is ticking inside him somehow. I don't remember any more what it was about, but (.) erm (…) yes I can't- don't REMEMBER any more. Well (.) he reacted very, so very sensitively and soft, like he perhaps wouldn't have done before."

Many family members found this incorporation of someone else's bodily tissue to challenge the identity of both donor and recipient. Some family members speak of bodily joining as leading to a positive psychological unification or unusual closeness between donor and recipient. For instance, the non-donor sister in the Minz family describes the close bond between the sibling who received and the one who provided bone marrow: "he saved her life and [there's] so much (.) similarity and [they're] so much the same that they now also share through the shared bone marrow, that is (.) something very special." However, others speak of being teased and feeling that it is upsetting or uncanny to know that one child's body now works as it does because of incorporating a functioning part of another family member. For instance, the bone marrow donor in the Minz family remarks "my Dad sometimes makes silly comments, if it's like (.) I dunno, if Malle, if there's some kind of opinion about Malle or Malle is supposed to make some kind of decision and isn't here, then he can- my Dad always says: yes, Marlena can do it, she has the same thoughts as he has, he has the same bone marrow or something like that." The donor in the Rohde family describes her uneasy response to having her bone marrow functioning in her sibling: "Sometimes I have moments when I (.) when I- when when it becomes so CLEAR to me or when I (.) suddenly realise that I am actually in my sister. And then erm (.) then I also ask myself how much of ME is now in her or (.) somehow? Does it now have different effects, I mean not just on her blood, erm but also somehow on (.) her herself or on her personality or something."

Several donor siblings speak of worry that their gift will not save their sibling, and could even make them worse, and children whose siblings died despite receiving bone marrow are left feeling guilt, even if they know they should not. The donor daughter in the Rohde family says: "it's also important to know that, if something goes wrong, that you yourself are not to blame. I mean (..) THAT could always happen and then (.) you should- I mean, and then (.) you really have to see that you somehow get rid of these feelings of guilt or whatever." Even those whose bone marrow helps to save their ill sibling can feel ongoing worry that their bodily tissue won't perform as it should in their sibling's body.

The consequences of being a seriously ill child who has received bone marrow from a sibling, or being the young sibling or parent of that child, are long-lasting. They could include resentment of a child who receives bone marrow from another family member but does not go on to behave or appreciate life in a manner expected by other family members. Fortunately, they may also include some positive developments such as enhanced family unity and greater appreciation for being able to enjoy mundane pleasures. The mother in the Speidel family says: "Other things are more important for us and erm, it's a pity that you have to learn something like that, but I think I can say that, since that first day of being ill, we as a family really have lived every day as if it were our last, every day. It IS like that."

8.2   Relational Autonomy and Informed Decision Making

Having discussed how families responded to the crisis they faced, relying often on their own words, I turn now to the first set of questions I wish to explore, with a focus on factors that can undermine or support informed decision making. In the passage cited directly above, the Speidel family mother draws attention to how quickly her family's life was transformed by diagnosis, from "that first day of being ill." This is part of a pattern of families understanding the temporal dimension of their child's serious illness as involving a shockingly sudden diagnosis, accompanied by the need to act swiftly to initiate treatment that might prove the difference between death and life, and the associated feeling that one's actions are scripted with no real choices are available. It usually takes time to adjust one's habits and expectations to a dramatically altered reality, and yet many of these families felt as if they had no time, and were expected both to quickly understand the nature of their child's illness and any treatment options, and to make speedy decisions. This often extended to the involvement of a donor minor child, who was expected to volunteer or assent to donation despite fear and confusion about what their role meant and what its long-term consequences would be.

We typically assume that informed consent to medical treatment requires understanding of an illness or condition, awareness of the options that could be therapeutic, along with a clear understanding of the consequences of refusing to use some or all of those options, and the risks acquired by making use of them (Beauchamp and Childress 2012). These are competency conditions. We also generally assume that decision-makers are deciding on their own for themselves or for somebody for whom they are serving as a substitute decision maker. Finally we assume that they are not acting in circumstances in which they are either coerced or so badly deceived that they cannot adequately pursue cares and commitments which they find personally meaningful. These are conditions related to the authenticity of their commitments. In the absence of evidence of coercion or deceit, medical personnel will typically assume that authenticity conditions have been met and worry only about their patients' competency.

However, the situation in these families reveals that often two individuals, the parents of the children involved, will be making decisions, and they will be making decisions that take into account not only their seriously ill child, but also their other children, both when they are tested to see who might be a good donor, and when one is chosen to donate. We have seen above that as a result of this complexity, frequently children feel pressured and uninformed, parents realize uncomfortably that they are expecting one child to make sacrifices in order to benefit another, and no or very little discussion takes place. Although the impact of the donation sometimes includes a sense of blurred boundaries between donor and recipient, and some significant fear and worry, in addition to short term pain and risk, families understandably do not focus on the negative impact on their donor children. Because parents feel rushed, pressured and incredibly worried about their sick children, it appears likely that their decision making might be less competent, and autonomy more compromised, than would be ideal and also less than would be feasible if they were given some time to reflect and some support with their decision making.

Most often, when we think of compromised autonomy in a context of medical decision-making we focus on the patients themselves and want to be sure they are able to make decisions about options they understand in a way that reflects what is important to them. We worry about factors that can make it difficult for them to understand their options, both in terms of medical risks and benefits, and how the different options fit with or could undermine things they value. Carel et al. (2019) speak of patients' epistemic deficiencies produced by pain, distress, and "the lack of sufficient time to probe the decision with a health professional." (377) However, entire families are likely to experience epistemic deficiencies, including parents who are expected to make decisions for more than one of their children.[2] Parents will typically be emotionally overwhelmed by a diagnosis that means their child might die, especially when they have not had time to adjust their understanding of what is happening to the family. Feeling as if they have no time to make decisions, let alone understand their risks and implications, is a source of epistemic deficiency and therefore compromised autonomy. Being expected to represent the potentially conflicting interests of minor children is another potential source of compromised autonomy.

Theorists of relational autonomy stress that we not only develop the capacities and resources we need to make informed and autonomous decisions by being raised by people who help us develop them, but also often need other people on an ongoing basis when we make major decisions, especially under stressful conditions. As one such theorist, Mackenzie, writes, an adequate understanding of the competence conditions for autonomy, must recognize "the extensive interpersonal, social and institutional scaffolding necessary for the development *and ongoing exercise* of the complex cognitive, volitional, imaginative and emotional skills involved in self-governance." (2014, 8, my italics) When we face overwhelming emotions, are

---

[2] Carel, Havi and Gyorffy recognize that families can face significant distress during their child's illness and treatment, and can vary in their knowledge and competence (see 381).

stressed, and need to make quick decisions, our identities are disrupted and our ability to become informed and to evaluate our options is almost certainly decreased. Access to emotional support, and to accounts of the experiences of other families who have faced similar circumstances, could facilitate more informed and collaborative decision making. It could also guide medical professionals to help families understand when the need to make a quick decision truly requires immediate action and when it can permit taking a brief time, even if only a few days or a week, before a family commits to a course of action.

The research project that prompted this volume, and other sources of access to people who have experienced what they have and are willing to share their experiences, could help provide highly relevant information to families making these difficult decisions. This could include learning what a child might be worried about, whether the ill child, the potential donor child, or other children in the family. In addition, medical professionals could learn more about the attitudes and concerns of the families they interact with, and more sensitively respond to their patients and their families, especially if they can draw upon external resources, such as experts in medical communication with children of various ages. This information could particularly help families who are already aware that their decision making is ethically fraught. For instance, the father in the Wahl family says: "Is it actually somehow permissible, erm, to use this- a child as a construction site for the other?" The donor child in that same family speaks of wondering if she was now a "spare parts depot" for her ill sibling. Since parents and children alike may be confused, pressured, and uneasy, their communities and healthcare teams have a responsibility to offer resources to help them better understand and cope with their situation, both to reduce their distress, and to enhance the autonomy of their decision-making.

8.3 The Ethics of Care and Meeting Needs Within the Family

Human beings are all vulnerable and dependent. Our needs for care vary throughout our lives but are always present; therefore detecting those needs and responding by providing care are among our most significant moral responsibilities. An ethics of care, also known as care theory, need not deny there are other significant moral categories that correspond to other major areas of moral responsibility. Indeed it is important to ensure that those who provide care are not unjustly burdened, with some providing far more unpaid care than others. Far from care and justice being in necessary tension, there are important connections between the two, and working to ensure that private, familial provision of care is supplemented by other forms of care is an important aim for an ethics of care.

An ethics of care can be an important resource to bring to bear in analyzing the families who are the focus of this chapter as not only does the ill child require care, but also their illness can increase their whole family's need for care. The entire family will face a dramatic and unwelcome transformation of daily life while the parents must make life altering treatment decisions. When I say that the family as a whole is likely to have increased needs for care, what is meant by 'care'? Care theorist Daniel Engster writes: "Care may be said to include everything we do directly to help others to meet their basic needs, develop or sustain their basic capabilities, and alleviate or avoid pain and suffering, in an attentive, responsive and respectful manner." (2005: 55) What are 'basic needs' and 'basic capabilities'? Needs refer to what we must have in order to function in a wide range of ways of life, and include not only things like having food, adequate shelter, and medical care sufficient to allow us to recover from significant ailments, but also feeling secure and attached to others. Basic capabilities are actual opportunities people have to do what they value. They include mobility, the ability to imagine alternatives, the ability to interact socially with others, and the ability to understand enough about one's circumstances to make choices that aim to realize one's goals. Capabilities can be understood in line with Martha Nussbaum (2011) and Amartya Sen's (2001) capability approach, but readers need not agree with the specific lists of capacities Nussbaum, or any other theorist develops. What is important is that thinking about capabilities required to function in a wide range of domains of life can help us identify the skills and resources people need to be able to do things – even if they choose not to pursue activities in some of those domains.

Engster builds attentiveness, responsiveness, and respect into his understanding of care but we can help others meet at least some of their basic needs in more or less attentive and respectful ways. We can care for another in a manner that flows from valuing the person we care for, but also in manners that do not. We can also value another person, and genuinely wish to improve their well-being, without respecting them, and taking their point of view into account when we strive to meet their needs.

The relevant sense of respect I have in mind is that captured by Robin Dillon in her discussion of care respect (1992). Dillon introduces the notion of care respect to remind her readers that we can respect people who are still agents even if not fully autonomous, and that a truly caring response to someone who has a point of view must take that point of view into account. This is not to say that it is only people with partial or compromised autonomy who should be treated with care respect since care respect involves valuing another person, seeking to meet their needs, and doing so in a manner that takes that other person's perspective into account. Nonetheless, it is not the same as more arms length respect for the autonomy of a person with fully developed capacities to understand her situation, evaluate her options, and make decisions and take actions that reflect her values. It involves active caring, or seeking to meet another's needs, but the determination to do so in a way that recognizes the person cared for is a person with a perspective or point of view. Care respect is something we can and should demonstrate for children. Moreover, demonstrating care respect for people who lack full autonomy does not mean that we merely consult with them as a source of information about what they think and care about. It means having an open mind as to the possibility that the person who is respected may have good insights into what would help them and what makes them feel worse. It also means recognizing that we cannot have a deep understanding of what helps others or harms them without knowing something about what matters to them. We acquire this kind of knowledge about others not only by asking them to verbalize it, which can be too demanding for many adults as well as children, but also by attending to what they do and the feelings they reveal.[3] Good care involves meeting another's needs in a manner that reflects care respect.

Since families are typically a primary site for meeting members' needs for care, especially emotional needs, the inability to do so can be very challenging. The inability to access support within the family for one's emotional needs, such as the needs for reassurance and connection, may be bewildering and upsetting not only for the siblings of the ill child but also for the parents. As a result, one of the most useful things we can do to support families in which all members have increased needs for care and decreased ability to provide it, is to challenge the idea that families are flawed when they cannot be self-contained about meeting one another's needs. As mentioned above, this is in keeping with seeking a more just distribution of the work involved in providing care. In virtue of this recognition, it is important to develop informal and formal mechanisms to make external support available to all family members for their needs for care to be met. Learning from families of seriously ill children what helped them and what made them feel isolated or rejected, could let the friends and acquaintances of affected families know what to do and what to avoid. Support groups that focus on particular needs, such as those of minor children with a seriously ill sibling, can try to support these children at a time when most attention will be directed towards that ill sibling.

There are certainly other situations, besides the fortunately relatively rare cases of seriously ill children who need bone marrow transplants, in which children, and family members more broadly, suffer when families are thought to have sole private responsibility for meeting most of the needs of their members. These include other situations of sudden disruption, as when an adult family member becomes seriously ill, physically or mentally, or loses a job that provided the sole family income. However, they also include more chronic circumstances, as when physical or mental illness will not end even while it may not threaten life. Challenging the idea that parents should be able to solve all their child's problems and meet all their needs can also address the unjust life prospects this attitude can generate for children, given how much some parents' resources, financial, social and emotional, vary from those of others.

As is clear from the interviews, and as could be predicted, the ill child becomes the primary, and almost the sole, object of parental attention. One parent may stop paid employment, and move to another city to be with the ill child if an appropriate hospital is not available nearby. Loss of employment will strain a family's economic resources, at precisely a time when they may be facing greater financial pressures, and this can impact other family members who perhaps can no longer afford to engage in activities they enjoyed. Even if finances are not affected, parental time and focus will be seriously absorbed, and so the other children may have to drop out of activities that were a source of pleasure, pride, and social engagement.

One of the non-donor children in the Molle family acknowledges both her acceptance of how her parents acted, which included very little attention for the healthy

---

[3] This is discussed in Mullin, A. (2014).

and non-donor siblings, and how difficult she nonetheless found it: "I think my parents couldn't really have done anything BETTER than what they actually did, …. it's a complete (laughs) shitty situation, like (.), anyway, WHATEVER you do, it's always going to be stupid." A non-donor child in the Minz family similarly expresses understanding for her parents and how difficult she found her own situation: "I COULDN'T have DEALT with things any other way, because if you believe you're losing a child then it's- then this child has a different status in the family. And after all I was ALL RIGHT, wasn't I? So I didn't have a problem with it, I was OK, despite everything (.) it was really (.) hard somehow."

The parents may resent the fact that a child's illness requires them to give up activities they had enjoyed, whether on their own, with the family as a whole, or with other children. Yet at the same time, they might feel guilty for missing cards night, or movies with friends, or watching their children do sports or act in a play, when they know the ill child is much more dramatically affected. Their marriage partner may be an important source of support, and yet also a source of stress and conflict. This is because the parents need to find a way to share the enhanced work-load associated with caring for a seriously ill child, and are expected to help their partner while under serious stress themselves.

As suggested above, the siblings of the ill child can realize that their parents' priorities must shift, and yet understandably would not like losing their parents' attention. The siblings also lose the security of knowing that things are going well in the family and that their parents can protect them from danger and difficulty. It must be frightening to feel like a crisis has hit the family that the parents cannot handle alone. Realizing that one's young sibling is the cause of that crisis, while also appreciating that the ill sibling is suffering and threatened, could be very diffi-cult. To compound the problem, the people to whom they often turn for help with emotional upset are much less available. Even if parents manage to support the emotional needs of the ill child's siblings, it could be very hard for those children to express sadness, resentment, or confusion. Nonetheless, if they are to be treated with care respect, those striving to meet their needs should aim to understand their point of view. If the parents cannot meet some of those needs, families should be offered support to ensure they are met.

While parental and broader community attention are likely to be more devoted to the seriously ill child than other children in the family, this does not mean that the ill child will welcome a strong focus on their illness. The bone marrow recipient in the Minz family remarks: "Exactly, yes, I'm not just the one, (.) exactly// not just the one who, like (.) was ill and did well despite that, but I also have a lot of other things that I (.) CAN do, rather than just being ill (laughs), (.) that sounds stupid, but // that's what it is." A seriously ill child is never just his or her illness, and having people in their lives so focused on that illness is likely to be unpleasant. Someone outside the family circle, especially a social worker or similar professional, might help the ill child access experiences that make them feel normal, and just a child among other children. Once again, the perspective of the child needs to be taken into account if they are to be treated not only with medical care, but also with care respect.

8.4 Gratitude and Indebtedness Within the Family

After the ill child's medical treatment has come to an end, questions about gratitude and indebtedness may come to the fore. The recovered child or their parents may be expected to be grateful for a donation that was potentially lifesaving. Interpersonal gratitude, I have argued elsewhere, is best understood as appreciation of a real benefit, provided by someone who gives that benefit at least partly due to a desire to help someone they value and respect (Mullin 2016).[4] For instance, a woman, motivated by love and concern for her sibling, notices that her brother is struggling at work and comes up with a plan to help. She makes the offer, and her brother suggests some changes to the plan. The two of them carry it out, and the brother is more successful in his job. A real benefit has been conveyed; the motivation for the help included care and concern for the recipient, and the recipient's perspective was considered and incorporated into the plan, evidencing respect for him. Sometimes, only some of the conditions that properly merit gratitude are present. For instance, the bone marrow donor may donate under pressure rather than truly willingly. They may act so as to please, or not worry and anger, their parents rather than because of valuing and respecting their ill sibling. In such situations, parents may appropriately be grateful but not the ill children if they are aware of their siblings' motivations. Tense relationships with siblings are common, including when a sick child is the primary parental focus. Alternatively, the bone marrow may be given to benefit a much-loved sibling, but it may not improve and could actually worsen their health. While everyone in the family may be grateful that the donor tried, and experienced pain, worry, and feelings of guilt at the failure of the transplant, the bone marrow would not be a real benefit. Any gratitude would be for the effort rather than the result.

When gratitude is appropriate because its conditions were met in a manner that the beneficiaries can recognize, this can have positive effects. There is considerable evidence that it can be life enhancing to experience gratitude in the aftermath of receiving a gift that provided a real benefit, and was provided because one was valued and respected (Wood et al. 2010). Positive impacts associated with adults' experiences of gratitude include increased life satisfaction, and studies of gratitude in children suggest that it has a similar impact on them (Froh and Bono 2011, Froh et al. 2008). Evidence suggests that gratitude expressed in early adolescence correlates with life satisfaction, and social integration (Froh et al. 2011, 289).

However, if one lives full time with one's benefactor, and this benefactor is a sibling with whom one has both joyful and more conflicted interactions, the recipient of the gift, in this case bone marrow, may occasionally end up feeling less grateful and more indebted. The distinction between gratitude and indebtedness is discussed in psychological literature (Tsang 2006; Watkins et al. 2006) and I have

---

[4]There are further conditions for gratitude to be merited. The recipient must be able to recognize the benefit received as truly of value, and the benefit provided should not have been immorally acquired by the benefactor, or owed to someone else. See Mullin 2016 for more details.

discussed it in previous work (Mullin 2016). When we are grateful, we feel not only that we have been provided a benefit, but also are valued by the person who gave it, and are disposed to value that person in return, because they helped us and did that partly or wholly for our own sake. We may be very pleased to be able to 'return the favour' but do not feel expected or morally required to repay our benefactor with goods or services of equivalent valued to what we received from them.

By contrast, when we feel indebted, we feel expected to pay off our debt, and do not feel that the benefit was provided to help us by someone who cares about our well-being, but instead that this was part of an expected quid pro quo. The recipient in the Kirstein family expresses resentment of her sibling's expectation that she owes him now: "I can't owe him erm (.) my whole life long erm- I mean that he like, I mean that I have a DEBT towards him or something. That can't be the case, can it".

Far from enabling well-being, feeling indebted can be an unpleasant burden, and can threaten a previously existing relationship. While people are generally happier when they notice and appreciate the good things that others have done for them, at least when those others were motivated to provide a benefit to someone they value, indebtedness is not so positive. It can hang over a person, always there, always owing, especially when the benefit is as significant as the provision of bone marrow. In this case, the donor, recipient and other family members may all feel resentful. For example, the bone marrow recipient in the Kirstein family was suicidal for a time, and this was resented by other family members, including the donor who says: "you see how erm the person whose life you've (.) well indirectly perhaps you've saved, (.) erm throws away their life, or tries again DELIBERATELY to destroy it, and you want to prevent that."

Fortunately, the other families studied did not struggle with resentment and feel owed or indebted. Instead many focused on the positive aspects of the bone marrow donation for the family as a whole. Gratitude, rather than indebtedness, seems relevant to their responses. Of course, motivation to do anything for others is almost invariably complex, and a mix of altruistic and self-serving motives may be present. But in the case of bone marrow donation, so long as one of the motives was a desire to help one's ill sibling, to have them feel better and recover, and the sick sibling was showed care respect, this should suffice to motivate gratitude.[5] Given what we know about the many positive effects of experiencing gratitude, both in children and in adults, it is important for families to have a chance to focus on gratitude and those they feel grateful to. If the family is encouraged to experience or discuss gratitude, it would be useful to contrast gratitude with indebtedness. No doubt any conversations on this complicated topic, or efforts to encourage gratitude, could be professionally facilitated. Bone marrow is a gift no one should expect to repay or be repaid.

Families should be counseled not to expect the child who received the bone marrow transplant, and survived, to feel they owe the donor. In particular, children who receive bone marrow from a sibling should not be expected to live their lives in ways

---

[5] If family members were to ignore the recipient's point of view and concerns this would be a failure of care respect.

that please their sibling or parents. Parents are very likely to have goals for their children's lives, and it would be difficult to see a child whose life had been saved develop poor health habits or suicidal thoughts. However, pressuring them not to do so because they should feel indebted, and duty bound to repay what they have received with good behaviour – is not only likely to backfire, but also is unfair. A child's illness is something that happens to them rather than being caused by their mature poor choices or bad behaviour, and they do not acquire a life-long responsibility to live in ways that please others as a result of receiving bone marrow. We all receive significant care as children in order to make it to adulthood, but do not thereby acquire a debt to be repaid.

8.5   Conclusion

As a philosopher I am trained to seek larger lessons from specific situations, but do not want to end on a note of generalizing from the experiences of the families interviewed in the interesting and important research project that generated the interview materials. Instead I would like to express my own gratitude to the people who participated in those interviews, sharing their experiences, good and bad. They have furthered our understanding of a situation which may have begun with some of them feeling like they were suddenly cast against their wills in the wrong movie, but in which they struggled forward to meet one of the most enormous and grueling challenges a family can face.

Literature

Beauchamp, Tom, and James Childress. 2012. *Principles of biomedical ethics*. 7th ed. New York: Oxford University Press.

Carel, Havi, Gene Feder, and Gita Gyorffy. 2019. Children and health. In *The Routledge handbook of the philosophy of childhood and children*, ed. Anna Gheaus, Gideon Calder, and Jurgen De Wispelaere, 373–383. London: Routledge.

Dillon, Robin S. 1992. Respect and care: Towards moral integration. *Canadian Journal of Philosophy* 22: 105–132.

Engster, Daniel. 2005. Rethinking care theory: The practice of caring and the obligation to care. *Hypatia* 20 (3): 50–74.

Froh, Jeffrey J., and Giacomo Bono. 2011. Gratitude in youth: Review of gratitude interventions and some ideas for application. *Communiqué* 39 (5): 26–28.

Froh, Jeffrey J., Robert A. Emmons, Noel A. Card, Giacomo Bono, and Jennifer A. Wilson. 2011. Gratitude and the reduced costs of materialism in adolescents. *Journal of Happiness Studies* 12 (2): 289–302.

Froh, Jeffrey J., William J. Sefick, and Robert A. Emmons. 2008. Counting blessings in early adolescents: An experimental study of gratitude and subjective Well-being. *Journal of Social Psychology* 46: 213–233.

Jürgensen, Martina, and Madeleine Herzog. 2018. *Care, responsibilities and integrity: Stem cell transplantations between siblings as social phenomena within and beyond families.* Institute for History of Medicine and Science Studies: University of Lübeck.

Mackenzie, Catriona. 2014. Three dimensions of autonomy: A relational analysis. In *Autonomy, oppression and gender*, ed. Andrea Veltman and Mark Piper. Oxford Scholarship Online. https://doi.org/10.1093/acprof:so/97801969104.101.

Mullin, Amy. 2014. Children, paternalism, and the development of autonomy. *Ethical theory and moral practice, special issue on "Private autonomy, public paternalism?"*, eds. Annette Dufner and Michael Kühler, 17(3): 413–426.

———. 2016. Dependent children, gratitude and respect. *Journal of Moral Philosophy* 13: 720–738.

Nussbaum, Martha C. 2011. *Creating capabilities: The human development approach.* Cambridge: Harvard University Press.

Sen, Amartya. 2001. *Development as Freedom.* Oxford: Oxford University Press.

Tsang, J.-A. (2006). The effects of helper intention on gratitude and indebtedness. *Motivation and Emotion* 30 (3): 199–205. https://doi.org/10.1007/s11031-006-9031-z

Watkins, P.C., J. Scheer, M. Ovnicek, and R. Kolts. 2006. The debt of gratitude: Dissociating gratitude and indebtedness. *Cognition and Emotion* 20 (2): 217–241.

Wood, Alex M., Jeffrey J. Froh, and Adam W.A. Geraghty. 2010. Gratitude and Well-being: A review and theoretical integration. *Clinical Psychology Review* 30: 890–905.

Open Access This chapter is licensed under the terms of the Creative Commons Attribution 4.0 International License (http://creativecommons.org/licenses/by/4.0/), which permits use, sharing, adaptation, distribution and reproduction in any medium or format, as long as you give appropriate credit to the original author(s) and the source, provide a link to the Creative Commons license and indicate if changes were made.

The images or other third party material in this chapter are included in the chapter's Creative Commons license, unless indicated otherwise in a credit line to the material. If material is not included in the chapter's Creative Commons license and your intended use is not permitted by statutory regulation or exceeds the permitted use, you will need to obtain permission directly from the copyright holder.

Chapter 9
Dwelling on the Past: Illness, Transplantation and Families' Responsibilities in Retrospect

Christoph Rehmann-Sutter

Abstract From family members' perspectives, a bone marrow transplant is the source and the focus of many responsibility-related considerations. The chapter searches for connections between responsibility, memory and time, in order to explain the complex meanings of "retrospective responsibilities". Story-telling within families and the emergence of family narratives is a place where responsibility is not just remembered, but also enacted. Families care about how things in the past are recounted in the present. One family case is discussed in detail, in which family members had to cope with the failure of multiple transplants and other therapies, and with the death of their daughter. The final part of the chapter considers problems of retrospective justification. With hindsight, what were the interests of the donor child? What were this young child's will and duties? Can the anticipated retrospective consent of potential donor children serve as an orientation and an ethically reliable justification for the decision taken by the parents, as proxies, to allow a young child to become a donor? The chapter advocates the perspective of an ethics of care.

Keywords Stem cell donation · Bone marrow transplant · Retrospective responsibility · Narrative ethics · Ethics of care · Anticipated retrospective consent

> Absence is present, Time doth tarry.
> *John Donne*[1]

Over the last couple of years, Martina Jürgensen, Madeleine Herzog, Christina Schües and I have conducted a qualitative study with 17 families who have lived

---

[1] John Donne (1573–1631): Present in Absence (last verse of second stanza).

C. Rehmann-Sutter (✉)
Institute for History of Medicine and Science Studies, University of Lübeck, Lübeck, Schleswig-Holstein, Germany
e-mail: christoph.rehmannsutter@uni-luebeck.de

© The Author(s) 2022
C. Schües et al. (eds.), *Stem Cell Transplantations Between Siblings as Social Phenomena*, Philosophy and Medicine 144,
https://doi.org/10.1007/978-3-031-04166-2_9

through bone marrow transplantation between siblings who were children at the time. The study is described in detail elsewhere in this volume (see Chap. 1: Introduction). Here I highlight that our focus was on these families' long-term retrospectives, with time intervals from the transplant ranging from just a few years up to 20 years. In the conversations (one-to-one interviews and family interviews) we heard stories about what happened at the time of the transplant and since. In their stories they revealed, with hindsight, how they saw these events and their own involvement in them.

These people had gone through a unique and sometimes difficult experience. All families in our study remembered the time of the disease and of its treatment as a major rupture. The fact that it was a sibling child who donated bone marrow was not the major issue for most of the families, compared to the deadly threat of the disease. In the interviews conducted a long time after the acute illness was overcome, or in a few cases, after the child patient had died, we see a general pattern: Illness as experience is not something that ends, but remains a lasting reality for a very long time afterwards, even if the physical illness has been cured.

We analysed the interviews because we wanted to learn from these experiences and from the families' views of them – with an eye to the ethics of decision-making in present and future cases. People who were actually involved have the advantage of being able to sort out what was particularly important in the long run. As well as recounting what they remember of their distress at the time of treatment, they are also able to tell how they dealt with it afterwards, how the events of the transplant shaped their subsequent family life, how responsibilities were re-allocated and re-negotiated, and how all this became part of their biographical memory.

In this chapter I focus on how family members retrospectively see their responsibilities throughout the process. As a philosopher I am interested in attaining a deeper understanding of the morally complex situations that emerge. There is something to learn about responsible decision-making, which might help parents and healthcare professionals who are at the beginning of a clinical journey. In addition to the interview material I will draw on two theoretical resources. First, hermeneutic and phenomenological work about responsibility, including Paul Ricoeur's philosophy of narrativity and Margaret Urban Walker's work on responsibility practices; second, Robyn Fivush and colleagues' psychological work on narrative biographical memory in families. In the first part of the chapter I search for connections between responsibility, memory and time, in order to explain the complex meanings of 'retrospective responsibility'. I will refer to examples from our interviews from family members who looked back on their experience of responsible decision-making. In the second part I will discuss one example of retrospective responsibility: dealing with failure. The third part refers to three models of justification that have been proposed for deciding on donation by a small child who cannot give proper and valid informed consent.

9.1 Responsibility, Memory and Time

9.1.1 Through Bone and Marrow

It has literally gone 'through the bone and marrow' of a family and its members, when one child becomes critically ill with a disease of the blood building system, and with the infused stem cells ultimately a whole new immune system is implanted. For the transplant, quite a large portion of bone marrow would have been extracted from one of the healthy siblings. This is an invasive procedure carried out in hospital. We have heard that once it was known that a sibling was a match, in most families the transplant was taken from the sibling without much hesitation, even if the 'donor' child was still very young. The parents just gave their consent. The intervention might be burdensome and also somewhat painful in the short term, but for most of the donors it has no serious risks or side effects beyond the risk of a general anaesthetic. And to the parents and physicians, the survival of the sick child was clearly and understandably at the centre of their concern.

Once the transplant was over – let us hope with a good outcome – the family was in a new situation. Parents were glad and grateful that the threat posed by the disease had been averted and that the sick child could recover. However, this was not the only thing that mattered. The survival of the sick child was dependent on the donor child's transplanted blood stem cells, which had previously been a functioning part of her/his body. After the donor's extracted bone marrow grew back, the formerly sick other sibling's life still depends on these donated cells, which are now part of the patient's body.

Afterwards the sibling is healthy and leading a normal life. In some cases, however, after a few years, a second transplant may be needed, or lymphocytes may have to be transplanted as well. Or the procedure does not work at all and the disease returns. Grieving family members who have lost a child at least know that they had tried everything they could.

Within the different possible scenarios following a bone marrow transplant, when looking back at that time, the decision to carry out a transplant remains important for the donor, as well as for the recipient, for the non-donating siblings, and for the parents. But there is more: the encounter with disease, the threat of death, the transplantation of body material from the other sibling, the special bond that developed from it, all the associated clinical procedures, all the logistical difficulties that a family may have encountered when being separated or displaced for a long time – all this will have changed a family's life. These experiences have changed something in the family relationships, in the identities of the family members and in the family narratives. These changes do not just go away afterwards but continue to contribute to the background from which each next step in their lives departs. Changes initiated further changes.

Time and time again, family members need to tell each other what happened in those days, and how they now see and understand what happened to them and to the others in the family. How they understood it at the time was also part of how they understood their responsibility then, and how they understand their responsibility for each other now. Family members also remember it silently, even when nobody talks about it. But they *do* talk about it. Brief references to it appear in everyday conversations. Family memory seems to be a remarkable, delicate and much more complex phenomenon than the passive process, which is suggested in Plato's famous parable in the *Theaetetus*, where memories are compared to impressions, traces in a block of wax (see Ricoeur 2004, 9ff). It is instead an ongoing social *activity* through which family members remain vulnerable in many ways.

9.1.2 Memory and Family Narratives

Using a modern parallel, we sometimes compare remembering with filming or tape recording. However, this comparison is as inadequate as was Plato's wax block. It can only explain the part of memory that works similarly to recording and replaying. Most of our memories just aren't like that. The closest to recording/replaying is perhaps the intrusive flashback memories that can be so distressing for a person after trauma. The primarily distressing excerpts from traumatic events can 'pop' into consciousness and overwhelm a person who suffers from post-traumatic stress disorder (PTSD: Brewin and Holmes 2003). We can also memorise images of excerpts of sequences from a movie that we have seen and imagine these parts of the film accurately, however selectively. Or I can try to remember what exactly I did yesterday before going to bed, and can then imagine myself walking through the rooms of our apartment. But I don't remember everything I have seen, heard, thought or felt yesterday. In strange ways, memory is productive, selective and dependent on forgetting. The phenomenology of our mnemonic faculties is certainly much more complex, as these examples suggest, and as is well documented in the philosophical literature (see Bergson 1950; Ricoeur 2004).

The point I want to make here is that remembering dramatic things in a family context needs to be addressed as a social activity that involves the family as a family. Of course it involves the capacity of each individual to recollect past events, but in the activities of recollection it also involves narrative practices and lived hermeneutics that reach beyond the individual's consciousness.

But from the individual's perspective as well, remembering involves activity in the present. Dwelling on the past is remembering some aspects of the past in present consciousness. We connect it with meanings that relate not solely to the absent past but also to the actual present. It is thus unsurprising that narrative recollections about the really important things in our lives do not always stay exactly the same when they are brought into or seen from a new perspective. They then provide stories from former times presented, in a new situation. The storytellers do not yet know how they will tell and re-construct the story next time because they do not yet know what demands will constitute the speaking situation in the future. What they do know for sure is that how they tell that story next time will in part depend on unforeseeable new events.

It will not change the whole story, however. What are believed to be hard facts, incontestable parts of memories will perhaps not be much altered. For example, to the families we visited it remained clear *when* the operation was performed, *by whom* and *where*. But what this operation *meant* for everybody, and which parts of that story were especially relevant, or what is now no longer important, will not always remain the same.

In the first part of his extensive study *Memory, History, Forgetting,* Paul Ricoeur offers a series of insights that are helpful for our discussion. I want to introduce two particularly relevant key distinctions. One distinction is between habit and memory, the other between evocation and search. The distinction between *habit and memory* had previously been elaborated by Henri Bergson (and Ricoeur draws on his book *Matter and Memory*). Habit and memory "form two poles of a continuous range of mnemonic phenomena. What forms the unity of this spectrum is the common feature of the relation to time. In each of the opposing cases an experience that has been acquired at an earlier point is presupposed; however, in the case of a habit what is acquired is incorporated into the living present without the mark of being a memory. Habits are often unremarked references to a past. In the other case, a noticeable reference is made to the anteriority of the prior acquisition. In both cases, however, it is true that memory 'is of the past'" (Ricoeur 2004, 24 f.).

For example, Marlena, the recipient in the Minz family, noted the changes in her personality brought about by the events of disease and transplant: "I just notice that myself, I – it did of course change me quite a lot, I'm (...) relatively mature really (compared) to other people of my age because I've realised a few more things, like, that you don't actually get to know at this age." (Minz, recipient) She said this seven years after the transplant, when she was nineteen years old. These changes in personal development contain habitual, unmarked and marked references to the transplant events. These two modes of memory might be difficult or even impossible to separate. The habitual part may influence the way she now speaks, reacts and feels in her life. Habitual references to past transplant events were also present when family members told us about the changes in family relationships and the redistribution of roles, of duties and tasks associated with illness and transplantation. Some of them are now just normal parts of everyday life, their being 'of the past' no longer noticed.

The other distinction that I want to mention, which Aristotle originally had introduced into the philosophical literature, is between the simple evocation of something in the past, which is a passion, and the search for the past, which is an active effort to recall. Ricoeur explains that Aristotle used the terms *mneme* and *anamnesis* (Ricoeur 2004, 15ff. and 26ff.) to describe these two ways in which the absent can be present. "And he defined *mneme* as *pathos*, as an affection: it happens that we remember this or that, on such and such an occasion; we then experience a memory. Evocation is an affection, therefore, in contrast to the search" (26). The contrast is "between laborious recollection and spontaneous recollection" (27). We will also find that element of labour in the analysis of family narratives, which can be described as narrative elaborations of the past.

Before we come to that, let us look at a few more examples from the experiences of transplantation. The first way of re-presentation is what happens when somebody says, for instance, that she has a very clear memory of how it smelled in the hospital corridors where she had been as a child. The second way of re-presentation involves, for instance, reminiscence of the events and circumstances that eventually led to the hospitalisation and the transplant. For the purpose of recollection, a former child-patient might need the help of parents and siblings who remember other things about the same past events.

The two kinds of memory can be closely interlinked. When Gino, the recipient in the Grohmann family, said in the family interview: *"There was a time like that, when we were really at loggerheads"* (Grohmann, family interview), this was probably a simple evocation of the quarrels within the family in the period after the transplant. But the words he chose to describe these quarrels to us, about eight years afterwards, in the presence of his other family members, and the emotion that these words conveyed, belonged to a more active search, recollection and re-presentation, involving effort on his side and likewise on the side of his listeners.

From time to time and under particular circumstances, important things that have happened need explicitly to be revisited. Memories are refreshed not just by a mental search but also in dialogue about the transplant events between the family members involved. The interview itself, which was purposefully organised after correspondence via e-mail or telephone calls, was such an occasion for explicit search. The process started with a family interview, where the family members met face to face and talked about the transplant. There, the interviewers were present in a very restricted way, since all the family members were able to ask each other questions and a conversation then developed which was less exclusively controlled by the interviewers. In such occasions (inside or outside the interview situation), memories of the past are revisited and reinterpreted in the context of new life circumstances. I think that this is the way in which absence becomes present, as John Donne has phrased it, not in a raw state but often elaborated, in both ways of re-presentation: as an affliction and as a search. In the recall and the reminiscence, both part of an elaboration practice, fragile presence of the absent is constituted.

Psychological research has spent some effort on understanding autobiographical memory. I can refer to an apt overview by Robyn Fivush, who defines autobiographical memory as "memories related to the self" (Fivush 2008, 50). Studies (and common experience) show that narratives play a crucial role: parental storytelling, family narratives, and the person's own storytelling: "through stories we understand our worlds and ourselves" (ibid.), since stories provide meaning, not just the enumeration of facts or events. "Autobiographical memories differ from simply recalling what happened to include information about why this event is interesting, important, entertaining, etc., essentially why this event is meaningful for the self" (ibid.). The transplant and the events around it were important in many ways, not just as a matter of life or death for one child. In different roles as caregiver or donor, others were involved in ways that crucially affected them. And therefore, these stories must be especially important within the family conversations. As Fivush suggests on the basis of broad research evidence, such stories shape how we see ourselves: "Narratives of past events provide the building blocks of a life story. It is as individuals create narratives of specific experiences that are then linked together through time and evaluative frameworks that individuals construct an overarching life narrative that defines self" (51).

The first autobiographical narratives begin when children start to talk about their past. According to psychological knowledge this is very early on, at about 16 to 18 months of age (52). Fivush et al. observed that children's capacity to tell stories about their past depends on how their parents tell stories. Mothers (or other family members) differ in their 'reminiscing styles', and some are more elaborated than others: "parents differ in their reminiscing style along a dimension of elaboration" (53). Elaboration, however, is already an interesting concept here (apart from a story being more or less 'elaborated') since, as we have seen in Ricoeur's phenomenological sketch of memory, the presence of the past in memory can involve more or less labour. Not all memory happens spontaneously; we are not merely passively affected by memories that come up. Narrative family research adds a social dimension to this labour: stories are told to others in certain ways, and the act of telling them is also relevant to the self of the storyteller. By asking questions, making responses, asking more questions, finding an overarching narrative etc., 'family narratives' are built, which are then typical of and constitutive for the identity of the family.

Robyn Fivush, Catherine Haden and Elaine Reese, who have studied narrative memories in families, refer to the reminiscing styles that are characteristic for family memories (Fivush et al. 2006, 1581). Reminiscing styles may be characteristically different for different family members. They also differ between families, depending on the family narratives and also on cultural contexts. Family narratives can cover shared emotional experiences and "are linked to self-understanding in at least three ways – in terms of self-definition, self-inrelation, and self-regulation" (Bohanek et al. 2008, 155). Narrative meaning-making of past difficult or even traumatic experiences plays an important role in self-development and well-being, as research shows (Sales et al. 2013).

This provides a perspective from which our interviews can be seen: How do family members narrate this past? In what reminiscence style? If we look for style, differences in more than one dimension can be observed: stories are not just more or less elaborated (they were), but also differentiated in the ways they defined and distributed roles and responsibilities. In analysing them, we can ask questions such as: How do they re-present the transplant events and their own or their kin's involvement in them? How do they see them as relevant for themselves and for each other in the present?

9.1.3   Responsibility and Responsiveness

In the interviews, topics related to responsibility were frequently raised when interviewees made judgments on the basis of being agents acting with free will who are
therefore accountable for their actions, or of having special duties. 18 years after the
transplant the mother in the Bahr family explained (Berit, the donor, was 5 at the
time of the transplant):

> As she says, I knew, I had to do it, I (.) she (.) sensed the PRESSURE, she HAD TO - she
> didn't have a choice. We asked her (.) and explained it to her, said to her, ARE you going to
> do this, do you want to do this, but actually everything was really obvious (.), she's got to
> do this, even if we ask her, it was a charade, (.) you see. (.) It was clear to all of us (.) and
> SHE sensed the pressure, yeah (.) great, (.) I am terribly scared, (.) No way could I dare
> say - I can't say no, like. (Bahr, mother)

Berit *was* asked whether she was ready to donate bone marrow to her older brother
Björn and she *said* yes. But the mother knew (i) that Berit had no other choice, and
(ii) that Berit knew what depended on her agreement and therefore could not say no.
She said that the situation was obvious to Berit and to herself: *"but actually everything was really obvious (.), she's got to do this (…)."* Berit explained her feelings
at the time of transplant in the corresponding family interview:

> …for me as a child I was still aware: if I don't do this, I'm to blame (…) if Björn dies. (Bahr,
> family interview)

Both for the mother and for Berit herself, the moral demand in the situation was that
Berit had to do this; and this was, as the mother said, 'obvious' to both of them.

What does 'obvious' mean here? Which epistemology was involved in this form
of seeing? What Berit and her mother describe, I suggest, is a form of *moral perception*, as theorised by Martha Nussbaum. I refer to Lawrence Blum's more systematic
definition of moral perception that he developed with reference to the work of
Nussbaum: "I am including under 'perception anything contributing to, or encom-
passed within, the agent's salience-perception of the situation before he deliberates
about what action to take" (Blum 1994, 37). The mother and the child Berit both
saw that there was one morally salient thing in the situation: Björn needed bone
marrow; and how the situation was told by the family,[2] he needed it from Berit and
Berit could therefore save Björn's life by donating it to him and agreeing to the
operation.

It would, however, be inaccurate to describe this moral perception as a judgment.
They did not judge that they 'had a duty' to donate. It is rather a form of understanding: they understood that Berit needed to donate. This difference between judging
and understanding refers, I think, to two models of moral decision-making, as
Margaret Urban Walker distinguished in her book *Moral Understandings* (2007).
These two models contain different epistemologies, i.e. different senses of obviousness. One – Walker called it the "theoretical-juridical model" – sees morality as an
action-guiding system of rules for an individual. The other – Walker called it the

---

[2] Families rarely mentioned the possibility of looking for an unrelated donor.

"expressive-collaborative conception" – "pictures morality as a socially embodied medium of understanding and adjustment in which people account to each other for the identities, relationships and values that define their responsibilities" (Walker 2007, 67 f.). In the second model, obviousness refers to an understanding of a responsibility, which is very concretely defined by their identity (as mother, as sister), relationships (to Björn) and values (the importance of saving a life).

At the beginning of his article on 'Moral Responsibility' in the *Stanford Encyclopedia of Philosophy*, Matthew Talbert refers exclusively to the first of Walker's two models, without even mentioning that there is a choice to be made here between different moral epistemologies: "Making judgments about whether a person is morally responsible for her behaviour, and holding others and ourselves responsible for actions and the consequences of actions, is a fundamental and familiar part of our moral practices and our interpersonal relationships" (Talbert 2019, 1). Responsibility, in this account, as a familiar part of our moral practices and our interpersonal relationships, is primarily a practice of judging whether somebody is morally responsible for actions and their consequences. In obvious ways, Berit's statement fulfils this criterion. She said that she knew she would be to blame for her brother's death if she did not consent to the donation. She therefore felt she had to do it. She felt 'the pressure', as her mother put it.

But something is missing in Talbert's statement that is at the centre of both Berit's and her mother's accounts, and is better captured in Walker's second 'model' or moral epistemology: the relatedness of the moral demand. *Björn* needed the bone marrow and would die without it, therefore Berit had to give it. When she said she would be to blame, she did not mention potential guilt about breaking rules or rejecting obligations, but stated very concretely that she would cause (and be to blame for) the death of Björn. Her donation was an attempt to rescue Björn, perhaps the only way, as she saw it as a child, to save him. Talbert of course also makes reference to responsibility within interpersonal relationships, but in the sense of making judgments about whether a person is responsible for an action and its consequences. In Talbert's account, responsibility seems to be something that is added to the action with its consequences, when questions about blame or praise arise and need to be answered, whereas in Berit's account, and in her mother's explanation of it, the act itself – the donation and everything that was involved with it – answered her brother's needs, and therefore are part of the responses that constitute responsibility. And of course, not agreeing to the donation, with the consequence of letting Björn die, would then be something for which she was to blame.

If this is to be captured by the term 'responsibility', the idea of responsibility must be made broader and richer than simply moral blame and praise. It must contain the relationships and the relatedness of actions. Berit said it would have been wrong not to donate. But this was not a way of avoiding blame. Rather, it was about avoiding Björn's death as a consequence of her refusal – in which case, she would not have been able to forgive herself.

When talking about morally relevant matters as connected, in manifold ways, to the transplant events, families did not solely 'judge' whether they were morally responsible for what they did and for the consequences of their actions. They were much more concerned with questions of why it was sensible to do what they had done in a situation of conflict. They evaluated their own roles in the interactions and discussed the duties, difficulties and sometimes the limited possibilities of care. If we were to reduce the term responsibility to the blame- or praiseworthiness of actions, and explain moral responsibility only with reference to the problem of free will, we would not be able to code under the category of 'responsibility' many interview passages that in reality clearly dealt with responsible (in the sense of sensible, attentive, responsive) behaviour.

The mother in the Zucker family, for instance, explained that she saw no other choice than to convince her 9-year-old son Zorro to become the bone marrow donor for his younger brother Zedrick: *"It was also clear to me, without us having a massive discussion with Zorro, that Zorro WILL donate whether he wants to or not"* (Zucker, mother, 26). For her, it was mandatory in that situation to override the will of one son, in order to save the life of her other son Zedrick. While Zorro only lost a small amount of freedom for a short time, Zedrick would have lost his life. By doing this, she acted, in her own view – we might perhaps disagree with her on this point – as a responsible mother.

These examples fit well into a care ethics framework (Conradi and Vosman 2016; Kittay 2006). The mothers in both the Bahr and the Zucker families acted as they did because it was how they could best care for their sick children. Berit acted as a consenting donor even as a 5-year-old, because donation demonstrated her care for the life of her brother. Zorro's problem was not that he was unwilling to donate, or did not care about Zedrick's life. His actual problem was that he was not heard by his family. He felt isolated, and expressed his need to be cared for too, not just to be silenced with presents.

Margaret Urban Walker, herself writing from a care ethics perspective, has suggested looking closely at the complex networks of relationships and 'charting' the responsibilities that constitute the moral understandings of those living these relationships. Responsibilities, in her view, are not fixed arrangements (like signed contracts) but rather, as she put it, *practices* – practices of responsibility. They involve assignment, reassignment, confirmation, negotiation and sometimes deflection. By charting responsibilities in relational networks such as families, family members understand the ethically bonding character of their relationships. "I suggest that we have an urgent need for *geographies of responsibility*, mapping the structure of standing assumptions that guides the distribution of responsibilities" (Walker 2007, 105).

In order to make explicit the content of the moral relation that Walker terms responsibility, or the moral practice that is involved in practices of responsibility, we need an account of responsibility that is relational and in tune with the narratives that family members provide. This does not need to be invented from scratch. There is another tradition of philosophical thought about responsibility that is not included in Talbert's review (nor in Williams, 2020), but is most forcefully represented in the twentieth century in the highly influential work of Emmanuel Levinas. Paul Ricoeur, in the context of his ethical theorising of narrativity and narrative identity, explicitly refers to Levinas' work *Otherwise than Being* when he proposes an understanding of responsibility as a relational capacity that reaches beyond causal responsibility and blameworthiness.

In Ricoeur's systematic interpretation, responsibility has two essential meanings: (i) The other to whom I am responsible *counts on me*: being responsible means behaving in such a way that the other can count on me; (ii) I am *accountable* to the other to whom I am responsible: I have to account to the other for my actions and omissions (Ricoeur 1992, 165). "Because someone is counting on me, I am *accountable for* my actions before another." The term 'responsibility', Ricoeur argues, unites both these meanings: 'counting on' and 'being accountable for'. It unites them by adding to them an idea of a *response* to the question 'Where are you?' asked by another who needs me. "This response is the following: 'Here I am!' A response that is a statement of self-constancy." (ibid.) Identity, in a Ricoeurian view, has two poles: one is the character by which a person can be identified and re-identified; the other is self-constancy, which is a prerequisite for the possibility that others can count on somebody. It must still be substantially the same person. Responsibility appeals to this self-constancy as it appeals to the needs of the other.

Ricoeur's account of responsibility does not exclude those aspects of responsibility that have been reviewed by Talbert and Williams. But it reverses the priority of the issues. Whereas in the latter account the issue of free will is seen as primary, followed by the issues of accountability and blameworthiness which then can be contextualised in human relationships, Ricoeur's ordering of the issues is the reverse: the asymmetrical relationship to the other who is asking me, 'Where are you?' is primary. The other is counting on me. I understand that I am counted on by the other. This leads to my being accountable for my response. And I can only be accountable if I see myself as a person with moral agency.

I want briefly to mention the closeness of this to the current discussion of 'relational autonomy' and how to reconstruct the concept of moral autonomy in the context of care ethics. This discussion starts from the hypothesis that moral autonomy and the relationality of the self cannot be contradictory. Andrea C. Westlund, while criticising liberal individualism, places answerability at the core of her relational account of autonomy. What she calls 'dialogical answerability' requires "that the autonomous agent actually have a certain kind of self-relation – namely, one in which she holds herself answerable, for her action-guiding commitments, to external critical perspectives" (Westlund 2008, 35). These external critical perspectives must include the perspectives of the other to whom the agent is responsible.

9.1.4 Looking Back – Responsibly

In the family interview from which I have already quoted, recipient Gino said: *"There was a time like that, when we were really at loggerheads"* – and he went on: *"and now it's actually, it's evened out again, probably because we were sitting on top of each other at that time"* (Grohmann, family interview). In this statement, as well as accepting his own share of the responsibility for those earlier quarrels, he also explained it by citing a difficulty that was beyond their control: they were sitting on top of each other at that time. Now, with more space available, things have evened out. The family shared a common fate in difficult times, when they had to act together and do the right thing, and quarrels were frequent. In hindsight, however, he wanted to stress that nobody is now to blame for the difficulties that emerged with the transplant.

Both Zorro's mother (see above) and Gino (in the last quote) are concerned about how to think about it now, how they should explain what happened in retrospect, when they already know the outcome. The act of telling their stories therefore comprises *two temporal layers*. Both are related to responsibility: one is the past that is told (the transplant events), and the other is the present in which the telling occurs (the act of telling and the teller's narrative identity). In both layers, responsibility contains appeals from others to which it responds. In Zorro's case, the mother in the past acted out of a moral conflict, which only arose because of her commitment to both her sons. They both appealed to her morally. The action she recounts in the interview (overriding Zorro's will in order to make the donation possible) was her response to the demands of the situation in which one of her children was under threat and the other child's body contained the means to avert the threat. In the present temporal layer, in the act of storytelling, she explained to the interviewer how she still believes that overriding Zorro's will was inevitable. She would perhaps have explained this to Zorro in similar terms. We don't know whether he would have been satisfied, or whether he would just feel disrespected again. This act of telling is perhaps an unsuccessful[3] response to Zorro's present need to restore meaning in his life, as a son and brother who felt he had been used.

What should be discussed in the temporally backward dimension of 'retrospective' responsibility therefore is not only who is responsible for what, who should be blamed or praised and for which reasons. It is also what these past choices mean in the present, or how actors relate to them in their actual present. In most cases, past actions and decisions cannot be undone. They did change things in the world; the dice have been cast. Parents and donor child did agree; bone marrow has been extracted, cells have been transplanted, and so on. The patient child did survive. But how and why the decisions were taken, what were the main motives and reasons to proceed as they did, are matters of explanation *in the present*. If feelings have been hurt, self-respect or memory has been wounded, alleviation might now be possible. Relationships can heal with time and effort. How the events are told or retold in different ways, opening more room for dissident views, can either contribute to this healing or equally, refresh old wounds. Corrective measures in the present are new interpretative and communicative actions, through which somebody may try to amend and repair something without being able to undo what has already been done.

Only in the aftermath can the full weight and significance of a decision or a course of action unfold. When we think about the moral implications of our past

---

[3] In the corresponding family interview, the interviewers witnessed a difficult situation in which Zorro clearly felt excluded and withdrew from the conversation. We discussed this situation from an research ethics perspective in Herzog et al. 2019.

practices, their temporal relations need to be considered, including how past, present and future are structured or modified in the context of this activity. Looking backwards in time is in many ways connected to and inseparable from our perspectives on the future.

Of these future perspectives of retrospective responsibility I want to mention two. First, at the time of the events, there was a perspective on a future that may or may not have materialised how it was anticipated: the anticipated future in the past. Present understandings of the past therefore also include how futures have been imagined or hoped for in the past. Second, present actors relate to a not-yet past when they think about how their actions will be seen and remembered in the future. They ask how what they do next will be judged from future points of view. These might be their own   points of view (how they will see it themselves), or the points of view of others considering their actions. For parents, the others will still be their children when they are older. Referring to narrative identity and to a hermeneutic framework of ethics, as it is explored by Paul Ricoeur in *Oneself as Another,* I want to stress that retrospective responsibility is *intrinsically connected* to prospective responsibility. We can read the retrospective interviews with family members post-transplant with a view to how they see this connection between the retrospective and the prospective, and how they explain the ethical relevance of both.

A further aspect of retrospective responsibility is connected to the concept of self-constancy, as described in Ricoeur's account of responsibility. Self-constancy is of course a temporal concept. We are the same person now and therefore accountable for what we have done in the past. However, in a narrative ethics it is important to see self-constancy as a broader concept than sameness over time. I can try to explain this point using Mary Midgley's account of human freedom:

Humans are responsible actors in the sense that they are capable of caring about what they are doing. This ability starts early in childhood. But what is involved in it? To care about what one is doing has to do with freedom. Midgley suggests a simple (but essentially non-reductionist) perspective to explain what is meant by this term of freedom. Humans evaluate their decisions and their activities in the context of how they understand themselves as a whole person. In a rather agent-centred perspective, Midgley explains the essence of human freedom as the ability "in some degree, to act as a whole in dealing with its conflicting desires." This wholeness can never be fully achieved, "yet the integrative struggle to heal conflicts and to reach towards this wholeness is surely the core of what we mean by human freedom" (Midgley 1994, 168). This freedom at the heart of responsibility is clearly not captured by reductionistic negative descriptions as being 'free from' (coercion or inducement), or as some sort of indefiniteness or vagueness in the neurological make-up of our brains. "This strangely negative idea misses the point altogether" (164). And this idea of wholeness can evidently not be understood as an atemporal or purely presentistic idea. Acting as a whole essentially includes our identity in relationships, which is contained in life stories. It includes how the family members lived on with their narratives about illness and transplant.

9.2 Dealing with Failure

With this in mind we now look more closely at one of the families who volunteered to share their stories with us. The Jaschkes were special in many respects. They lived through three different kinds of transplant and had to cope with the failure of all attempts to save the life of the young patient Jennifer. After she first became seriously ill with acute myeloid leukaemia (AML) and was treated with chemotherapy for quite a time, at the age of 12 she received bone marrow from her older sister Janine who was then 15. But the transplant had no lasting effect, the treatment failed and the disease returned. Two years later, Jennifer received a second transplant, this time with bone marrow from her mother Jutta. After this attempt also failed, a third transplant was carried out with bone marrow from an unknown and unrelated donor. But Jennifer could not be saved by this third attempt either. After experiencing several complications she died of her disease at the age of 17.

The Jaschke family's story is complex, highly dramatic and of course very emotional. The first interview was (as always in our study) the family interview. The father had previously refused to take part in interviews, and so he was not present. It was said that he generally refuses to speak about his daughter's illness and death. The interviewer therefore met the donor sister Janine and her mother. Both gave us extended and rich individual interviews after the family conversation was over.

The family interview took place in Janine's apartment, since she was the one who had contacted us and organised the meeting. Janine and her mother Jutta sat at the table in the living room with the interviewer, over coffee and cake. Also present was Janine's fiancé, who also sat at the table for about half the interview, but remained quiet.

The opening part of the conversation mainly discussed the question, 'Who can talk about what happened?' First of all Jutta explained that her husband did not want to talk about what had happened to Jennifer. She said that she herself had hesitated, but was encouraged by her daughter Janine to participate in the study and to share their stories. After a warning that she might walk out of the interview if she could not take it any more, she and Janine started to talk. Janine placed a photo of Jennifer on the table, taken during her last holiday in Turkey.

Janine, who was 28 at the time of the interviews, offered a series of comparisons between herself and Jennifer. In Janine's view, Jennifer, who was four years younger, had a more beautiful name, was cleverer than Janine (a point her mother confirmed), and had learned how to do sums earlier. Jutta confirmed that Janine had always glorified her younger sister. But, as they went on to say, Janine had other qualities: for example, she was better at literature and more able to analyse poems. Then the interviewer asked why Janine wanted to talk about Jennifer, the illness and the transplants. Janine vigorously made the point that she thought it absolutely necessary to talk about this, and that, in contrast to her parents, she wanted to and dared to talk about it. Janine said that she was the only family member in psychotherapy, and stressed this point to her mother. This therapy, however, was necessary because Janine had serious psychological troubles that started after the second transplant, when she had stopped eating, isolated herself from her friends, and suffered from anxiety. Her anxiety was probably triggered by the enormous suffering her younger sister had to live through.

After a long phase in the family interview, dominated by the recollection of Jennifer's pain and suffering, the interviewer tried to clarify the events, asking about the diagnosis and how long the chemotherapy took up to the first transplant. To support their memory, and in a surprise for the interviewers, Janine exposed the skin of her lower back, where she carried a tattoo. She had had Jennifer's name, birth date, the dates of all the transplants, and also the date of Jennifer's death tattooed – in an artistic design. Janine's explanation for the tattoo was that she had always wanted to do tattooing herself but could no longer do it. But she had drafted the tattoo's design herself.

The tattooed dates on Janine's body supported the memory of this difficult time, with all the fighting and setbacks. It is perhaps no coincidence that the tattoo was placed on her lower back, near the spot where the bone marrow was extracted from Jennifer's hip bone. This place symbolises an intercorporeal connection between the two sisters that she emphasised several times, both in her own individual interview and in the joint interview with their mother Jutta. When her narrative reached the point of her HLA test, she said:

> Then I also asked myself, because the first transplant, well, it was my bone marrow, and we were so similar, like 99.99999 point 9 percent or whatever, and it was kind of, at first I thought: 'HEY, (.) REALLY COOL'. That was kind of like, well you felt (.) like one of those heroes. (.) Like (..), it's a nice feeling, when you're, ehm, the one who can, ehm, turn the whole thing round (.) an- and I sort of gave HER LIFE, if you can (.) put it like that, (.) then I thought: 'HEY [delighted], it's me (.) the saviour.' (.) Well, it didn't work out all that well. (Jaschke, donor)

The nearly ideal match between the two sisters was something she felt very happy about. The power to turn things around and to save her sister gave her very positive feelings, even if it did not work out in the end. She said she had hoped that the test would turn out this way and that she could be the one donating the bone marrow to her sister. She continued:

> (…) when it really was like that, it was really, ehm, like – I can't describe it now, the feeling, it was really like (.) BADASS. I'm really the one and because we were so SIMILAR as – as well, I can only EMPHASISE this, that we were really (.), I don't know whether the DNA is then really so similar or what exactly the similarities are, (.) that it – it was just relatively rare too, that siblings are quite so similar (.) and I did find that kind of cool. I found it REALLY cool, because in terms of character we were fundamentally different (.), but inside (.) we were kind of THE SAME (..). I thought that was so fascinating, how you can be so different on the outside, but so much the same inside, that's why I could never explain why I have blonde hair and she had brown, like, [laughs] I never understood how that could be, but it was probably that zero point something 1% difference that accounted for us perhaps (.) something like that. I mean, it really was like that (.), yeah, (.) pretty insane, (.) that it was really LIKE THAT and then of course the chance that we were similar, (..) the chance was higher that the body would say, like: 'HEY, I KNOW THIS (.), I'VE SEEN THIS BEFORE.' (Jaschke, donor)

The interviewers then asked how she felt about the failure of the transplant. She explained the failure with their 'inner' similarity, as she put it. Her immune cells were too similar to Jennifer's, and therefore were no better able to fight the cancer cells than Jennifer's own immune cells.

> The only stupid thing was that we were so similar, that MY cells didn't twig either that cancer cells would come back, they said it (.) like that and didn't recognise it bec- because were so similar. (.) Of course that was DUMB as well, (.) but it had a good and a [laughs] bad side somehow and of course that was another strange feeling, that (.) I thought at first, like: now everyone's blaming me a bit (..), it's my fault that my cells haven't managed it, but I couldn't influence that AT ALL, //but// (Jaschke, donor)

Thoughts about guilt were there. She herself thought about it, at least 'from the first moment', but she had not told anyone in the family, in order not to burden them even more. After all, she had done everything she could, and she could not change her body, nor their 'inner' similarity. This gave her relief:

> (...) so I thought like: okay, (.) thanks a lot, my body is [laughs] just the same, it's also the weaker one a bit, but (.) I couldn't- what was I supposed to do, I couldn't go in there and fight with her (.), I couldn't do anything at all, apart from donating it to her (.). That was the only possibility there was and if it doesn't work (..), it's - (.) well, then it doesn't work. (Jaschke, donor)

When conversation touched on the failure of the first transplant and Janine's possible bad feelings about it, the interviewer asked whether they had ever talked about it. Jutta replied:

> She did say that sometimes, yes, that she thought it wasn't great ehm, or she was very disappointed that it hadn't worked, (.) but there – that doesn't make sense (.) and I always said, perhaps you were just too similar. (Jaschke, mother)

Jutta said that she has 'always said' it was because of their close similarity. From the perspective of narrative, retrospective responsibility, it is significant that Jutta characterised the explanation as something she had always told in this way. It was her narrative for this problem which she used in talking to the sisters, and especially Janine. We heard in her own words how Janine echoed this narrative. She could believe it, because it resonated with her own explanation of the closeness of the HLA match ('99.99999 point 9 percent') with their 'inner' similarity despite external differences. This narrative of resemblance was something she could live with. It accommodated the failure as not being Janine's fault but rather a consequence of their being too closely alike 'inwardly'. And she could not sneak into Jennifer's body and fight the cancer cells herself – to use Janine's graphic wording. She had done what she could.

In contrast to another unlucky donor in our sample – Zorro in the Zucker family – she was able to believe this narrative explanation and did not say that she felt guilty. Zorro could not believe it, despite having his parents frequently tell him that it was not his fault. He was only 10 and a half years old when talking about the unsuccessful first transplant in his individual interview he said:

> I: So how was it actually for you, when you found out that (..) Zedrick became ill again even after the first donation?
> D: Erm I blamed myself, (4) because my bone marrow, or I thought, my bone marrow must be bad. (6)

I: Did your parents say anything about this?
D: No. (Zucker, donor)

In the family interview, however, Zorro's parents had told us that they found this self-blaming 'nonsense' and that they *had* explained it to him: *"M: Which is OF COURSE nonsense, which I also tried to explain to Zorro, that it's nonsense"* (Zucker, family interview). In the Kunow family too, the donor Kira felt guilty because the transplant was unable to save her sibling's life: *"because it was my bone marrow, which worked against his cells"* (Kunow; donor). Her narrative differs from Janine's in the essential point that she thought that her cells "worked against his cells", whereas Janine thought her cells were too similar to Jennifer's own immune cells to be effective against the cancer cells.

In this example of a typical problem-centred narrative we can identify the different temporal layers that we have mentioned above: (i) the past events of the transplant going awry; (ii) the present time where the story about that past is told, (iii) the future in the past, when Janine's mother 'always', i.e. consistently and from a perspective of Janine's feelings in the future, said that her cells could not heal Jennifer because of their inner similarity and closeness. It was a responsible story since it resonated with Janine's own feelings of closeness to Jennifer, and with her ideals of having done everything that she could for her. It created a presence of that deeply troubling past Janine could again live in.

9.3 Justification in Retrospect

The discovery of serious illness in one of their children and the subsequent fight for survival led all the families we talked to into an extreme situation, where danger was high and threats came from unlikely quarters. For the parents, the illness and the necessary therapeutic measures, including the transplant, first came as a shock and then developed in a very unpredictable way. The whole family was affected, directly or indirectly, and everybody struggled to stay upright in that storm. Keeping the family together during the crisis was a major challenge. The fight also welded members in some families together, while roles within the family had to be at least partly rewritten. Duties and tasks were redistributed between parents and among or between the children. New tasks emerged that could not be fully foreseen: for instance, doing justice to all family members to meet the needs not only of the sick child but also those of the donor child and other siblings as well. It was mainly the mothers who said they suffered from the sheer impossibility of this task, which resulted in feeling guilty if they neglected one child over a period of time. The non-donating siblings sometimes struggled with the feeling of being superfluous, as one non-donor sibling in the Minz family said: *"I had nothing to do, I wasn't a donor, I wasn't a donor match, so I was in a way, spare"* (Minz family; non-donating sibling). The storm also shook the non-donating siblings.

The disease itself, and sometimes also the too-reductionist approach of healthcare professionals who focused only on the disease and the sick child, caused a variety of intra-family injuries. The battle created a tight network of solidarity within the family who tried to keep together in order to get through the storm intact. This is the overall picture we formed from our interpretation of the interviews.

Looking back at the decision from a point when the events were past, we can scrutinise the arguments used by physicians and parents at the time to justify their decision to let one child become a stem cell donor for a sibling. My question here is less about how convincing these arguments were at the moment of decision-making, but rather how they match the long-term experiences with the decision and its consequences.

Based on the ethical literature on hematopoietic stem cell donation between siblings and our own findings, we can distinguish three possible models of justification (Schües and Rehmann-Sutter 2014): (a) the interests of the child, (b) the will of the child, if he/she had been able to decide at the time, and (c) the will of the child in retrospect (see also Chap. 3 in this book). I will discuss them one by one.

9.3.1   The Interests of the Child and the 'Benefit' of Donation

None of the families we spoke to, not even those where the transplants had failed, questioned the decision for a sibling child to donate. But self-interest justifications for making this decision feel odd afterwards. Yes, some of the donors said that they benefited by being able to be a 'saviour', to be the one who could turn the disease around (as Janine said, for example). But they did not use it as a justification of their decision to donate. To have done it for self-interest, for their own psycho-social benefit, feels wrong.[4]

In the families' stories, it became obvious that, in retrospect, most donors rated the donation positively also with regard to themselves: they were proud to have helped their sibling to survive. This was the case even in those two families in our sample where the sick child had severe side effects or died. They had done everything they could, and this gave them a feeling of pride and also the more short-term benefit of getting their parents' attention again.

However, from an ethical perspective I would hesitate to claim that the psycho-social benefit (not losing the brother or sister, to be able to help in healing, pride, attention) even retrospectively *justified* the extraction of bone marrow from a child. The justificatory argument of benefit does not work because it would also be a benefit *not* to be taken as a donor (benefit in other respects), although this completely disappears from the comparison as soon as a tissue compatibility test is done, showing that one child could be a donor. The psycho-social benefit can certainly help to cope with the burden that must be accepted, and is therefore an important aspect. But as a justificatory argument, I believe it cannot work. If we imagine the child has

---

[4] Psycho-social benefit is an argument that frequently appears in the medical ethics literature about paediatric stem cell transplant from siblings. See for instance AAP 2010; Pentz 2004.

a say in this decision we would find it awkward if the child decides to donate *because* she wants to feel pride and get attention. The reason for the donation is other-related: the attempt to help the sick sibling. It is solidarity or responsibility of the donor for the sibling, and not a trade-off between individual pain and loss of body material versus psycho-social benefit.

For this reason I argue that psycho-social benefit should not be part of the inventory of justificatory arguments for a proxy (i.e. parents) deciding whether to allow a minor to donate. Rather, a proxy needs to determine, to the best of their knowledge and in good conscience, what the potential donor would decide if she or he could. According to our data, it seems reasonable to assume that a child *would* consent to donate, as soon as histocompatibility is established, because it is lifesaving for the sick sibling – but not because it provides psycho-social benefits. It is the will of the child (if able to decide) that is the salient reason, rather than the interests of the child in being a donor and saviour.

9.3.2 The Child's Will and Duties

The argument of the child's will if able to decide, however, does not work to justify the exclusion of a search for unrelated donors. The families' stories reveal that, at least in Germany, there was considerable encouragement by the medical professionals to first test within the family and then look for an unrelated donor as a backup. Donation within the family was presented to them as advantageous and, if possible, as good luck. We can find many indications of this in the transcripts, as well as parents and donors saying they had preferred to do it within their family. But this retrospectively stated preference in those families who actually carried out a transplant from a sibling donor cannot support the claim that families would always prefer to use a sibling or that it is ethically preferable to use the sibling.

Families may spontaneously think first of a possible sibling donation, because they want to mobilise all their resources to help the sick child, and this includes the ordeal of bone marrow extraction. They may also first perceive an unrelated donor as being more risky. So their preference for the donation from a sibling can be triggered both by the doctors and by their own motivation to be practical and do everything necessary, even if it hurts, to save the life of the child patient.

Similarly problematic is using the idea of the donor child's duty to justify the donation.[5] The Jaschke family is very interesting in this respect. As we have seen, there were three transplants, first from the older sister, then from the mother, and finally from an unrelated donor, before the child patient eventually died. The first two donations did not really involve a 'decision', as they told us. As most of the other families also said, consent to the donation was a matter of course; experiencing the situation made it clear. The alternative of refusing a donation was not

---

[5] We have made this argument theoretically in Schües and Rehmann-Sutter 2017.

considered a realistic alternative. We can call that a situational duty, in the sense that the families saw only strong and good reasons to do it, either as a sibling, or, in the Jaschkes' case, as a mother.

Nevertheless, we should distinguish sharply between a duty that is used to *justify* the extraction of bone marrow from a healthy child's body and this situational duty, which is part of moral perception and guides the donors' own narratives. It explains why it was essentially a no-choice situation for them. But then the Jaschkes had unrelated donation as well, before the child had a second relapse – and then died. The mother had considered contacting the donor, and wanted to get to know her. But after the treatment failed, she decided not to contact her, because the knowledge of failure would only burden the donor.

This is an important point: there is an additional and morally relevant advantage of unrelated donation. In the case of failure or relapse, the donor is protected from having to deal with it. The sibling in this family had serious after-effects and needed psychotherapy for panic attacks, anxiety and depression. Nevertheless, she did not regret having donated and she felt no lasting guilt, as we have seen.

9.3.3 The Anticipated Will of the Child and the Child's Retrospective Consent

In difficult situations, where we are unsure about which of several possible chains of activity is right, we often ask ourselves, 'Can I live with it?' or 'Can we live with it?' We then imagine ourselves being past the decision and looking back on it. Christina Schües and I had discussed this idea as one element of the ethics of decision-making before actually doing the empirical study (Schües and Rehmann-Sutter 2014). We called it in a formal way 'anticipated retrospective consent'. It would, as we thought, capture the temporality of bone marrow transplantation within families better than the standard framework of 'free and informed consent' in decision-making, because the free and informed consent's temporal focus is primarily on the present, without considering the present as seen from the future as past. We hypothesised that for parents who act as responsible proxy decision-makers about stem cell transplantations between siblings, who at the time of the transplant are children, their thoughts about their future matters most: How will our children, when they are older, see what we as parents decide to do now? How will they judge us? How will they see their own involvement? If there is burden and harm involved: Will they be able to absolve us?

We felt that when taking a proxy decision as parents in the present, the temporality of the child's future must be taken into consideration. The parents should try to take this into consideration, while letting the donor child participate as far as possible, to make it more likely that the child will in future be able to agree with what happened. This is the idea of anticipated retrospective consent – anticipated consent in the temporal mode of *futurum passatum*. Parents *hope* that their children will, when they are old enough, understand the situation and approve of what had been done to them. This model of the decision based on anticipated future approval as a criterion has the advantage, we claimed, of appreciating temporality and allowing for the child's participation in the long term (not just at the moment of decision-making). The alternatives against which we discussed the retrospective consent model were the child's best interests and the hypothetical will of the child.

When we now critically revisit this idea in the light of the interviews and the discussions we have had since, the idea of 'anticipated retrospective consent' remains to be defensible in some respects, but it covers not the whole story. In at least two aspects the moral implications of the decision are more complicated than we had assumed.

(i) The model of retrospective consent, used as a model of the decision-making situation pre-transplant, was not sufficiently aware of the unpredictability of events and the impossibility of the parents anticipating how things would be for the child afterwards, in the long term. Hence, it cannot really be a clear criterion for their decision. Used as a criterion, it would almost certainly exclude all plans that involve a procedure that would never be acceptable to a child, and could therefore not be approved in retrospect, for instance, foreseeable exploitative schemes of repeated extraction of bone marrow or other organs. But the bone marrow transplant about which the parents were actually deciding was not of this kind. The consequences were more fine-grained. They could not reasonably assume knowledge of how it would appear to the child afterwards, and base their decision upon such an assumption.

(ii) Therefore the retrospective consent model needs an addition. Apart from taking the right decision at one point in time, it is rather a *continuous task* in the families to act in such a way that it will indeed be acceptable to the child when she/he is old enough to understand. This is a continuous task that provides an orientation for how the parents care for all their children, not just the donor child.

The decision to allow stem cells to be taken out of the body of a little brother or sister is based on a desperate attempt to save the life of the sick child by doing all that is reasonable. This is how we can understand the lesson that the families' stories contain. They very clearly say that there was no real choice to be made. By their own description it was a no-choice situation, not because physicians put them under pressure or did not mention alternatives, but because the situation demanded it. And it demanded it very powerfully. The reason for this demand is an ethical one: the attempt to get through the storm with everybody alive.

When we look at what these donors cared about most – their 'carings', to use Claudia Wiesemann's beautiful term[6] – it was not only the stem cell transfer itself, the medical procedure, but also how they themselves were treated in the process, whether their own will was respected, whether they had been asked beforehand, whether they were paid attention to during the procedure and afterwards, in that complicated and evolving family situation.

---

[6] See her chapter in this book.

An 'ethics of care' view of this kind of caring for the donor child's carings emphasises that it is key to care for the child in a way that the child's concerns, thoughts, feelings, self-respect, subjectivity, experience and so forth *matter*. These are not only the carings the child *will have* later in life, but the carings of the child in the present. It would be wrong to treat the child in such a way that its future carings always automatically overrode the present ones. The child's life happens in the present, with a view of the future, but with a stronger concern for present needs.

We must keep in mind, then, that if the medical team constructs the situation in such a way that after testing the siblings for HLA compatibility, the family can donate, the parents will have no choice other than to agree. This means allowing the life-saving motive to override all other concerns, and certainly also to override some of the donor child's short-term carings or fears. This is not a morally trivial matter. It should be seen as a strong reason for prioritising an unrelated donor and for expanding donor registers everywhere, to make it more likely that a suitable unrelated donor can be found.

Literature

American Academy of Pediatrics (AAP), Committee on Bioethics. 2010. Policy statement. Children as hematopoietic stem cell donors. *Pediatrics* 125: 392–404.

Bergson, Henri. 1950. *Matter and memory*, transl. Allen and Unwin: Nancy M. Paul and W. Scott Palmer. London.

Blum, Lawrence A. 1994. *Moral perception and particularity*. Cambridge: Cambridge Univ. Pr.

Bohanek, Jennifer G., Kelly A. Marin, and Robyn Fivush. 2008. Family narrative, self and gender in early adolescence. *Journal of Early Adolescence* 28 (1): 153–176.

Brewin, Chris R., and Emily A. Holmes. 2003. Psychological theories of posttraumatic stress disorder. *Clinical Psychology Review* 23 (3): 339e376.

Conradi, Elisabeth, and Frans Vosman (eds.). 2016. *Praxis der Achtsamkeit. Schlüsselbegriffe der Care-Ethik*. Frankfurt/M.: Campus.

Fivush, Robyn. 2008. Remembering and reminiscing. How individual lives are constructed in family narratives. *Memory Studies* 1 (1): 49–58.

Fivush, Robyn, Catherine A. Haden, and Elaine Reese. 2006. Elaborating on elaborations: Role of maternal reminiscing style in cognitive and socioemotional development. *Child Development* 77 (6): 1568–1588.

Herzog, Madeleine, Martina Jürgensen, Christoph Rehmann-Sutter, and Christina Schües. 2019. Interviewers as intruders? Ethical explorations of joint family interviews. *Journal of Empirical Research on Human Research Ethics* 14 (5): 458–461.

Kittay, Eva Feder. 2006. The concept of care ethics in biomedicine. In *Bioethics in cultural contexts*, ed. Christoph Rehmann-Sutter, Marcus Düwell, and Dietmar Mieth, 319–339. Dordrecht: Springer.

Midgley, Mary. 1994. *The ethical primate. Humans, freedom and morality*. London: Routledge.

Pentz, Rebecca D., Ka Wah Chan, Joyce L. Neumann, Richard E. Champlin, and Martin Korbling. 2004. Designing an ethical policy for bone marrow donation by minors and others lacking capacity. *Cambridge Quarterly of Healthcare Ethics* 13: 149–155.

Ricoeur, Paul. 1992. *Oneself as another*, transl. Kathleen Blamey. Chicago: University of Chicago Press.

———. 2004. *Memory, History, Forgetting*, transl. Kathleen Blamey and David Pellauer. Chicago: University of Chicago Press.

Sales, Jessica M., Natalie A. Merrill, and Robyn Fivush. 2013. Does making meaning make it better? Narrative meaning-making and Well-being in at-risk African-American adolescent females. *Memory* 21 (1): 97–110. https://doi.org/10.1080/09658211.2012.706614.

Schües, Christina, and Christoph Rehmann-Sutter. 2014. Retrospektive Zustimmung der Kinder? Ethische Aspekte der geschwisterlichen Stammzelltransplantation. *Frühe Kindheit. Die ersten sechs Jahre* 2: 22–27.

———. 2017. Has a child a duty to donate hematopoietic stem cells to a sibling? In *New issues in ethics and oncology*, ed. Monika Bobbert, Beate Herrmann, and Wolfgang U. Eckart, 81–100. Freiburg: Alber.

Talbert, Matthew. 2019. Moral Responsibility. In *The Stanford Encyclopedia of Philosophy* (Winter 2019 Edition), ed. Edward N. Zalta, https://plato.stanford.edu/archives/win2019/entries/moral-responsibility/, Accessed 19 Oct 2020.

Walker, Margaret Urban. 2007. *Moral understandings. A feminist study in ethics*. 2nd ed. Oxford: Oxford Univ. Pr.

Westlund, Andrea C. 2008. Rethinking relational autonomy. *Hypatia* 24 (4): 26–49.

Williams, Garrath. 2020. Responsibility. In *The Internet Encyclopedia of Philosophy*, ISSN 2161–0002, https://www.iep.utm.edu/, 11.03.2020.

Open Access This chapter is licensed under the terms of the Creative Commons Attribution 4.0 International License (http://creativecommons.org/licenses/by/4.0/), which permits use, sharing, adaptation, distribution and reproduction in any medium or format, as long as you give appropriate credit to the original author(s) and the source, provide a link to the Creative Commons license and indicate if changes were made.

The images or other third party material in this chapter are included in the chapter's Creative Commons license, unless indicated otherwise in a credit line to the material. If material is not included in the chapter's Creative Commons license and your intended use is not permitted by statutory regulation or exceeds the permitted use, you will need to obtain permission directly from the copyright holder.

Part IV
Processes of Decision Making

Chapter 10
Processes of Decision Making: Report from the Qualitative Interview Study

Martina Jürgensen and Madeleine Herzog

Abstract This chapter describes in some detail how complex family decision-making processes were made and how they have been and will be judged by families (members), both at the time of the illness and in retrospect. With one exception, all families said that the decision to conduct a BMT was not experienced as an option but as another step in the therapeutic process, to which there was no alternative. They felt they had no other choice. The decision to have family members typed and, if they match, use them as donors, was not interpreted as a "decision" either, but was considered a matter of course for the family members. Families preferred a sibling donor over an unrelated one. Parents felt that they needed to talk to the (potential) donor about the donation; the child was usually also "officially" asked whether she or he agreed to the donation. However, everyone knew that a negative answer to this question was not possible. In retrospect, only one family (out of 17) doubted that they had taken the right decision.

Keywords Descision making · Sibling donation

Medical decision making is often complicated. Ideally, full and comprehensive information and exploratory discussions enable the patient to make an informed and balanced decision regarding her or his health care. This ideal of informed consent often seemed unattainable in the families we studied, due not least to the immense time-pressure because treatment of the sick child had to start immediately.

In paediatrics, making decisions about medical interventions is far more complicated than in adult medicine – as there are major ethical, legal and personal challenges. In general, the role of parents is to make decisions for their minor children that are in the child's best interest (present and future). Their responsibility towards the ill child generated the strong wish for a BMT and a sibling donation in many families.

M. Jürgensen (✉) · M. Herzog
Institute for History of Medicine and Science Studies, University of Lübeck,
Lübeck, Schleswig-Holstein, Germany
e-mail: martina.juergensen@uni-luebeck.de

© The Author(s) 2022
C. Schües et al. (eds.), *Stem Cell Transplantations Between Siblings as Social Phenomena*, Philosophy and Medicine 144,
https://doi.org/10.1007/978-3-031-04166-2_10

But parents are equally responsible for their other children, the donor and non-donor siblings. For the potential donor, donation involves an invasive intervention with no medical indication or justification for the donors themselves. That is one reason for having enduring ethical and juridical discussions about sibling donations by minors.

The purpose of this section is to examine in more detail how family decisions were made, and how they have been and are judged by family members, both at the time of the illness and in retrospect.

10.1 Decision Making About Treatment

In view of the severe life-threatening illness of the child, none of the parents who took part in our study hesitated to begin medical treatment immediately. Their goal was the survival of the sick child, and to reach this goal, some parents explicitly advocated choosing the strongest possible therapeutic option. Overall, however, parents did not have the impression that deciding about therapeutic issues was in any way an option. This impression was also due to the fact that the treatment of cancer (the diagnosis in many families in our study) followed strictly standardized protocols. Accordingly, there *were* in reality few decision-making options for parents. Many of them therefore found it superfluous and almost absurd to be asked for their consent over the many subsequent steps of the treatment. In their view, they had no alternative in their situation and they would have signed anything, even if they did not fully understand the risks and side-effects of the therapy.

> Mother: She HAS to have it, she has to have thrombocytes too and by the time of the BMT she was having it every day. Then you don't think erm at ALL, you HAVE to sign it every time, yes, I say (.) WHAT FOR? I say, why don't we do this on the first day and on the last day, because she has to have it anyway, what CHOICE do I have. I don't have any other choice. Then you also think, you're not allowed to think about it at all any more. Even erm (.) side effects of some medications, I didn't read it. I say, what kind of CHOICE do I have? She HAS to have it, WHATEVER they give her, I have no other choice, or I let her die, I mean, I would like her to live, so I have to accept all that they give me, I don't have any other choice and that's why you don't think about it any more. (Jaschke)

10.1.1 Decisions Under Time Pressure

A particular difficulty arises from the fact that all decisions – both about therapy and about the new design of everyday life (who takes on which task) have to be made under immense time pressure.

The family had no opportunity to familiarize themselves with the diagnosis, to obtain medical information or a second opinion, or to discuss the needs of individual family members. This contributes to the fact that the parents did not even feel they were making decisions at all, but instead found themselves in a situation in which they could only consent to what was now presented to them as necessary and without alternative.

Several families in our study describe their feeling of finding themselves in a "race against time", in which every day, every minute counts and any hesitation ultimately presents a threat to the life of the sick child.

10.2   Decision Making About the Transplant

With one exception, all families said that deciding to conduct a BMT was not considered as a *decision* but as just another step in the therapeutic process, without alternative. At this point, parents usually referred to the doctors who presented a transplant as essential.

> Recipient: [We] had no other choice I mean from the medical side (Kötter)

The only family who described a very intensive decision-making process about BMT stands out from our sample in two ways. First, this family was interviewed shortly *before* the planned BMT, and second, in this family an unrelated donation was planned (sibling donation was impossible for medical reasons). We do not know whether the other families who were interviewed after their BMT had previously undergone a similar decision-making process about it.

However, unlike the other cases, this family did not think solely in terms of "survival" or "death", but also raised questions about potential limitations on quality of life as a result of the BMT. Against the background of a rather small chance of curing their daughter's disease, these parents weighed up the consequences of BMT. On the one hand, the procedure would increase the chance of curing or at least halting the progression of the disease; on the other, the BMT would mean a severely reduced quality of life for their child, who at that point was almost unaffected by their illness.

10.2.1   The Decision About Sibling Donation

Like the decisions about medical treatment and conducting a BMT, the decision to have family members typed and – if they match – used as donors was not interpreted as a "decision" by the family members. Medical staff and the families themselves considered it self-evident that the family members would do so.

In the narratives of the families it became very clear that they preferred a sibling donor over an unrelated donor. This was strongly supported by the fact that doctors referred to sibling donations as being superior to third-party donations. Many families said that the medical staff congratulated them if a sibling was found to be compatible as a donor, and spoke of winning the jackpot. To label it that way made it almost impossible for the families not to seize this "great opportunity".

In some families, the parents had thought in advance about the problems that donation could present for the donor. Possible physical issues and mental consequences, especially if the BMT were to be unsuccessful, were addressed. They anticipated that the donor child might feel guilty if the transplant failed to have the hoped-for success. But only a few families spoke to their children about this possibility before the transplant.

10.2.2   The Rationale: The Advantage of Sibling Donation

Apart from the medical benefits, there were other reasons behind the families' view that a sibling donor was preferable. In particular, it was the security of having the donor child available: the risk of withdrawal of consent is much higher for third-party donors than for sibling donors.

The advantage of a sibling donation seemed so overwhelming to the parents that they sometimes treated medical risks to the donor child as secondary, as the following quote illustrates:

> Interviewer: But that means, an unrelated donor for David wasn't up for discussion at all?
>
> Father: No. Look, it was quite clear that it would work with Dorothea, now I'll have to think, did they, I don't remember at all whether they erm looked further as well, because the problem was that Dorothea was relatively small and that they, let's say, needed a particular amount and erm yes, then erm (.) yes it wa- it was a bit borderline, didn't- don't know how many millilitres they erm were ALLOWED to take of this bone marrow. It was specified precisely, it was erm was also a situation like, Dorothea had to (swallows) was supposed to donate and then there was a kind of- kind of consultation and then a erm a doctor was there who was basically well, on Dorothea's side and then erm well, who was basically supposed to represent [her], that erm yes, well she's small and erm you can't just take vast amounts (laughs) of bone marrow from there and well, he saw it from her side, and I, said, of course we'll take and erm and if- I dunno, if you're allowed to take 40 ml but we need 60, we'll take 60, like, that's clear. You want to help another child and you hope that erm nothing happens to the other one. (Dietrich)

A further advantage was that some families hoped that donations within the family would strengthen the bonds between the whole family and/or the siblings.

10.2.3   Involving Children and Adolescents in Decision-Making Process?

In the literature and in the accounts of clinical practice that we heard, there is an enduring debate about whether and to what extent children and adolescents could and should be involved in medical decisions relating to themselves.

The way in which information is handled and the extent of involvement in decision making of course depend on the age and developmental status of the child(ren). Beyond that, we could see a recurring pattern in nearly all families we interviewed in which families and medical staff framed the sibling donation as a matter of course, as following an unstated rule. The risks to and side effects on the sick child and the donor were weighed against each other, and after consideration the parents concluded that a BMT with sibling donation should be carried out. Family members pointed out that the donation process itself may be unpleasant for the donor, but the burden overall was seen as very small. It was seen as more than justified by the goal of saving the life of the sick sibling. This interpretation of the situation implied that the parents had to talk to the (potential) donor about the donation, and the child was usually also "officially" asked whether she or he agreed to donate. However, everyone knew that a negative answer to this question was not possible. Many parents stated that they secretly thought about what they would have done if the potential donor had refused the donation. Parents were aware that they were putting pressure on the donors, and several parents made it very clear that if the child had refused to donate, they would have been prepared to override the refusal.

In our study, two siblings refused donation at first. Later, however, both children donated, saying that the pressure on them had been too great and that they saw no chance of carrying out their refusal. In the interviews, which took place some years later, both said that they were happy to have donated.

It sounds as if the donors were retrospectively justifying the pressure to donate that was exerted on them and the coercion that they felt.

Donor: and then in that situation my parents had no better idea than to pressure me: come on, DO IT, and that is your brother. I mean sometimes that sort of pressure isn't such a bad thing, because it can also simply (..), well sometimes it can lead to something good, because the- because the parents do always know best, what's good the the children and what isn't. And in retrospect I do have say it was GOOD: I mean for one thing it was really good for me that they pushed me towards it and said, come on and erm, do it now, because I shudder to think how it would have been if they hadn't applied any pressure at all and I'd said I don't want to do it. (Kunow)

10.2.4 Evaluation of Decision-Making Options and the Decision Made, in Retrospect

In retrospect, families depict a situation in which they had little decision-making latitude. They felt as if they had to fit into the medical system and its scripted logics. Some families found the lack of real choices difficult and unsettling, but others felt relieved.

Only one family in the interview expressed doubts that the decision to conduct a BMT had been the right decision. Interestingly, this was one of the families whose child died years after the BMT as a result of GvHD.

Father: The bone marrow transplant, that really gave us hope, but when it went on with the the GvHD, I sometimes asked myself: was that the right thing, the bone marrow transplant? (..) because we'd already it was erm was my brother-in-law (sniffs), the er the- the the brother whose son also had leukaemia. He was in (.) in city F in paediatric oncology unit or the hosp- in the children's hospital, he didn't need a bone marrow transplant. (Kunow)

The correlation between the assessment of the outcome of the disease / BMT and the appropriateness of the decisions made at the time is obvious and not very surprising.

Donation within the family was considered by many family members in retrospect as very positive.

> Mother: so now in retrospect I'm somehow glad that it wasn't a stranger, because that's a person who we maybe never get to know. You can of course get to know them afterwards, but even, if maybe you never get to know them it's still someone who suddenly belongs to the family, regardless of who it is and (..) that's how it would be at least for ME and to be honest I'm now really glad that I don't have to deal with a total stranger and I always think: who was that and who is that actually? (.) very glad, to be honest, that it stayed in the family. (Rohde)

Open Access This chapter is licensed under the terms of the Creative Commons Attribution 4.0 International License (http://creativecommons.org/licenses/by/4.0/), which permits use, sharing, adaptation, distribution and reproduction in any medium or format, as long as you give appropriate credit to the original author(s) and the source, provide a link to the Creative Commons license and indicate if changes were made.

The images or other third party material in this chapter are included in the chapter's Creative Commons license, unless indicated otherwise in a credit line to the material. If material is not included in the chapter's Creative Commons license and your intended use is not permitted by statutory regulation or exceeds the permitted use, you will need to obtain permission directly from the copyright holder.

Chapter 11
Deciding About Child Bone Marrow Donation – Procedural Moral Pitfalls

Tim Henning

Abstract This chapter focuses on two morally significant procedural issues that arise in decisions about intra-family bone marrow donations. 1.) There is a danger of violating what moral philosophers refer to as the separateness of persons, and of viewing the children as mere "value receptacles." 2.) There is a special danger to the child's autonomy – the danger of using the burdens of autonomy to undermine autonomy. These dangers are described, and possible ways to avoid them are explored.

Keywords Bone marrow donation · Ethics · Child's autonomy · Separateness of persons · Manipulation

When a child's life is at stake and parents have to decide whether to let a sibling donate bone marrow, it is easy to be concerned with the outcomes of one's decisions only. The only relevant question, it may seem, is this: Which alternative is to be preferred, which is less harmful and dangerous, etc.?

This outcome-focused point of view anticipates what we will think in retrospect. And in the cases under discussion in this volume, it is easy to anticipate that everyone, the donor child included, will be happy about the decision to donate. This is confirmed by some of the interviews:

D: only in retrospect we're now actually just happy that everything went so well and (.) that- that we were somehow able to help and yeah. (Grohmann, donor, 41)

M: (sighs) //that's how it was// a burden of choices (...). YES and then we did it and it was OK that we did it and I believe, (.) yes.

I: You'd do the same thing again?

M: Definitely, I'd do the same thing again, of course, (.) yeah yeah. So (.) definitely. (Bahr, mother, 149)

T. Henning (✉)
Department of Philosophy, Johannes Gutenberg University of Mainz, Mainz, Germany
e-mail: thenning@uni-mainz.de

© The Author(s) 2022

C. Schües et al. (eds.), *Stem Cell Transplantations Between Siblings as Social Phenomena*, Philosophy and Medicine 144,
https://doi.org/10.1007/978-3-031-04166-2_11

Understandable as it may be, the focus on beneficial outcomes overshadows other significant issues. What matters, I want to argue, is not just whether the best outcome is achieved but *how* it is achieved. Decisions about intra-family BMD not only lead to better or worse outcomes, they are also made in right and wrong ways. It is possible to make a decision that is correct, but do so for questionable reasons, and *vice versa*. This chapter focuses on two morally significant procedural issues.

1. Even if the benefits of a donation outweigh the burdens, all things considered, there is still a question as to whether those who decide have *responded* to the values at stake in the appropriate way. Specifically, there is a *danger of viewing the children as mere "value receptacles."*
2. The issue of the child's autonomy is especially virulent in the cases at hand, and while it is not entirely clear what respect for this autonomy demands, in these cases there is a special danger of misuse. It is the *danger of using the burdens of autonomy to undermine autonomy.*

11.1   Value Receptacles and the Separateness of Persons

In typical cases of intra-family BMD, we have to weigh the burdens on one child (surgery, fear, etc.) against the benefits to another child. It is natural to conclude that the benefits outweigh the burdens. But the ease with which we seem to perform such calculations deserves some suspicion.

It is well known that some economists and philosophers (most notably Nobel-laurate Kenneth Arrow) have claimed that such *interpersonal comparisons of well-being* do not make sense. Their point is not an epistemological one; it is not just that it is often hard or impossible to know who is better off and who is worse off. The problem is conceptual in nature. When we compare something that is bad for an individual A but good for a different individual B, it makes no sense to ask whether it is, on the whole, good or bad – or so they claim. Attempts to say that it is good on the whole invite the question: "Good for *whom*?" But we have already answered any reasonable version of this question – it is, we said, bad for A and good for B. Once we try to summarize our person-bound findings by a further evaluation on some "common scale," we are, they say, just confused.

I do not think that this worry is compelling. But there is a different problem in the vicinity. Whether or not there is a conceptual problem with interpersonal comparisons of well-being, there is often a *moral* problem with decisions that aim to maximize an interpersonal sum of well-being.

One of the first people to articulate this worry was John Rawls. Rawls observes that "the most natural way [...] of arriving at utilitarianism [...] is to adopt for society as a whole the principle of choice for one man" (1971, 26 f). To see what he has in mind, contrast the following claims:

Intrapersonal trade-offs:

People are often required to accept a small burden for themselves in order to attain a greater benefit for themselves.

Interpersonal trade-offs:

People are often required to accept a small burden for themselves in order to attain a greater benefit for others.

It will often be that case that you should forego certain opportunities for enjoyment in order to benefit more greatly later. Quite similarly, utilitarians will say that you should forego these enjoyments if doing so secures greater benefits, not for yourself but for your neighbor. Now, it may be correct that you should indeed do the latter. But what is counterintuitive is that according to utilitarianism, both claims are descriptions *of the very same moral phenomenon*. And this is surely far from clear. Intuitively, in cases of intrapersonal trade-offs the person who carries the burdens is also the person who is compensated by the greater benefits. And this will not be the case with interpersonal trade-offs. And utilitarianism does not offer us the resources to mark this difference. So, Rawls says: "Utilitarianism does not take seriously the distinction between persons" (1971, 27).

Robert Nozick (1974) presses the very same problem in the following passage:

> Individually, we each sometimes choose to undergo some pain or sacrifice for a greater benefit or to avoid a greater harm... In each case, some cost is borne for the sake of the greater overall good. Why not, similarly, hold that some persons have to bear some costs that benefit other persons more, for the sake of the overall social good? But there is no *social entity* with a good that undergoes some sacrifice for its own good. There are only individual people, different individual people, with their own individual lives. Using one of these people for the benefit of others, uses him and benefits the others. Nothing more. [...] To use a person in this way does not sufficiently respect and take account of the fact that he is a separate person, that his is the only life he has. (1974, 32 f)

This objection has come to be known as the *separateness of persons objection to utilitarianism*. Briefly, the objection is that in aiming for a maximal interpersonal sum of well-being, we fail to acknowledge the fact that there will typically be some who benefit and others who pay the cost for their fellows.

We find instances of this form of moral neglect in striking passages in the interviews, e.g.:

> M: [...] Speaking for myself I always thought, it's a- it's not such a major intervention. OF COURSE, you're interfering with a perfectly healthy child, Zorro is basically healthy, erm but when you look at the BENEFIT of it, then that is NOTHING. (Zucker, mother, 26)

Here, one wants to say: "Well, if the benefits and burdens accrued to one and the same individual, it would indeed be safe to say that the burdens pale in comparison with the benefits. But you ignore that *here*, there is *one* person who benefits and a *different* person who is being left to bear the burden."

Take a trivial example: If you can buy some great bread for an extremely low price, you might say that the cost, compared to what you receive, is "nothing." But you would certainly hesitate to say the same thing to someone else who just bought the bread for you. Low as the price may be – since this other person paid the price in order that you, another person, benefits, that is *not* nothing.

Most people recognize that there is, in fact, a moral problem here. But it is worth spelling out what exactly the problem is, and to find a theoretical rationale for the intuition. After all, the problem at hand will require a practical solution. So we need to know what exactly the moral mistake that is being made here amounts to, how serious it is, and how we can strive to avoid it.

As the wording in the above quote suggests, Nozick thinks that the separateness of persons objection consists in a charge of treating people in an *instrumental* fashion, as mere means to others' ends or as resources to be used by others. In a recent paper, R. Yetter Chappell (2015) explains in what sense there is an instrumental stance in play. As he observes, it makes no sense to compare how two persons, A and B, fare in terms of *A's* well-being. So if we weigh A's and B's well-being, we treat them as instances of a *general* property of well-being, which either of them can instantiate equally well. Given this, then if we strive to maximize that general property, we treat the *particular* well-being of A, and B, as means to an end with regard to which they are *replaceable*. The well-being of A and the well-being of B matter only insofar as they help to constitute a certain amount of the general property. Chappell calls this "constitutive instrumentality." In consequence, both A and B could come to feel that they are being treated and seen as mere receptacles for well-being, or value.

The separateness of persons can be put into focus when we imagine other kinds of trade-offs. It is natural to assume that most persons would be willing to sacrifice a limb, if this is required to save their own lives. Within one person's life, this is a trade-off that pretty clearly makes sense. On the other hand, I suspect that few of us would say that *other* people should be willing to sacrifice a limb to save *our* lives. Of course, we may wish that other people are so heroic. But that is very different from the view that we can *expect* them, in a normative sense, to do such things for us.

This becomes especially clear once we describe cases with the concept of a moral claim-right. J. Thomson gives examples that show this clearly. One of her (deliberately absurd) cases is this:

> If I am sick unto death, and the only thing that will save my life is the touch of Henry Fonda's cool hand on my fevered brow, then all the same, I have no right to be given the touch of Henry Fonda's cool hand on my fevered brow. It would be frightfully nice of him to fly in from the West Coast to provide it. It would be less nice, though no doubt well meant, if my friends flew out to the West Coast and carried Henry Fonda back with them. But I have no right at all against anybody that he should do this for me. (Thomson 1971, 55)

So the concept of a right brings the separateness of persons into sharp focus. Even when a person has to do something that is not very costly to save our life, we do *not* think that we have a right to this. Correspondingly, we would not want to say that they *owe* this to us. Of course, we do not do justice to the complexity of the case if we say *merely* that the protagonist has no right against Fonda. Thomson herself makes this clear numerous times, stressing, e.g., that it would be nice of Henry Fonda to help. We might add that we would find it callous and selfish if he refused to do it. So the case is not supposed to suggest that helping is morally neutral. It would be virtuous, laudable, and so on. It is important to stress this. But it is *also* important to consider the full range of moral concepts at our disposal, and of the fine discriminations that they allow us to make. And Thomson's example suggests that there are circumstances in which we do not have a moral right to others' help, even if our lives are at stake and even if the help could be provided easily.

What is required by respect for the separateness of persons, and for the fact that individuals cannot be treated as so many locations for a general commodity of well-being? One important part is the reactions that are fitting responses to the value of an individual's well-being. It is important to be aware of, and explicit about, the fact that any interpersonal trade-offs have to leave aside something that is not commensurable. Thus, attitudes of ambivalence and doubt are apt responses to what is, of necessity, an attempt to treat different person's fates as exchangeable commodities.

We find examples of this kind of awareness in some of the interview materials in this book:

> "M: Now this really is always an issue: here we have a healthy (.) PATIENT, (.) and (.) to do the bone marrow donation, they administer a general anaesthetic (.), when they put the central line in (..) they also administered a general anaesthetic, it always involves some sort of (.) risk, which probably might also put some other families off, but what that means right now, that we need to administer something to a healthy human being, (.) not for their own benefit, rather so that they have to, so to speak, help someone else. (Preuss, mother, 20)

> F: This exact issue (.) has cropped up in several places. Is it actually somehow permissible, erm, to use this – a child as a construction site for the other? (Wahl, family interview, 224–229)

Secondly, the separateness of persons should be understood to at least influence the proper *exchange rate* of well-being, so to speak. As I said, we can expect that one and the same person will be willing to sacrifice a limb in order to save her own life. But we *cannot* expect the same across different individuals. That does not mean, however, that we cannot legitimately expect *anything* from others. While it is unreasonable to demand that others should be willing to give a limb, they can definitely be expected to suffer certain inconveniences if someone else's life is at stake. As A. Voorhoeve (2014) puts it, we do seem to have a standard of "a permissible degree of self-concern", and of its limits. These intuitions should inform our decisions, although they will, of course, be vague. The idea would then be that the exchange rate for well-being transfers should be sensitive to our moral view of permissible self-concern. If we would not think it wrong for someone to refuse to bear a certain burden in order to secure a certain benefit for us, then we may not just impose it on her.

There is, at any rate, one further practical upshot that is certain: If *the law* specifies regulations for child donations, and if these laws seem at least reasonably well attuned to the fact of the separateness of persons, then respect for the separateness of persons definitely requires that the law be taken strictly and seriously. In light of this, the following example reveals a serious problem:

> I don't remember at all whether they erm looked further as well, because the problem was that Dorothea was relatively (.) small and erm (.) that they, let's say, needed a particular amount and erm yes, then erm (.) yes it wa- it was a bit borderline, didn't – don't know how many (.) millilitres they erm were ALLOWED to take of this bone marrow. It was specified precisely, it was (.) erm was also a situation like, Dorothea had to (swallows) (.) was supposed to donate and then erm there was a kind of- kind of consultation and then a erm a doctor was there who was basically (.) well, on Dorothea's side (.) and then erm well, who was basically supposed to represent [her], that erm yes, well she's small and erm you can't just take vast amounts (laughs) of bone marrow from there and well, he saw it from her side, and I (.), said, of course we'll take and erm and if – I dunno, if you're allowed to take 40 ml but we need 60, we'll take 60, like, that's clear. You want to help another child and you hope that erm nothing happens to the other one. (Dietrich, father, 54–55)

This passage illustrates that in the attempt to save a child, parents are easily tempted to ignore laws that are designed to protect the interests of their other child. Importantly, the point is not to blame the father (or the parents). In a situation of desperation, we cannot hold parents to high standards of conscientiousness. But it was of the utmost importance that a medical professional should take the side of the donor and argue against the donation. Arguably, it would have been even better if the official regulations had been enforced and followed.

11.2   The Burdens of Autonomy, and Their Misuses

We routinely assume that parents have the authority to make most of the decisions that affect their children. Usually, this authority is backed by the law. The same holds true in the cases discussed here. Whether a child donates bone marrow for a sibling is not, ultimately, up to him- or herself.

In the interview material, we find some very explicit expressions of parental authority:

> [I]t was clear to me, without us having a massive discussion with Zorro, that Zorro WILL donate whether he wants to or not. And as a result this matter was, er, initially not debated with Zorro much at all, rather, like, it was ACTUALLY already CLEAR for us, whatever Zorro wanted. (Zucker, mother, 26)

Although not everybody would be so frank about it, few people doubt the presumption of parental authority. Yet it is surprisingly difficult to say what justifies it. The main lines of justification that come to mind do not draw the line between children and adults in quite the way they would have to, if they are to vindicate our current practices. Consider some typical defenses of the presumption:

1. *Lack of Competence*

In many important areas, children lack the knowledge and foresight to make the decisions that are in their own best interest.

2. *Lack of Prudence*

Children often irrationally prefer smaller short-term benefits to greater long-term benefits.

3. *Special Relations*

The close relations of love and trust within a family render permissible acts that would, in other contexts, be impermissible intrusions.

4. *Responsibility*

In having a child, parents take on a special responsibility for their well-being. This special responsibility makes it permissible to assume authority over their decisions.

Again, the problem with all of these typical defenses is that they do not draw the line where it needs to be drawn. It is a sad fact, but a fact nonetheless, that many adults are lacking in foresight, knowledge, and prudence, and therefore are prone to make decisions that are against their own best interest. People gamble away their money and home, eat and drink so much as to seriously endanger their health, leave or neglect their families on spontaneous and selfish impulses or out of a lack of concern – only to find later that they have ruined their lives in entirely predictable ways.

This happens with an awful lot of people – but nobody thinks that this gives other people the right to interfere in their decisions. If we know someone who makes lots of bad and imprudent decisions, we may offer our advice (and if we know them rather well, do so rather insistently). But that is not at all the same as *taking away their authority*. I may find a lot to criticize in other adults' decisions, but that does not mean that I may take the freedom to make their decisions for them.

So all of the deficiencies that we find in many children can be found in a depressing number of adults as well. If these deficiencies were sufficient to establish that others can assume authority over their lives, that would change our practices and relations among adults in very drastic ways. But in fact, we do not think that our fellow adults' deficiencies make their authority questionable. On the contrary, many of us even feel that even trivial restrictions (like laws requiring helmets or safety belts) come very close to objectionable paternalism. With children, we lack these scruples.

True, some deficits may occur in children more regularly, and as a matter of biology. But why does this matter? The question of whether a child should have the authority to make certain decisions should depend only on that child's competences and deficits, not on their statistical distribution over a population. And as far as biological determinants are concerned, I consider it very well possible that many comparable deficiencies in adults are biologically determined as well.

What about the special family relations? They cannot do the required justificatory work either. I am close with my adult sister, but that does not give either of us authority over the other.

What about the final point, the special responsibilities that parents have assumed by having children? Even this point does not provide the required justification, or so I think. First of all, the fact that a person's parents chose to have her will remain true as long as the person exists. So if parents have a special responsibility for those they have created, and if this responsibility gives them authority, then parents should have the authority to make even the decisions of their adult children (*at least* in those cases where their adult children would decide against their own interest). We clearly do not think that this is true. So our moral view does not, in general, seem to say that this kind of responsibility generates authority. Secondly, it is not clear why parents' responsibility should generate this form of authority. It may be plausible to say that this authority generates strong positive duties of beneficience, aid, and support. But why does it give parents the right to systematically execute power in matters that concern their children, against their children's will?

There is, however, one important difference between children and adults. It does not have to do with the general level of competence. Again, I do not believe it is true that all children are less competent than all adults, and yet we do grant full authority to all of the latter (pathological cases aside). The important difference is that children will *change* over time, in a way and to a degree that is greater and more certain than it is with typical adults. And when they face the consequences of their decisions, it will often be from a perspective of an older and very different individual. This is something that matters, and something we have a rather general reason to expect. Here is why.

Derek Parfit has argued that certain facts about personal identity over time may have important ramifications for the issue of paternalism. I cannot argue for Parfit's position here. (Nor do I have to; Parfit's own arguments can be found in Parfit 1984, Part III.) But I want to suggest that if we take his position seriously, this makes it possible to provide a more convincing argument for our practice of letting parents decide whether their children donate bone marrow to siblings.

As Parfit famously argues, the continued existence of a person over time does not consist in the continued existence of a certain entity, a Cartesion Ego. When we speak of the continued existence of one and the same person over time, this can in fact be fully explained in different terms – that is to say, in terms that do not invoke the continued existence of any kind of entity at all. The facts that are really picked out by our talk of identity over time is really the instantiation of certain *relations* of psychological and physiological continuity and connectedness across time. To put it simply, to say that one and the same person exists both now and then is to say that between the person that exists now and the person that exists then, there are certain close physiological and psychological connections which can be traced over time. But these connections are a matter of degree, and they can be instantiated in degrees that do not quite suffice for the existence of one person over time. Hence our relation to ourselves in the future and in the past is *not necessarily categorically different* from our relation to *other* persons – or so Parfit's arguments suggest.

As Parfit argues, this fact has a number of normative and moral implications. And in part, they concern the issue of paternalism. Suppose we intervene in someone's decision because we predict (correctly, we may suppose) that this decision is strongly against the interests of that person at a later time. Typically, we think of this as an intervention in the name of that person's self-interest. And the difficulty with paternalistic interventions of this kind is that *practical irrationality* as such does not seem to license them. But now suppose that the person who is about to make the decision will predictably change a lot. Consequently, the physiological and psychological connections that underwrite identity over time will hold only to a lesser degree. And even though we may still speak of the same person at the later time, this simply masks the fact that the relation between the stages is a lot more like the relation between distinct persons than it is in other cases.

And this, Parfit argues, means that the normative restrictions on such a choice may change as well. When we intervene with a decision because it will have bad consequences for the person later, the objection to this may be *moral* in nature. The case may no longer be categorically different from a case in which a person makes a decision that will have bad consequences for *another* person later on. Again, this is because, again, there is no categorical difference between our relation to later stages of ourselves and our relations to other people. The difference is more a matter of degree, and therefore some of the moral objections that are apt in the latter case may be apt in the former.

Parfit agrees that this may be hard to swallow at first. But he goes on to explain:

> It may be easier to believe this if we subdivide a person's life into that of successive selves. As I have claimed, this has long seemed natural, whenever there is some marked weakening of psychological connectedness. After such a weakening, my earlier self may seem alien to me now. If I fail to *identify* with that earlier self, I am in some ways thinking of that self as like a different person. (Parfit 1984, 319)

Importantly, Parfit's view is that this perspective is not pathological, or some kind of distortion. On the contrary: A failure to "identify" in cases of weakened psychological connectedness *correctly* registers that the existence of one and the same person is, in effect, a manner of talking, and a way to summarize facts in an absolute fashion that are really gradual and vague in nature. A failure to "identifiy" in these cases is, so to speak, better attuned to the real metaphysics of personal identity.

What follows from such a stance? Consider the following example:

> Reconsider a boy who starts to smoke, knowing and hardly caring that this may cause him to suffer greatly fifty years later. This boy does not identify with his future self. His attitude towards his future self is in some ways like his attitude towards other people. This analogy makes it easier to believe that his act is morally wrong. He runs the risk of imposing on himself a premature and painful death. We should claim that it is wrong to impose on *anyone*, including such a future self, the risk of such a death. More generally, we should claim that great imprudence is morally wrong. We ought not to do to our future selves what it would be wrong to do to other people. (Parfit 1984, 319 f)

This normative difference in how we see imprudent decisions also makes a difference for the question of paternalism. Once great imprudence is seen as morally akin to *wronging another person*, we have a very different justification for interference in imprudent decisions. Parfit puts it thus:

> We do not believe that we have a general right to prevent people from acting *irrationally*. But we do believe that we have a general right to prevent people from acting *wrongly*. [...] Since we ought to believe that great imprudence is seriously wrong, we ought to believe that we should prevent such imprudence, even if this involves coercion. (Parfit 1984, 321)

To sum up, if we accept the view that imprudent decisions about one's future are not categorically different from decisions that are harmful for other people, there is a whole new rationale for paternalistic interventions. We do not need to think of paternalism, and of parental authority, as intervening in the name of rationality and the person's self-interest. We can think of it as the legitimate attempt to prevent great *moral* wrong. On the one hand, the smoking boy from the above example may be onto something when he views his future self almost like a different person. But on the other hand, it is for precisely this reason that his harmful action is a case of *moral wronging*.

I return to the main thread of the discussion. I have criticized some typical defenses of parental authority above; I have now described one possible defense that I consider more promising. The defense is that a child, in making a decision, will often impose burdens on him- or herself later in the future. And in the case of children (unlike the case of adults) we have very much reason to expect the subject to undergo much change in between. The relation between the child who decides and the older person who has to bear the consequences will often involve weakened forms of psychological and physiological connections. This may lead the child to see his or her future self as a different person. But by the same token, we should view the case much like one in which we keep a person from wrongfully imposing burdens on someone who is, to some degree, like a different person. And if a wronging threatens, interference and coercion may be legitimate.

However, we must now face the most serious issue. *All* of the justifications of parental authority have claimed that this authority must be based *on the interest of the child*, or her future self. To the extent that these justifications work, they suggest that exercising authority over our child is legitimate because and insofar as it is done *for the child's sake*, or *for the child's own good*. The crucial problem is that in the cases we are discussing here, parents seem to use their authority over one child to serve the interest *of a different child*. Parents are here urging their children to do things that are *against* their own, narrow self-interest. As it stands, none of the above justifications cover *this*.

For example: If a child would wish to refuse to donate bone marrow, does that reveal a lack of competence that endangers the child's own good? This is certainly far from clear. Or does the child show a lack of prudence – and thereby a tendency to wrong her own future self? Again, this is far from clear. On the face of it, a refusal to donate seems to be very much in the child's interest.

At this point, I want to introduce a further important consideration that is often neglected. To give someone authority over something is *itself* to impose certain burdens on him or her. In some cases, I think, parents may have sufficient moral reason to spare their children these burdens.

A number of authors have observed that having certain options, and the authority to choose them or not, can in fact be a disadvantage. One of the earliest discussions of this kind is to be found in the work of economist Thomas Schelling (1960). He observes that is can often be a strategic advantage *not* to have certain options. (E.g., it can be good for the bank clerk not to know the code for the safe, and thus not to have the option of opening it.) Other authors stress that having an option may increase social pressure, and it may increase the need to justify and defend oneself. G. Dworkin (1988), e.g., observes that not all couples will be better off when their society adopts liberal regulations for prenatal screenings and abortions. Having the right to check for disabilities and to abort a fetus that is likely to be disabled is not simply having an additional option, which everyone is free to either take or leave. Instead, it means that having a disabled child now becomes a conscious choice, whereas it was beyond choice earlier. And this means that social pressure, demands for justification etc. increase. D. Velleman (1992) makes similar points about the effects of liberal regulations for assisted suicide. But he also gives a more mundane example: If a professor invites his student to his home for dinner, he gives this student an additional option. The student now has the option to visit his professor's home. And of course, he also still has the option of not doing so, if he declines the invitation. Still, it would be a mistake to think that the student's menu of options has simply increased, in a way that could not possibly disadvantageous. As Velleman observes, there is *one* option that the student no longer has, namely the option of not visiting his professor's home *without having to decline his invitation*. Due to the invitation, what was previously the default now becomes something for which one needs an excuse.

Now, this matters in our examples as well. Parents who have to decide will certainly feel the pressure, and the need to reassure themselves that what they decide can be justified. The question, "Am I doing the right thing? Will I be able to defend this choice against those concerned later on?" will be itself felt as an enormous burden, keeping them pondering day and night. This experience makes clear what it would mean to impose this burden on a child. Note that the point is not that the child will experience the burden in this same way at present, although this may be true as well. Rather, the point is that the child will later have to cope with the fact that the outcome of the decision is on her. If she refuses to donate, that not only means that her sibling may not survive. In addition, it means that her sibling's death is *her* responsibility, something *she* decided to allow.

Being in this position is an enormous burden. By giving the authority to decide to one's child, one not only places the relevant burden on the child *now*. One also risks that the child, by making a certain decision, will impose on her later self the burden of having to live with the responsibility.

This, I think, is the valid moral reason why it is permissible for parents to make the decision for their children, not allowing them to decide the matter themselves. As I have just argued, the justification for this can follow the more common patterns after all. Properly understood, it may be in the child's own interest (and in the interest of her later self) after all to suffer the surgery now rather than to have the burden of the decision on her own shoulders now and in the future.

Once we see this justification of parental authority, however, we can see a very particular danger of misuse. In some cases, parents may be tempted to use the burdens of authority to *undermine* authority. That is to say, they let their children feel the responsibility and the guilt they would have to carry if they made the wrong choice, to manipulate them into choosing differently:

F: The bone marrow transplant issue came up at once. Yes and then everything hap- happened to both of them but, what kind of procedure for that child or for the sibling, THAT,
er, of course trying somehow, you try, to persuade them somehow and whatever and 'no, no,
no'. Yes, I'm telling you it sounds stupid, I always said silly [things], I'd say: 'Kira, you're
the only chance', I'd say, 'do you want your brother to die?' Yes fine, I'm also using psychological pressure, not DELIBERATELY, on on her, or rather on Kira. That still cuts me
to the quick TODAY, that we said that. (Kunow, father, 72)

In the interview material, the daughter of the same family recalls the pressure
that was put on her:

D: because then I got so much PRESSURE from (.) my parents: come on, and you have to
do this, he's your brother after all and erm (.), if you don't do this, then erm (..), yes, then-
you you won't forgive yourself for the rest of your LIFE and come on, just do it. And then
at some point I'd been put under such emotional pressure that I just said: OK, you know
what, (.) you're not going to give up anyway and I don't want afterwards to have to take
responsibility, I didn't donate bone marrow to my brother, now – now you can go here and
there and you can visit him, can't you. (Kunow, donor, 17)

This is a document of an instance of a very serious form of manipulation – and an
instance that all the parties concerned still seem to remember as extremely hurtful.
There is a good reason for not giving the authority to make these decisions to the
children. This good reason is that the pressure, and the anticipated need to justify
their choice, is too burdensome for them to carry. What we find here is a family in
which this pressure is *used* – deliberately invoked in order to get the daughter to
consent to the decision. In view of this, it actually seems preferable *not* to put children into the position of having to make, and to defend, the choice at all, and instead
be frank about the fact that the decision is not for the child to make.

Literature

Chappell, Richard Yetter. 2015. Value receptacles. *Noûs* 49: 322–332.
Dworkin, Gerald. 1988. Is more choice better than less? In *The theory and practice of autonomy*,
     ed. Gerald Dworkin. Cambridge: Cambridge University Press.
Nozick, Robert. 1974. *Anarchy, state, and Utopia*. New York: Basic Books.
Parfit, Derek. 1984. *Reasons and persons*. Oxford: Clarendon Press.
Rawls, John. 1971. *A theory of justice*. Cambridge: Harvard University Press.
Schelling, Thomas. 1960. *The strategy of conflict*. Harvard: Harvard University Press.
Thomson, Judith Jarvis. 1971. A defense of abortion. *Philosophy and Public Affairs* 1: 47–66.
Velleman, David. 1992. Against the right to die. *The Journal of Medicine and Philosophy* 6:
     665–681.
Voorhoeve, Alex. 2014. How should we aggregate competing claims? *Ethics* 125: 64–87.

Open Access   This chapter is licensed under the terms of the Creative Commons Attribution 4.0 International License (http://creativecommons.org/licenses/by/4.0/), which permits use, sharing, adaptation, distribution and reproduction in any medium or format, as long as you give appropriate credit to the original author(s) and the source, provide a link to the Creative Commons license and indicate if changes were made.

The images or other third party material in this chapter are included in the chapter's Creative Commons license, unless indicated otherwise in a credit line to the material. If material is not included in the chapter's Creative Commons license and your intended use is not permitted by statutory regulation or exceeds the permitted use, you will need to obtain permission directly from the copyright holder.

Chapter 12
A Decision-Making Approach for Children to Ethically Serve as Stem Cell Donors

Lainie Friedman Ross

Abstract In this chapter, I explore the limits of the best interest standard and the role of third-party oversight for some medical decisions even when the parents' decision is not abusive or neglectful. The American Academy of Pediatrics (AAP) policy statement, "Children as Hematopoietic Stem Cell (HSC) Donors" proposes a role for a living donor advocacy team (third-party oversight) for paediatric HSC donation between siblings. The AAP recommendations are supported by data from the medical literature and from the qualitative empirical study on HSC transplantation between siblings that was conducted from 2016 to 2019 by members of the Institute for the History of Medicine and Science Studies (University of Lübeck).

Keywords Siblings · Pediatric decision-making · Best interest standard · Guidance principle · Intervention principle · Living donor advocate · Stem cell transplant · Donor benefit

12.1 Introduction

Consider the case of a young child with newly diagnosed leukemia. The treating pediatric oncologist explains to the parents that once the child is in remission, it is in her medical best interest to undergo a hematopoietic stem cell [HSC] transplant. Depending on the disease and other clinical factors, the options may include one or more of the following: autologous HSC transplant (where donor and recipient are the same person); bone marrow or peripheral stem cells from an unknown source or family member; or umbilical cord stem cells (obtained from either the child's own cord blood procured postnatally, a sibling or an unknown source) (Khandelwal et al. 2017). Depending on the medical condition, there are pros and cons for the donor to

L. F. Ross (✉)
Department of Pediatrics and the MacLean Center for Clinical Medical Ethics, University of Chicago, Chicago, IL, USA
e-mail: lross@peds.bsd.uchicago.edu

© The Author(s) 2022
C. Schües et al. (eds.), *Stem Cell Transplantations Between Siblings as Social Phenomena*, Philosophy and Medicine 144,
https://doi.org/10.1007/978-3-031-04166-2_12

be the patient him- or herself versus a sibling versus an unknown source and for the source of the stem cells to be bone marrow versus peripheral blood versus umbilical cord blood (Talano et al. 2014; Styczynski et al. 2012; Khandelwal et al. 2017). Within the family, siblings are the most likely to be histocompatible (match at 10 of 10 human lymphocyte antigens [10/10 HLA-match]), and a sibling donor often facilitates the logistical issues.

In this chapter, I will explore the ethical issues surrounding decision-making regarding allogeneic HSC donation by a minor (non-infant) to his or her sibling. I focus on the sibling donor for several reasons. First, although the most common HSC transplants in the US involve an autologous donation (~57%) or a non-related donor (~22%), siblings are the most likely related donor because they are more likely to be an HLA-match than other genetically related family members (Center for International Blood and Marrow Transplant Research n.d.), In the US, siblings account for ~10% of all donors (Center for International Blood and Marrow Transplant Research n.d.); Second, almost 20% of related donors are minors (Center for International Blood and Marrow Transplant Research n.d.) which raises important moral questions regarding parental authority, the moral underpinnings of their decision-making, and the role of the minor. To examine these moral questions, I explore a framework for decision making in pediatrics as outlined by Buchanan and Brock (1990). I then examine whether the parents must be guided by the "best interest" standard and what this means for both the child donor and recipient, and I discuss why Brock and Buchanan are correct to argue for third-party intervention for HSC transplantation when the potential donor is a minor sibling. Finally, I describe the recommendations we developed for the American Academy of Pediatrics [AAP] Committee on Bioethics statement (2010) "Children as Hematopoietic Stem Cell Donors" which provides the sort of oversight that Buchanan and Brock proposed. I show that the AAP recommendations are supported by data from the medical literature as well as interview quotations from the qualitative empirical study on bone marrow transplantation between siblings that was conducted from 2016 to 2019 by members of the Institute of History of Medicine and Science Studies, University of Lübeck (PIs: Madeleine Herzog, Martina Jürgensen, Christoph Rehmann-Sutter and Christina Schües) [Hereinafter referred to as "the Lübeck study"], and the citations are sourced from the Interview Material [IM] which can be found in the appendix.

12.2   Pediatric Decision Making

In *Deciding for Others: The ethics of surrogate decision making,* Buchanan and Brock (1990) offer a four principle framework for surrogate decision making for pediatric and adult patients. The four principles are: (1) underlying ethical values; (2) authority principle; (3) guidance principle and (4) intervention principle.

Buchanan and Brock state that the underlying ethical values (principle #1) for decision-making for those who cannot make decisions for themselves include both well-being and self-determination. When the patient is a child, they add parental interests as a third underlying value. They offer four justifications for adding this third value: (1) the child is unable to speak for him- or her-self, and parents will do a better job than others; (2) parents will bear the consequences; (3) parents, within limits, have the right to raise their child according to their own values; and (4) the family is a valuable social institution that promotes intimacy which requires, "within limits, to make important decisions about the welfare of its incompetent members" (Buchanan and Brock 1990, pp. 233–4).

The framework also establishes who is (are) the appropriate authority figure(s) (principle #2) and what principle(s) should guide them (principle #3). Adults who have decisional capacity can choose who will speak for them if and when they are no longer able, and their decision-makers should make decisions, when possible, that they would have made if they were still capable (either by following an advance directive or applying the principle of substituted judgement) (Buchanan and Brock 1990, p. 94). In contrast, in pediatrics, parents are the presumed decision-makers, and they are supposed to be guided by the best interest standard (Buchanan and Brock 1990, pp. 232–7).

The most obvious reason to intervene in a surrogate's decision making (principle #4) is because the surrogate's decision is abusive or neglectful—what is referred to as the "harm principle" (Diekema 2004, 2011). While decisions or actions that meet the criteria of abuse or neglect justify state intervention, Brock and Buchanan propose intervention for a broader array of cases and sanction a broader set of agents or institutions to intervene. According to Brock and Buchanan, third-party intervention can be justified in three sets of cases for both children and adults: (1) conditions that disqualify the family (e.g., abuse and neglect, conflicts of interest, or if the family "is incompetent to decide"); (2) cases deserving special scrutiny (e.g., the vulnerable position of the incompetent patient; the momentousness of the decision; or high likelihood of conflicts of interest); or 3) cases outside the scope of reasonable medical practice (e.g., parents who demand treatment that is not medically indicated or parents who refuse treatment that has high benefit and low harm) (Buchanan and Brock 1990, pp. 142–151). Buchanan and Brock also sanction other agents or institutions, such as ethics committees, to intervene (Buchanan and Brock 1990, pp. 148–151). (This decision-making framework and how it is similar and different for minors and adults who lack decisional capacity are detailed in Table 12.1).

One of the cases in which Buchanan and Brock support third-party intervention is in the case of a child sibling HSC donor (Buchanan and Brock 1990, p. 142). They support third party intervention because the parents are conflicted: while it is best for the ill child to undergo an allogeneic HSC transplant from a 10/10 HLA-matched sibling, it is not clear that it is in the healthy sibling's best interest to serve as an HSC donor. In the 30 years since the publication of their book, the medical and psychological risks experienced by HSC donors have been further characterized by empirical research. First, there are medical risks regardless of the source of the stem cells. Bone marrow donation is painful, requires anesthesia, and may lead to nerve damage or a need for a blood transfusion (Bosi and Bartolozzi 2010; Styczynski

Table 12.1 The primary ethical framework developed by Buchanan and Brock (1990) in *Deciding for Others*[a]

	ADULT without decisional capacity	MINOR
Ethical value principles	1. Respect for individual self-determination 2. Concern for the individual's well-being	1. Child's well-being 2. Child's self-determination 3. Parents' interest in making decisions concerning their children
Guidance principles	1. Advance directive 2. Substituted judgment 3. Best interest	1. Best interest
Authority principles	1. "Family" defined as whomever the individual is most closely associated with" 2. (To be replaced by advance directives)	1. Parents 2. State-appointed guardian

Intervention principles (Attempts to specify conditions that rebut the presumptive authority of the family)	1. Conditions that disqualify the family
	  a. Abuse or neglect
	  b. Serious conflict of interest
	  c. Family incompetent
	2. Certain classes of cases deserving special scrutiny by virtue of…
	  a. Vulnerable position:
	    i. Incompetent as organ donor
	  b. The momentousness of the consequences of the decision:
	    i. Result in preventable and considerable shortening of life
	    ii. Decisions that result in permanent and avoidable loss or impairment of important physical or psychological functions (e.g., sterilization)
	  c. High likelihood of conflicts of interest
	    i. Cases where strong familial attachments do not exist, and some treatment alternatives would impose great burdens on the surrogate
	3. Decisions outside of the range of medically sound alternatives	

[a]Table based on text developed in Allen E. Buchanan and Daniel W. Brock, *Deciding for Others: The Ethics of Surrogate Decision Making* (New York: Cambridge University Press, 1990). This table is reprinted with permission from Lainie F. Ross. Better than Best (Interest Standard) in Pediatric Decision Making. *Journal of Clinical Ethics* 2019;30(3):183–188 at p. 184. ©2019 by The Journal of Clinical Ethics. All rights reserved

et al. 2012). Peripheral stem cell donation requires pre-treatment with granulocyte-colony stimulating factor [G-CSF] to increase the number of peripheral stem cells. While the long-term increased risk of cancer has been shown to be unfounded, (Shaw et al. 2015) G-CSF injections are painful and can cause bone pain, headache and flu-like symptoms (Pulsipher et al. 2005). In addition, peripheral stem cell collection involves large bore catheters and the associated risks of clots or infection, and some children need blood transfusions post-donation (Styczynski et al. 2012). The risk of umbilical cord stem cells procurement should be nil provided that the birthing process is unchanged (American College of Obstetricians and Gynecologists

2009). However, when the child is conceived to donate to an older sibling, the cell dose may be insufficient (Locatelli 2009) and this may lead to a second collection of bone marrow from the child as a toddler (Chang 1991).

One could try to argue that the donation is in the child donor's best interest because despite the physical risks of HSC donation, it is psychologically and emotionally best to have a living sibling. If the recipient were to die, at least the donor and family are able to say that they "did everything". And yet, more recent data show that there are serious psychological risks of being a donor (Packman et al. 1997, 2010; Wiener et al. 2007; Pentz et al. 2014; Switzer et al. 2017). So, whether or not it is in the donor's best interest, all things considered, is ambiguous at best today as it was in 1990, when minimal to no data existed.

Even if the donation is not in the donor's best interest, all things considered, I believe that parents may still be justified in authorizing the donation. Elsewhere I have argued to respect broad parental discretion provided that their decisions do not sacrifice the basic needs and interests of any child, even if some compromises may be necessary (Ross 1998, 2015). I have also challenged the best interest standard as the appropriate guidance principle (Ross 1998, 2015, 2019) despite the fact that it is the prevailing guidance principle in policy statements around the globe (United Nations 1989; British Medical Association 2019; Larcher et al. 2015; Canadian Paediatric Society 2004; Royal College of Physicians and Surgeons of Canada 2013; Weise et al. 2017; Katz et al. 2016). I have challenged the best interest standard because it is too demanding a guidance principle for parents in an intimate family setting (Ross, 1998). Taken literally, it would require that parents sacrifice their own significant interests and needs for a small benefit to their child. It would also require that parents do what is best for each child which may not be possible if the siblings' needs and interests conflict. Buchanan and Brock also challenge using the best interest as an actual goal asserting that "as a guidance principle, the best interest principle is to serve only as a regulative ideal, not as a strict and literal requirement" (Buchanan and Brock 1990, p. 236). Parents need greater flexibility than such a principle allows.

However, even if best interest is the appropriate guidance principle, Buchanan and Brock do not support state intervention if the parents' decision is not the "best", but argue for a distinct "intervention principle":

> [U]tilizing our distinction between guidance principles and intervention principles, we noted that—except perhaps where the most basic interests of the child are at issue—a mere failure on the part of the parents to *optimize* the child's interest is not sufficient to trigger justified intervention by third parties, or even a challenge to the parent's decision-making authority (Buchanan and Brock 1990, pp. 235–236).

Buchanan and Brock support broad parental discretion and even argue that parental interests are a legitimate ethical value in their decision making model: "the interest of parents in making important decisions about the welfare of their minor children" (Buchanan and Brock 1990, p. 226). They argue that parents require significant freedom from oversight, control and intrusion in balancing the needs and interests of each family member and the family as a whole. Some refer to the gap between

Table 12.2 A visual aid representing guidance and intervention principles

Guidance (in principle)	Best interest standard
Guidance (in practice)	Zone of Parental Discretion or Good Enough Standard
Intervention	Abuse or Neglect Standard (and special circumstances that merit third-party consideration)

Adapted and reprinted with permission from Lainie Friedman Ross. Reflections on Charlie Gard and the Best Interests Standard from both sides of the Atlantic Ocean. *Pediatrics,* 2020; 146 (Supplement 1): Table 2

best interest and harm as "the zone of parental discretion" (Gillam 2016); others refer to parents whose decisions fall in this zone as "good enough" parents (Winnicott 1953) or refer to their decision as "good enough" or meeting a "good enough standard". While in principle guidance aspires to what is in the child' best interest (what Buchanan and Brock call a "regulative ideal"), in practice, guidance gives wide leeway to parental discretion for decisions that meet a good enough standard. Both of these guidance principles are distinct from an intervention principle that empowers third-party intervention (See Table 12.2).

12.3   HSC Transplantation: A Case That Deserves Special Scrutiny

Even if HSC donation is determined to meet the child's best interest, or at least good enough, standard, Buchanan and Brock assert that HSC donation by minors is one of the special cases for which oversight (intervention) is always appropriate. Children are vulnerable and the decision to authorize an HSC donation should require a process that requires serious reflection. I was the lead author of the 2010 AAP statement that created a process to determine if a child should be permitted to serve as an HSC donor for an intrafamilial stem cell transplant (AAP 2010). The process required evaluating whether five criteria were met:

(1) there is no medically equivalent histocompatible adult relative who is willing and able to donate;
(2) there is a strong personal and emotionally positive relationship between the donor and recipient;
(3) there is some likelihood that the recipient will benefit from transplantation;
(4) the clinical emotional, and psychosocial risks to the donor are minimized and are reasonable in relation to the benefits expected to accrue to the donor and to the recipient; and
(5) parental permission and, where appropriate, child assent have been obtained (AAP 2010, p. 396).

To ensure that these criteria were met, we required the involvement of a living donor advocate (LDA) or living donor advocate team (LDAT). The concept of an LDA(T) comes from the solid organ transplant setting (Rudow 2009; Hayes et al. 2015). It became a mandatory component of solid organ transplantation after several high profile deaths of living liver donors (Department of Health and Human Services, Centers for Medicare and Medicaid Services 2007). We argued that the inclusion of the LDA(T) in pediatric HSC transplantation would help ensure that the donor's well-being is considered independently and that the concerns and needs of the potential child donor are addressed. We argued for the inclusion for the LDA(T) from the onset—even before HLA testing is done (AAP 2010).

The first criterion requires that adults, who can consent for themselves, be considered as HSC donors before children. Now, again, the most likely HLA identical relative is a sibling but also other relatives are sometimes a 10/10 HLA-match. In the AAP statement, we considered whether all adults (parents, adult siblings or other adult biological relatives) should be HLA-tested and excluded based on histo-incompatibility before any minor siblings were HLA-tested, and decided against sequential testing because of the time urgency that an HSC transplant often involves. While we conceded that screening of potential children and adult donors should proceed simultaneously, we did argue in favor of selecting an adult over a child to be the HSC donor if both were 10/10 HLA-matches, all other things being equal. The AAP also considered whether a search of the international bone marrow registry which had over 6 million adult registrants at the time of the statement should be required before engaging child and adult family members. We argued no because of the time it takes, the greater possibility that a match may renege, and the possible benefits from additional minor histocompatibility antigens and because "it ignores the fact that authorization of a stem cell donation by a minor is within the proper realm of parental decisionmaking" (AAP 2010, 396, references omitted).

However, one point that we emphasized in the statement is that the decision to do HLA testing should not be seen as a simple blood test that can be done automatically, because the implications are anything but simple. The failure to consider the significance of HLA testing can be seen in the empirical data provided by the Lübeck team where the father of an almost 13 year old with myelodysplastic syndrome, whose 18 year old sister served as the donor, explained:

> F: YES, well (.) there was no discussion in any case that I can remember, but it was just clear that you have to do something for your (.) little sister and for your daughter.

(Minz, father, 28) 31 of 66

Similarly, the mother of a two year old child with acute myeloid leukemia (AML) whose 7 year old sister served as the donor is quoted as saying

> M: But also as part of the testing. It was just like, now the family will [go] first.
> I: Yes.
> M: You weren't asked. They just said, "Who wants to go first?" like. (laughs)
> I: Everyone line up.
> M: Yes, basically

(Kelling, family interview, 317–321

This lack of reflection about the significance of HLA-testing explains why it is critical to involve an LDA(T) independent from the team caring for the ill sibling from the time the idea of donation is being discussed—that is before HLA testing is performed. Once a family member (child or adult) is identified as a 10/10 HLA-match, it is hard for the individual (or family) to decide against that individual serving as an HSC donor. Parents and children describe being identified as a match as resulting in "no choice". The mother of a young child who required 2 bone marrow transplants from a sibling brother who was 9 and 10 at the time of the transplant explained:

> And because of that it was clear to me, without us having a massive discussion with Zorro, that Zorro WILL donate whether he wants to or not.
> (Zucker mother 26)

A 15 ½ year old sister who served as a donor for her younger brother explained:

> D: because then I got so much PRESSURE from (.) my parents: come on, and you have to do this, he's your brother after all and erm (.), if you don't do this, then erm (..), yes, then- you you won't forgive yourself for the rest of your LIFE and come on, just do it. And then at some point I'd been put under such emotional pressure that I just said: OK, you know what, (.) you're not going to give up anyway and I don't want afterwards to have to take responsibility, I didn't donate bone marrow to my brother, now – now you can go here and there and you can visit him, can't you.
> (Kunow, donor, 17)

That is, when a child's life is threatened and the health care providers recommend intrafamilial donation as the only or best option, if a potential donor is located within the family, the families feel compelled to move forward. This is why it is so important to engage an LDA(T) prior to HLA-testing. The LDA(T) engages with the potential donors, making sure that their needs, interests and concerns are expressed and addressed. The LDA(T) should also discuss that there may be alternatives (e.g., in the form of a stranger donation from one of the international HSC transplant registries or even a non-HSC treatment plan for the ill family member). Under extreme circumstances, the LDA(T) must be empowered to either delay or prevent a donation if the harms are so great as to overwhelm the potential family benefit (see criterion 5 below).

This sense of "no choice" can lead to disturbing situations. Consider for example the case described by Opel and Diekema (2006) in which a sibling is tested to be an HSC donor for a sibling who raped her. She is found to be an excellent HLA match and the mother then consents for her daughter (the rape victim) to be the donor to her son who is in jail for the assault. The girl, LR, undergoes only a cursory evaluation of her psychosocial and emotional well-being and an inadequate discussion about her willingness to serve as an HSC donor (she undergoes a single psychological evaluation that was done with her mother in the room). Ross and Glannon (2006) wrote that the first error was in HLA testing without a more complete discussion of whether the half-sister would be an appropriate donor if found to be HLA-compatible.

The second criterion states that the donor and recipient must have a positive relationship—this would exclude parents from seeking out siblings who are non-intimate (e.g., if they are genetically related but estranged due to adoption, donor gametes, or other social circumstances). For example, consider again the case of LR who served as HSC donor for her sibling who was in jail for raping her (Opel and Diekema, 2006). If this criterion had been in place, LR would not have undergone HLA typing. In the case of Curran v Bosze (1990), the judge ruled against HLA-typing due in part to non-intimacy. In this case, Mr. Tamas Bosze petitioned to have the twins he fathered with Ms. Nancy Curran to be HLA tested for potential HSC donation to a son born and raised by a different partner whom, he admitted, they barely knew. Ms. Curran, who had sole legal custody of their twins, objected to HLA testing as she stated she would not authorize the bone marrow procurement due to the risks to the twins even if they were a match for their half-brother. The Court sided with Ms. Curran. These cases influenced the AAP policy writers to argue for the need for a donor advocate (or a similar mechanism) for all child donors (except newborns donating umbilical stem cells) *prior* to HLA-testing (AAP 2010, p. 397).

The third criterion focuses on the likelihood that the recipient will benefit. Given the psychological trauma felt by the donor if the recipient dies (Butterworth et al. 1992; MacLeod et al. 2003)—even when the donor is a stranger (Billen et al. 2017; Wanner et al. 2009)—performing a HSC transplant should only be undertaken with a minor donor if there is a reasonable likelihood of success. Regardless of what the health care team or the parents say, the donors often blame themselves if the recipient dies or has serious complications like graft-versus-host disease [GVHD] (MacLeod et al., 2003). This sentiment was heard in interviews with several of the Lubeck donors: In the first example, the brother donated twice to his sibling--once at age 9 and again at age 10 years.

> I: So how was it actually for you, when you found out that (..) Zedrick became ill again even after the first donation?
> D: Erm I blamed myself, (4) because my bone marrow, or I thought, my bone marrow must be bad. (6)
> I: Did your parents say anything about this?
> D: No.
> (IM Zucker, donor, 309–312)

In this second example, the mother, then the sister and finally a stranger donated to a child with AML who subsequently died:

> D: of course that was another strange feeling, that (.) I first thought like this: now everyone is blaming me a bit (..), I'm to blame that my cells didn't manage it, but I really couldn't influence that.
> (IM Jaschke, donor, 82)

Finally, in this third example, a 15 ½ year old sister donated to her younger sister who subsequently died.

> I: At first it worked very well with the (.) with the transplant (.) and then there were problems in the end. How was THAT for you?
> D: That was (..) um, if I (.) put it in plainly: it was SHIT, (..) because erm, well for me it really wasn't good, because I then partly blamed myself, erm (.) that I'M to blame because in the end it was MY bone marrow that then erm (.) worked against his cells and destroyed them.
> (IM Kunow, donor, 84–85)

In the AAP statement, we suggested that the LDA(T) "should ensure that the likelihood of success is above some threshold to justify imposing the risks of donation on the minor sibling (AAP 2010, p. 397)." In order to avoid donor self-blame, we also stated what role the LDAT can play:

> The donor advocate should be involved from the onset, starting with the decision about whether the minor should undergo HLA testing. When older children and adolescents are being considered as hematopoietic stem cell donors, they should be included in all stages of the decision-making process to the extent that they are capable. Discussions that involve the potential minor donor must be developmentally appropriate. The psychological as well as medical aspects of the donation should be discussed in language that is understandable to the potential donor. Consistent with his or her capacity, the minor needs to be aware that the donated stem cells may not engraft or may fail after engraftment, the recipient may develop severe or even fatal complications of the transplant (e.g., GVHD), or the original disease may recur. The minor needs to be aware that the outcome is beyond his or her control (AAP 2010, p. 398 [references omitted]).

The fourth criterion requires minimizing the risks to the donor and ensuring that the risks to the donor and recipient are reasonable compared to the benefits to the donor and the recipient. Some of the psychological and emotional risks can be minimized by appropriate donor preparation. This does not always happen as seen by a quote from the mother of a 7 year old who donated to her 2 year old sister with AML:

> M: and then access was established and I just DIDN'T know. The doctor just said "OK, do you need anything else or shall we just get straight on with it". Like, oh God. And they hadn't prepared her for it, not properly I felt, that now she- and that was really bad for her, so she was afraid of falling asleep and it hurt and actually there was nothing in there but she's a child and there was still that feeling there was a needle in her.
> (Kelling, family interview, 327)

In our AAP statement, we suggested preparation could include "medical playacting, allowing them to ask questions, and by including them in the decision-making process to the extent of their ability" (AAP 2010, p. 397). A recent European study shows, however, that this is still not standard practice at all centers (Wiener et al. 2019).

The fifth criterion supports involving the child sibling in the decision making process when capable. And yet, the document also states that "the parents' consent alone may be sufficient, unless state law or institutional policy requires the minor's active assent (AAP 2010, p. 398)." In the AAP statement we discussed the importance of engaging the child even if his or her refusal could be overridden, and we explored under what circumstances it might be binding:

> a donor advocate should explore the reasons for the refusal and determine if further education and discussion can modify the minor's refusal. A child mental health professional and/ or an ethics consultant/ethics committee may also need to be involved to help clarify the child's concerns. The donor advocate, child mental health professional, ethics consultant, or ethics committee must have the authority to suspend or prohibit a donation if it is determined that the donation is likely to have a serious and sustained long-term adverse effect on the donor. The recipient should not begin myeloablative preparation for bone marrow infusion (conditioning) unless there is a clear decision to proceed with the donation (AAP 2010, pp. 398–9).

In the Lubeck study, two children did initially refuse but eventually donated because the parental pressure had been too great. It is unknown what would have happened had they persisted in their refusal. And yet, despite the fact that the children did not believe they could refuse, the children were glad to have been asked. Here is a 23 year old woman reflecting on her donation at age 5 ¾ years to her older brother (9 1/3 years at the time of transplant) for adrenoleukodystrophy:

> D: Then my parents also asked me, erm (..) I have to say I really don't know what (.) might have happened, (.) if I'd said no, whether my parents would have in any case decided or not for my brother, (.) but erm that was important at the time, to get my opinion on it and not simply to take decisions completely over my head. (.) I'm still OK with that (.).
> (Bahr, donor, 9)

In sum, parents can modestly thwart some of the interests and needs of the donor sibling for the benefit of the family provided that they do not sacrifice the child's basic interests and needs (Ross 1998, 2015). The transplant team should engage minors in discussions to the extent that the minors are able to participate, and minors should have an LDA(T) to provide them with a voice and support throughout the process.

12.4 The Importance of the Living Donor Advocate/Living Donor Advocate Team (LDA(T))

The requirement for an LDA(T) in the AAP policy statement was controversial in the US when first published, with concern expressed by some that it failed to respect parental autonomy and would delay, if not impede, life-saving stem cell transplants (Revera and Frangoul 2011; Joffe and Kodish 2011; Wells 2011). The criticisms were surprising because (1) Joffe had played a major role in writing the statement and only withdrew at the eleventh hour (Ross 2011); and Wells' institution had an advocacy program (Ross and Antommaria 2011). It is important to correct several inaccuracies stated by our critics. First, the intent of the LDA(T) was not to impede sibling donations, but only to ensure that the child was treated as a patient in his or her own right. Data that came out shortly after the statement was published showed that the majority of programs did not have separate teams for donors and recipients (for both children and adults) (O'Donnell et al. 2010). Furthermore, data from the US show that pediatric stem cell transplants have increased annually despite this recommendation. (Health Resources Service Administration n.d.). Second, although we asserted the importance of engaging the child in the process, we were clear that a child's refusal was generally not dispositive, but the reasons for the refusal should be explored and that in rare cases "it would not be appropriate for health care providers to permit a child to serve as a bone marrow donor, despite parental permission."(Ross 2011, p. 520).

Chan and Tipoe from The University of Hong Kong criticized the document from the other direction. First, they argued for the importance of the child's right to decide whether or not to participate and focused on Gillick competency. (Chan and Tipoe 2013). Second, they also criticized our policy to permit all potential donors to be HLA tested simultaneously and argued that "unless a recipient sibling will suffer from serious complications or die without the transplantation and no other medically equivalent donors are available, there is no moral or legal basis to violate the donor sibling's right to bodily integrity."(Chan and Tipoe, p. 1). I agree with their second criticism and in fact, the first criteria of the AAP policy clearly states that a child should only serve as a stem cell donor if: "there is no medically equivalent histo-compatible adult relative who is willing and able to donate". The AAP Committee on Bioethics was willing to allow HLA typing of minors and adults to be performed simultaneously only because in many cases, time is of the essence. In cases where this is not the case, (e.g. the use of transplant for non-malignant, not time-sensitive conditions), we would agree that adults should be tested first. But I strongly disagree with the first argument given by Chan and Tipoe. I do not believe that the minor child should have final authority in deciding whether or not to be a bone marrow donor for a sibling. As argued in the AAP statement it was the responsibility of the LDAT to decide whether the child's refusal had merit and then to override the parents (and not have the child be the one who decides to override the parent(s)). The importance of this distinction is clearly explained in Tim Henning's essay in this book (see Chap. 11. Deciding about Child Bone Marrow Donation—Procedural Moral Pitfalls). Professor Henning explains why it is morally "permissible for parent to make the donation decision for their children, not allowing them to decide the matter themselves." His argument is based on the moral need to protect the child and to avoid burdening the child in both the short- and long-term, with the weight of a present-day refusal to provide a possible life-saving donation: "it may be in the child's own interest (and in the interest of her later self) after all to suffer the surgery now rather than to have the burden of the decision on her shoulders now and in the future".

In the same year as the AAP statement was published, The World Marrow Donor Association (WMDA), which describes itself as "an international organization fostering collaboration in clinical transplantation and promoting the interests of unrelated stem cell donors", decided "that it is important to collaborate with those involved with family donors, to standardize the care" (Van Walraven et al., 2010, p. 1269). The WMDA published a document entitled: "Family donor care management: principles and recommendations)." Which stated that "[i]t is an important requirement that unrelated donors always have a specified independent donor advocate …Independent donor assessment is equally necessary for family donors (Van Walraven et al. 2010, p. 1270). The document was even more adamant about the importance of the LDA(T) when the donor is a child (Van Walraven et al. 2010, p. 1270). In its more recent statement in 2016, the WMDA argued in favor of separate teams for stem cell donors and recipients, whether the donor was a child or adult, and regardless of the relationship. (Bitan et al. 2016, pp. 97–98). The WMDA supported our idea of a donor advocate for minor donors but disagreed with our wording of condition # 2, that there be a "strong personal and positive relationship, or in the case of directed cord blood transplant, that a strong personal and positive relationship has to be anticipated". The WMDA proposed to modify this criteria to ensure the avoidance of psychological harm" (Bitan et al. 2016, p. 98). They concluded: "All siblings should be screened for seriously negative relationships as they go through the donation screening process, preferably before HLA typing as well." (Bitan et al. 2016, p. 98). Given that the WMDA interprets a non-relationship (as was seen in the case of Curran v. Bosze) as a negative relationship, our conclusions are virtually identical.

In sum, then, there is broad consensus of the need for an LDA(T) for child sibling donors.

Why do I digress to discuss the living donor advocate? While situations in which a minor's refusal to serve as an HSC will be (and should be) uncommon, a minor's refusal should alert the transplant team that the presumption of parental authority must be questioned and the LDA(T) must evaluate the appropriateness of compelling the child to donate. The decision not to permit a sibling stem cell donation will be (and should be) rare. I have no reason to believe that an LDA(T) would have sought to delay or reject any of the donors in the Lubeck study, but I would encourage all stem cell and bone marrow transplant programs to adopt this requirement.

12.5 Concluding Remarks

Buchanan and Brock's framework for pediatric decision making requires third party intervention for HSC donation to ensure that the child donor is treated as a patient and respected as a person who has needs and interest of his or her own. An LDA(T) is an appropriate third party mechanism for intervention in HSC transplantation involving minor donor children. The AAP guidelines provide a set of criteria that, if followed, can help establish the boundaries of ethical HSC transplantation involving a minor donor sibling.

The family is a valuable institution and parents have broad (but not infinite) discretion on how they raise their children and the health care decisions they make on their behalf. The case of HSC donation by a minor for his or her sibling helps clarify the guidance principle to which parents are held and the proper scope and forms of intervention that limit parental decision making.

Acknowledgements This chapter was funded in part by a National Library of Medicine grant: (NLM) G13LM013003. Sibling Obligations in Health Care.

Literature

American Academy of Pediatrics Committee on Bioethics. 2010. Policy statement: Children as hematopoietic stem cell donors. *Pediatrics* 125 (2): 392–404.

American College of Obstetricians and Gynecologists (ACOG) Committee on Genetics and ACOG Committee on Obstetric Practice. 2009. ACOG Committee opinion no. 771. Umbilical cord blood banking. *Obstetrics and Gynecology* 133 (3): e249–e253.

Billen, Annelies, J. Alejandro Madrigal, Katrina Scior, Bronwen E. Shaw, and Andre Strydom. 2017. Donation of peripheral blood stem cells to unrelated strangers: A thematic analysis. *PLoS ONE* 12 (10): e0186438. https://doi.org/10.1371/journal.pone.0186438.

Bitan, Menachem, Suzanna M. van Walraven, Nina Worel, et al. 2016. Determination of eligibility in related pediatric hematopoietic cell donors: Ethical and clinical considerations. Recommendations from a working group of the worldwide network for blood and marrow transplantation association. *Biology of Blood and Marrow Transplantation* 22 (1): 96–103.

Bosi, Alberto, and B. Bartolozzi. 2010. Safety of bone marrow stem cell donation: A review. *Transplantation Proceedings* 42 (6): 2192–2194.

British Medical Association: 5. Best interests. Last updated: 28 February 2019. https://www.bma.org.uk/advice/employment/ethics/children-and-young-people/children-and-young-peoples-ethics-tool-kit/5-best-interests

Buchanan, Allen E., and Daniel W. Brock. 1990. *Deciding for others: The ethics of surrogate decision making.* New York: Cambridge University Press.

Butterworth, Victoria A., Roberta G. Simmons, and Mindy Schimmel. 1992-3. When altruism fails: Reactions of unrelated bone marrow donors when the recipient dies. *Omega* 26(3):161–173.

Canadian Paediatric Society. 2004. Treatment decisions regarding infants, children and adolescents. *Paediatrics and Child Health* 9 (2): 99–103.

Center for International Blood and Marrow Transplant Research. n.d. *Transplant activity report covering 2013-2017 and reported as of December 2018.* On the web at: https://bloodstemcell.hrsa.gov/data/donation-and-transplantation-statistics/transplant-activity-report#summary

Chan, Tak Kwong, and George Lim Tipoe. 2013. The policy statement of the American Academy of Pediatrics – Children as hematopoietic stem cell donors – A proposal of modifications for application in the UK. *BMC Medical Ethics* 14: 43. https://doi.org/10.1186/1472-6939-14-43.

Chang, Irene. 1991. Baby girl's bone marrow transplanted into sister: Health: Parents conceived the child in an attempt to provide a donor for leukemia-stricken sibling. *The Los Angeles Times.* June 5, 1991. On the web at: https://www.latimes.com/archives/la-xpm-1991-06-05-mn-212-story.html

Curran v Bosze, 566 NE 2d 1319 (Ill 1990)

Department of Health and Human Services, Centers for Medicare and Medicaid Services. 2007, March 30. Medicare program; hospital conditions of participation: Requirements for approval and re-approval of transplant centers to perform organ transplants. Final rule. Federal Register 72(61): 15197–15280

Diekema, Douglas S. 2004. Parental refusals of medical treatment: The harm principle as threshold for state intervention. *Theoretical Medicine* 25 (4): 243–264.

———. 2011. Revising the best interest standard: Uses and misuses. *The Journal of Clinical Ethics* 22 (2): 128–133.

Gillam, Lynn. 2016. The zone of parental discretion: An ethical tool for dealing with disagreement between parents and doctors about medical treatment for a child. *Clinical Ethics* 11: 1–8.

Hayes, Rebecca E., D. LaPointe Rudow, M.A. Dew, et al. 2015. The independent living donor advocate: A guidance document from the American Society of Transplantation's Living Donor Community of Practice (AST LDCOP). *American Journal of Transplantation* 15 (2): 518–525.

Health Resources and Services Administration. n.d. Transplant Activity Report. On the web at: https://bloodstemcell.hrsa.gov/data/donation-and-transplantation-statistics/transplant-activity-report#year.

Joffe, Steven, and Eric Kodish. 2011. Protecting the rights and interests of pediatric stem cell donors. *Pediatric Blood & Cancer* 56 (4): 517–519.

Katz, Aviva L., Sally A. Webb, and The American Academy of Pediatrics Committee on Bioethics. 2016. Informed consent in decision-making in pediatric practice. *Pediatrics* 138 (2): pii:e20161485. https://doi.org/10.1542/peds.2016-1485.

Khandelwal, Pooja, Heather R. Millard, Elizabeth Thiel, et al. 2017. hematopoietic stem cell transplantation activity in pediatric cancer between 2008 and 2014 in the United States: A center for international blood and marrow transplant research report. *Biology of Blood and Marrow Transplantation* 23 (8): 1342–1349.

Larcher, Vic, Finella Craig, Kiran Bhogal, Dominic Wilkinson, Joe Brierley, and on behalf of the Royal College of Paediatrics and Child Health (RCPCH). 2015. Making decisions to limit treatment in life-limiting and life-threatening conditions in children: A framework for practice. *Archives of Diseases in Childhood* 100 (Suppl. 2): s1–s26.

Locatelli, Franco. 2009. Improving cord blood transplantation in children. *British Journal of Haematology* 147 (2): 217–226.

MacLeod, Kendra D., Stan F. Whitsett, Eric J. Mash, and Wendy Pelletier. 2003. Pediatric sibling donors of successful and unsuccessful hematopoietic stem cell transplants (HSCT): A qualitative study of their psychosocial experience. *Journal of Pediatric Psychology* 28 (4): 223–231.

O'Donnell, Paul V., Tanya L. Pedersen, Dennis L. Confer, on behalf of the Donor Health and Safety Working Committee from the Center for International Blood and Marrow Transplant Research (CIBMTR), et al. 2010. Practice patterns for evaluation, consent, and care of related donors and recipients at hematopoietic cell transplantation centers in the United States. *Blood* 115 (24): 5097–5101.

Opel, Douglas J., and Douglas S. Diekema. 2006. The case of A.R.: The ethics of sibling donor bone marrow transplantation revisited. *Journal of Clinical Ethics* 17 (3): 207–219.

Packman, Wendy L., Mary R. Crittenden, Evonne Schaeffer, et al. 1997. Psychosocial consequences of bone marrow transplantation in donor and nondonor siblings. *Journal of Developmental & Behavioral Pediatrics* 18 (4): 244–253.

Packman, Wendy L., S. Weber, J. Wallace, and N. Bugescu. 2010. Psychological effects of hematopoietic SCT on pediatric patients, siblings and parents: A review. *Bone Marrow Transplantation* 45 (7): 1134–1146.

Pentz, Rebecca D., Melissa A. Alderfer, Wendy Pelletier, et al. 2014. Unmet needs of siblings of pediatric stem cell transplant recipients. *Pediatrics* 133 (5): e1156–e1162.

Pulsipher, Michael A., Arnon Nagler, Robert Iannone, and Robert M. Nelson. 2005. Weighing the risks of G-CSF administration, Leukopheresis, and standard marrow harvest: Ethical and safety considerations for normal pediatric hematopoietic cell donors. *Pediatric Blood and Cancer* 46 (4): 422–433.

Revera, Greg, and Haydar Frangoul. 2011. Comment on the American Academy of Pediatrics Policy statement – Children as hematopoietic stem cell donors: A parent's point of view. *Pediatric Blood & Cancer* 56 (4): 515–516.

Ross, Lainie Friedman. 1998. *Children, families and health care decision making*. Oxford: Oxford University Press/Clarendon Press.

———. 2011. In defense of the American Academy of Pediatrics policy statement – Children as hematopoietic stem cell donors. *Pediatric Blood & Cancer.* 56 (4): 520–523.

———. 2015. Theory and practice of pediatric bioethics. Special symposium issue: The interface of child rights and pediatric bioethics in the clinical setting. *Perspectives in Biology and Medicine* 58 (3): 267–280.

———. 2019. Better than best (interest standard) in pediatric decision making. *Journal of Clinical Ethics* 30 (2): 183–195.

———. 2020. Reflections on Charlie Gard and the best interests standard from both sides of the Atlantic Ocean. *Pediatrics* 146 (Suppl 1): S61–S65.

Ross, Lainie Friedman, and Armand H. Matheny Antommaria. 2011. Letter to the editor: In Further Defense of the American Academy of Pediatrics Committee on bioethics "children as hematopoietic stem cell donors" statement. *Pediatric Blood & Cancer* 57 (6): 1088–1089.

Ross, Lainie Friedman, and Walter Glannon. 2006. A compounding of errors: The case of bone marrow donation between non-intimate siblings. *Journal of Clinical Ethics* 17 (3): 220–226.

Royal College of Physicians and Surgeons of Canada, Bioethics. Section 1: medical decision making. 1.5.1 Medical Decision-Making and Children. Samantha Brennan, PhD. Updated December 11, 2013. http://www.royalcollege.ca/rcsite/bioethics/cases/section-1/medical-decision-making-children-e

Rudow, Dianne LaPointe. 2009. The living donor advocate: A team approach to educate, evaluate, and manage donors across the continuum. *Progress in Transplantation* 19 (1): 64–70.

Shaw, B.E., D.L. Confer, William Hwang, and Michael A. Pulsipher. 2015. A review of the genetic and long-term effects of G-CSF injections in healthy donors: A reassuring lack of evidence for the development of haematological malignancies. *Bone Marrow Transplantation* 50 (3): 334–340.

Styzcynski, Jan, Adriana Balduzzi, Lidia Gil, on behalf of the European Group for Blood and Marrow Transplantation Pediatric Diseases Working Party, et al. 2012. Risk of complications during hematopoietic stem cell collection in pediatric sibling donors: A prospective European Group for Blood and Marrow Transplantation Pediatric Diseases Working Party study. *Blood* 119 (12): 2935–2942.

Switzer, Galen E., Jessica Bruce, Gabrielle Pastorek, et al. 2017. Parent versus child donor perceptions of the bone marrow donation experience. *Bone Marrow Transplantation* 52 (9): 1338–1341.

Talano, Julie-An M., Michael A. Pulsipher, Heather J. Symons, et al. 2014. New frontiers in pediatric allogeneic stem cell transplantation. *Bone Marrow Transplantation* 49 (9): 1139–1145.

United Nations (UN). 1989. Convention on the rights of the child. 1577 UNTS 3.

Van Walraven, S.M., G. Nicoloso-de Faveri, U.A.I. Axdorph-Nygell, on behalf of the WMDA Ethics and Clinical working groups, et al. 2010. Family donor care management: Principles and recommendations. *Bone Marrow Transplantation* 45 (8): 1269–1273.

Wanner, Martina, Sandra Bochert, Iris M. Schreyer, Gabi Rall, Claudia Rutt, and Alexander H. Schmidt. 2009. Losing the genetic twin: Donor grief after unsuccessful unrelated stem cell. BMC Health Services Research 9:2. https://doi.org/10.1186/1472-6963-9-2. On the web at: http://www.biomedcentral.com/1472-6963/9/2

Weise, Kathryn L., Alexander L. Okun, Brian S. Carter, Cindy W. Christian, and on behalf of the American Academy of Pediatrics Committee on Bioethics, Section on Hospice and Palliative Medicine, Committee on Child Abuse and Neglect. 2017. Guidance on forgoing life-sustaining medical treatment. *Pediatrics* 140 (3). https://doi.org/10.1542/peds.2017-1905.

Wells, Robert J. 2011. The American Academy of Pediatrics Policy statement: Children as hematopoietic stem cell donors. *Pediatric Blood & Cancer* 57 (6): 1086–1087.

Wiener, Lori S., Emilie Steffen-Smith, Terry Fry, and Alan S. Wayne. 2007. Hematopoietic stem cell donation in children: a review of the sibling donor experience. *Journal of Psychosocial Oncology* 25 (1): 45–66.

Wiener, Lori, Jennifer A. Hoag, Wendy Pelletier, et al. 2019. Transplant center practices for psychosocial assessment and management of pediatric hematopoietic stem cell donors. *Bone Marrow Transplantation* 54 (11): 1780–1788.

Winnicott, Donald W. 1953. Transitional objects and transitional phenomena. *International Journal of Psychoanalysis* 34: 89–97.

Open Access   This chapter is licensed under the terms of the Creative Commons Attribution 4.0 International License (http://creativecommons.org/licenses/by/4.0/), which permits use, sharing, adaptation, distribution and reproduction in any medium or format, as long as you give appropriate credit to the original author(s) and the source, provide a link to the Creative Commons license and indicate if changes were made.

The images or other third party material in this chapter are included in the chapter's Creative Commons license, unless indicated otherwise in a credit line to the material. If material is not included in the chapter's Creative Commons license and your intended use is not permitted by statutory regulation or exceeds the permitted use, you will need to obtain permission directly from the copyright holder.

Part V
Constructing Familial Bodies

Chapter 13
Constructing Familial Bodies: Report from the Qualitative Interview Study

Martina Jürgensen and Madeleine Herzog

Abstract After a bone marrow transplant between siblings, another family members' cells live on in the recipient's body. This connects family members in a variety of ways. Some families saw it as an essential change in the recipient's body and identity, while others saw it as a unification of two separate individuals. Some families described the donor's body as a "spare parts depot"; being seen as a life-saving resource then created a lasting responsibility in the donors. This relation was typically seen as creating one system, one familial body.

Keywords Transplantation medicie · Body boundaries · Exchange of body materials · Familiar bodies

This part of the book deals with the meanings of stem-cell transplants that relate to the fact that another's body material lives in the recipient. Transplantation medicine transcends body boundaries by connecting bodies that are compatible with each other through the exchange of body materials. In doing so, it correlates people and their bodies in a specific way, creating new material and social relationships between them. When body parts (tissues, cells) become a treatment for another family member, how does it affect ideas of being "whole" and "integral", for both the individual and the family? Can the family itself be seen as a "body"?

In the cases we encountered in our family study, the sick children were treated with the body materials of their siblings. This is a medical therapy that, in the experience of the participants of this study, had a very different connotation and symbolic meaning than using chemical medications. Most families were happy that the "problem" – the disease – could be solved from within the family. Yet others reported feelings of unease about the exchange of body materials both in general and within the family.

M. Jürgensen (✉) · M. Herzog
Institute for History of Medicine and Science Studies, University of Lübeck,
Lübeck, Schleswig-Holstein, Germany
e-mail: martina.juergensen@uni-luebeck.de

© The Author(s) 2022
C. Schües et al. (eds.), *Stem Cell Transplantations Between Siblings as Social Phenomena*, Philosophy and Medicine 144,
https://doi.org/10.1007/978-3-031-04166-2_13

The act of transplantation and its consequences for the body of the recipient child generated many ideas, images and notions in the families' narratives. For most families, the bone marrow/body material which "heals" the sick child was associated with images and ideas about transplantation and the transplant that go beyond the idea of a drug.

Injecting the bone marrow intravenously into the sick child's body, for example, was described by most families as the turning point, the moment of rebirth and new life – provided the BMT worked out and the child survived. In the two families of our study in which the sick child had died, the BMT was viewed differently, and the treatment of a sick child with heterologous body materials from a sibling was not seen as solely positive.

Furthermore, knowing the donor's gender, looks and personality opened up a space in the recipient's imagination for speculations about perceived changes in character or in gender-assigned behaviour. Bone marrow does not seem to be an impersonal or characterless medication, but for many families in this study carried a symbolic and character-giving meaning. Many families refer to the day of the transplant as a second birthday.

On the other hand, the transfer of body material also has some frightening scary aspects.

> Non-donor sister: that was kind of funny, to know that the cells are taken out of one of them and PLANTED into the other one, let's say. It was a bit spooky. (Rohde)

13.1 Incorporation of Another's Body Substances

13.1.1 Seen as a Change of Nature or as Unification?

In relation to this, the first thing that stands out from the interviews was that respondents found it very difficult to think about or to put into words the "physicality" of the transplant process. The first spontaneous answer to a question about the subjective meaning of the transfer of body material was often that it does not matter to them and that they do not think about it.

However, most family members also remembered what they have seen in crime films, that after a bone marrow transplant the blood DNA of donor and recipient match and that this can be problematic. In many families the topic of bodily exchange was addressed only in the form of jokes: *"there goes your bone marrow!"*

What was often brought up often is the notion that the two siblings involved, donor and recipient, were particularly strongly connected, in some narratives even before the transplant, such that the similarity was seen as a marker for a suitable donation, in other families just as a result of the bone marrow transplant.

In some families, changes on a physical and behavioural level in the recipient child were connected to the transplantation. For example, one recipient powerfully described how he has become like his brother after the transplant of his brother's blood stem cells, even developing the same hobbies.

It is noticeable that the idea of a physical and psychological "approximation" of the recipient to the donor emerges particularly frequently in those families where the donation was between children of the opposite sex. This may indicate that the transfer of body materials activates ideas about the bodily basis of human nature – and thus also latent fears about how a human character could be affected by the transfer of body material from one to another. Parents from two families claimed that their son became significantly "softer" and "more feminine" after his sister's stem cells were transplanted – and attributed this directly to the transplanted material and not to the experience of the disease or the new situation as a whole.

> Father: and after the illness erm or (coughs) or after this whole story, I always said, "bloody hell", I say, now, he got very different hair. His hair became different and his whole nature, I say, "now you're becoming a girl!" "Shut up you arsehole!" he says, "are you actually completely bonkers?" Because suddenly he got such fine, he got such fine hands. Before, he was a blacksmith, I should say, he had erm (sniffs) wh- wh-when I was tinkering with the car, he also had to tinker with something and make and do something and then he became quite, then he became quite different. I mean he he had a fine-manual thing, he assembled things and erm. He was a Lego Star Wars fan. (Kunow)

Several families also emphasized that there was a similarity between the siblings on a physical level. But most families also made it clear that they rejected the idea that the recipient would take on the physical or behavioural characteristics of the donor through the donation – which nevertheless does not mean that they did not care about this point.

> Donor: Sometimes I have moments when I (.) when I - when when it becomes so CLEAR to me or when I suddenly realise that I am actually in my sister. And then erm then I also ask myself how much of ME is now in her or somehow? Does it now have different effects, I mean not just on her blood, erm but also somehow on her herself or on her personality or something, but I mean it's actually not the case, those are actually – it's just her immune system (laughs), but then I really do sometimes ask myself like that (..), I mean, I think it's, perhaps it also contributed to some special bond with my sister. I mean at that time I did feel somehow very attached to her, because I knew that we are so much the same and then that [part] of me that is in HER, I mean that was somehow (..), I mean I ask myself, yes, that's a very strange feeling somehow and (..) yes (..) yes. (Rohde)

13.1.2 *"Spare Parts Depot" (Ersatzteillager)*

Being used as a "means to the end" of serving the sick sibling with their own body was mentioned by several of our study participants. This touches on issues of physical integrity, of family responsibility and its limits, and in particular of who owns bodies and who has the authority to dispose of (children's) bodies.

In this context "spare parts depot" (Ersatzteillager) is a resonant term that was brought up by a few interviewees. The notion generates questions about whether and how long the donors must keep themselves ready for further donations, be it stem cells or other body materials. Some donors never questioned the need to be ready to donate to their sibling, others reported feeling used and exploited in the process of the bone marrow transplant.

Donor: so I remember that time with the with the glands (..), that THEN for the first time ever this thought CAME to me, that now I – if I now was a (.), like at some point I expressed it really badly, whether I was now a SPARE PARTS DEPOT for him. Erm ah like NO, exactly, there was once this this thing with the glands, when I had these thoughts, whether it's like that or not, and maybe if it is, then that's OK if that's the way it is. (Wahl)

Being seen as a life-saving resource created a lasting responsibility for the donors as family members, including keeping their body available for future "donations".

13.2 Transplantation: Concepts, Metaphors, Ideas

When speaking about the transplant, many families used vivid metaphors and comparisons, symbolizing the transformative act of the BMT: rebirth and new life were recurring characterizations in this context. Some families viewed the transplant as a "spiritual moment".

13.2.1 Question of "Sameness" and "Otherness"

Looking more deeply into the interviews it became clear that the question of personal uniqueness, "sameness" and "otherness" played a role in the thoughts of the study participants.

According to the interviews, most families had not previously thought about this topic: they responded to our question with great surprise, and emphasized that they had never thought so before, but that it was an interesting question.

For some families, the bone marrow is interpreted only as a kind of drug that was given to the recipient's body. There it becomes a part of this body. In these cases the recipient's personal integrity and uniqueness is not challenged or damaged. Other families however articulated ideas and images that indicate they see the recipient's personal uniqueness as changed because of the transplant. Interestingly, they generally saw no danger in this. With only one exception (father Kötter), most families saw it rather as a positive and unifying thing.

13.2.2 Family as a Body: One System

We have already described how the donation of bone marrow was seen as a "matter of course" in families. To be a part of a family system entails special duties, tasks and benefits which, in the view of the families we studied, included the donation of bone marrow.

A distinctive feature of families is that the members are usually connected by a generative aspect, physically related to each other. Apart from socialization, family members share features of their bodies and genetic configurations – a fact that is used in the search for a donor.

These similarities in genetic makeup go together with the psychological and social dimension of the family system and strengthen the family as a unique unit. Finding a donor within the family affirms the feeling of shared strength, as the family is able to solve its problems by their own means. Many families in our study emphasized how proud this made them. Knowing who the donor is and the fact that they were so close to the recipient child seemed to be comforting, whereas the idea of an unrelated-donor had connotations of bringing something alien into the family.

The view that the donation was a natural thing to do was based on the idea of a family as one body. From that point of view, the family was seen as a single system in which the individual parts work together hand in hand.

> Donor: even if you think it maybe sounds a bit odd but I KNOW who that person is, a BIT of whom my brother is carrying around in him and (…) I don't know. Maybe that might have changed more of his character of it if you knew that it was a stranger like in- in the place of my brother, so that it was a stranger- or an unconnected part and whether that maybe would have changed something for him or for someone in the family. (Bahr)

13.2.3 Inscribing Family History in the Body: Tattoos

To our surprise several family members – donors, recipients, parents, and non-donor siblings – revealed that they tattooed the memory of the bone marrow transplantation onto the skin of their body using symbols, dates and words. With this act of inscription others become aware of a certain importance assigned to the bone marrow transplant, making it something that happens not only in a hidden, interior place but that is also visible to others on the outer surface of the body.

It is interesting that the tattoos were not just personal, individual tattoos, but that often a community act emerges from them: in several families, siblings devised a motif that they shared and that served as a sign of their solidarity and shared history. In their accounts of this it became clear that for these families, the illness of one child and the transplantation of blood stem cells from a sibling were deeply relevant family experiences for the long term.

> Interviewer: And you really thought of the tattoo together?
> Recipient: Exactly, then there was the idea that in the meantime we had grown together SO strongly as siblings that we would like to record that in some way and a tattoo offers that, because it lasts a lifetime. Erm, then we thought about, yes, a sibling tattoo is simple, I think, it's something very good, that would connect us even, even more closely and then we thought of what motif we could have, something that all three of us like very much erm the three of us like so much that we want to have it. That somehow [connects] us to one another or that marks us out, that connects us to one another and without necessarily [focussing] on this story erm of the illness erm, yes without putting the focus on that, we nevertheless came up with this date and then we jointly decided that that was simply THE most important, or one of the most important things that determined our life and that we wanted to record, exactly. (Speidel)

Open Access   This chapter is licensed under the terms of the Creative Commons Attribution 4.0 International License (http://creativecommons.org/licenses/by/4.0/), which permits use, sharing, adaptation, distribution and reproduction in any medium or format, as long as you give appropriate credit to the original author(s) and the source, provide a link to the Creative Commons license and indicate if changes were made.

The images or other third party material in this chapter are included in the chapter's Creative Commons license, unless indicated otherwise in a credit line to the material. If material is not included in the chapter's Creative Commons license and your intended use is not permitted by statutory regulation or exceeds the permitted use, you will need to obtain permission directly from the copyright holder.

Chapter 14
Stem Cell Transplantation, Microchimerism and Assemblages

Margrit Shildrick

Abstract The exploration of stem cell transplantation (SCT), especially as a socially situated phenomenon, demands a combination of empirical, biological and bioethical insights. Questions of identity, of gifting, and of mortality abound, and in kin SCT where the whole process happens within the complex relationships of a single unit, the intertwined impact on lived experience is highly concentrated. In looking at everything involved in the understanding of SCT – the biomedical procedure, the individual and collective experiences of the family, the data collected, the expertise and expectations of the researchers, and the varying analyses applied – what emerges, building on a Deleuzian framework, is a knowledge assemblage.

Keywords Biophilosophy · Deleuze · Assemblage · Hybridity · Microchimerism · Self-identity · Immunology

In the discussion of matters pertaining to stem cell transplantation (SCT), especially as a socially situated phenomenon, it is always necessary to abandon a singular perspective in favour of bringing empirical, biological and bioethical insights into conversation. In crossing the boundaries between those familiar forms of enquiry, I want to explore and reflect on some recent concerns in the realm of biophilosophy. My own approach to SCT is solidly related to my involvement in a collaborative heart transplantation project that sprang from my identification as a body theorist with a strong commitment to postconventional philosophy and critical cultural theory. Solid organ grafts are materially very different to bone marrow transplants but there is considerable overlap in the phenomenological aspects of the procedure as it differentially affects recipients, donors, and families alike. Questions of identity, of gifting, and of mortality abound, and in kin SCT where the whole process happens

M. Shildrick (✉)
Department of Ethnology, History of Religions and Gender Studies, Stockholm University, Stockholm, Sweden
e-mail: margrit.shildrick@gender.su.se

© The Author(s) 2022
C. Schües et al. (eds.), *Stem Cell Transplantations Between Siblings as Social Phenomena*, Philosophy and Medicine 144,
https://doi.org/10.1007/978-3-031-04166-2_14

within the complex relationships of a single unit, the intertwined impact on lived experience is highly concentrated.

A great deal of empirical research is already to hand around the topic of transplantation – though not so much in relation to SCT – both in strictly biomedical texts that have little place for speculation on the implications of the results and in the social sciences, which are generally more open to providing a theoretical approach to research data. But beyond that, the systematic enquiry into reported lived experience requires, I think, a philosophical approach to complement the sociological and biomedical material. Rather than relying on an additive model to produce new knowledge, what is required is a mode of analysis that intends to interweave many areas of expertise – social, biomedical, legal, psychological – with diverse methodologies that reflect the complexity of the object of enquiry,[1] in this case SCT involving siblings. In looking at everything involved in the understanding of SCT – the biomedical procedure, the individual and collective experiences of the family, the data collected, the expertise and expectations of the researchers, and the varying analyses applied – what emerges is a knowledge assemblage. That term reflects my own methodological approach in this chapter and views the significance of transplantation itself through the framework of Deleuzian assemblage.[2]

Like heart transplantation, the event of a bone marrow transplant – which is the main form of stem cell transplant under consideration here – speaks to a radical encounter between self and other, and is the site where the conventional boundaries of what constitutes a singular self are deeply problematised. In the case of living kin donation, with which the umbrella project on SCT and the child's well-being is concerned, the collision of life and death is less prominent than it might be in other scenarios, but nevertheless provides the underlying motivator for action. What I want to focus on is that in the experience of stem cell transplant, the relation of self to other is no longer binary but also reflects an irreducible intertwining that produces a somewhat unstable sense of self for both recipient and donor. At very least, and whatever the empirical connection between the two, the procedure and its aftermath is shot through with some ontological uncertainty. For recipients of donor stem cells, the lived experience arouses complex emotions, not only about the relation between self and the other, but also about the presence of the other within the self. In a powerful way it is a relationship of hybridity, or even spectrality in the philosophical sense intended by Jacques Derrida.[3] Of course any exercise in life-saving procedure, which SCT may be, raises awareness of personal mortality,

---

[1] See 'Messy Entanglements' (Shildrick et al. 2018).

[2] Briefly, the term refers to an epistemological and ontological tool developed by the postmodernist philosopher, Gilles Deleuze, initially together with Félix Guattari. Assemblage theory provides a way of understanding social relations and being-in-the-world through a dynamic nexus of interconnections between human beings, other living beings, technologies, events, expressions and so on. There is no fixed point in an assemblage but rather constant fluidity, interchangeability, and heterogeneous forms of capacity. See Deleuze and Guattari (1987).

[3] See Derrida's exposition in *Spectres of Marx* (1994), which lends itself to the implementation of spectrality in many different guises.

insofar as biotechnologies increasingly intervene into terminal conditions that once seemed natural and inevitable. As with other types of transplantation, success in averting death is relatively high, so that the hope for better health and prolonged life is soundly based, albeit living on is not as unproblematic as might be expected. Both recipients and their sibling donors may be significantly disturbed by the procedure, but are afforded little opportunity to explore and try to make sense of any negative emotions that they may experience. As some of the project transcripts make clear, this seems particularly to be the case in the context of intra-familial donation, where the well-being of the family as a unit may be privileged above individual disturbance.[4] Given, moreover, that the transaction is between siblings, the majority of whom were children at the time, the imposition of a unified narrative of hope might be even harder to resist.

> F: [T]hat what's nice about the whole thing, that a family like that can solve something like this, these problems. (Kötter, father, 130)

Stem cell donation rightly generates public debate around questions of consent and the exploitation of so-called spare parts, but what are given far less time are the wider ethical and philosophical implications of incorporating another's genetic material. Based on my own participation in a multi-dimensional research project on heart transplantation – The Process of Incorporating a Transplanted Heart (PITH)[5] – I believe those aspects should be a site of specific attention and perhaps merit primary concern, particularly in the context of the emergent understanding of the phenomenon of microchimerism, which I will go on to explore in detail. There is little doubt that all organic transfer is symbolically complex, such that stem cell donation – like other forms – swiftly moves beyond the functional repair or spare parts metaphor and may seem to constitute the gift of life (though few of the respondents in the SCT project explicitly referred to the transfer as such). Nonetheless, the seemingly laudable metaphor of the gift frequently underlies family understanding of the process, but it raises its own problems and specifically amplifies the potential disturbance to the relation between self and other. Moreover, unlike the case of deceased organ donation – as with heart transplantation – where the spare parts discourse is positively encouraged as less disturbing, in scenarios where there are

---

[4] The interchange between a donor and her mother in the Bahr family interview spells out the pressure:

> D: I still think it was right, but (…) for me as a child I was still aware: if I don't do this, //I'm to blame//

> M: //Exactly, if Björn dies, exactly//. (450–455)

Many parents determined to push ahead with familial donation and simply overrode their children's hesitations. (See also Kunow donor, 17; Rodhe father, 66–68; Jaschke, mother, 100; Preuss, father, 47.)

[5] The PITH (The Process of Incorporating a Transplanted Heart) project [REB # 07-0822-BE] was established in Canada in 2008; the GOLA (Gifting Life: Exploring donor families' embodied responses to anonymous organ donation in Canada) project followed on in 2014.

living familial donors – as in SCT – the reverse is true and the notion is silenced as being highly insensitive. But whichever the type under consideration, few of those intimately involved feel the transaction to be a simple replacement of faulty components for better-working ones. Far from being a neutral and depersonalised procedure, or even the expression of disinterested altruism, the organic material takes on the sense of a real and symbolic gift that binds the giver and receiver together in an economy of exchange. Respondents do not need to be familiar with Marcel Mauss' theory of the gift (1990) to recognise that the transplanted object carries with it intangible aspects of the other and expectations of reciprocity. The often burdensome but usually inexpressible relation between the two parties centres on the discourse of having been given something precious, the acceptance of which generates certain supposed obligations to the donor.

At the same time, the relation between recipient and donor is more or less existentially loaded in terms of personal identity, as is plainly exemplified in many of the SCT transcripts. The Wahl family mother remarks of her recipient son: "it is something (…) something (…) VERY existential and important for him, that it's also from his SISTER, because actually he is very attached to her and even more because of this" (65), while the Rohde donor reflects: "now my sister is (*laughs*), yes, the same as me, how stupid, now I'm no longer unique or something" (102). In the field of heart transplantation, very few of the respondents gave extravagant accounts of felt changes to their sense of personhood, but many felt themselves to be no longer the people they had previously been, in tastes, temperament or behaviour. The researchers in the stem cell study suggest that it is having a close knowledge of the donor – who is after all a sibling relation – that generates such disturbing reflections, but research in the wider field of organ donation shows that complete anonymity is no bar to speculation about hybrid identities (Kaba et al. 2005; Poole et al. 2009). The ontological question 'Who am I now?' is a central concern in either case. Although the degree of palpable distress expressed by heart recipients in their newly embodied states was more strongly evident (Poole et al. 2009), it is clear that many stem cell recipients too felt themselves now entangled with the donors beyond the level usually expected of siblings. Certainly there were deep feelings of obligation, or perhaps even guilt in that the prolongation of their own lives depended on not just generosity but the potential discomfort and anxiety endured by very specific others, but it is the intimation of shared attributes that is the most remarkable. In the Spiedal family mother's account: "it was like this, he [the recipient] gets his brother's blood, so he BECOMES his brother" (26), while the recipient himself confirms her view: "I mean, I dunno, it's just a feeling, you've got your brother's blood actually IN you. Like and, mh, yes, it's FUNNY to describe. It's as if you were linked even more closely than you would be anyway" (31–32).

The empirical findings from the SCT study interviews reiterate that the experience of bone marrow transplantation can indeed invoke an unfamiliar sense of hybridity. The initial understanding of that disturbance relies on the phenomenological claim that as the self is always embodied, then any changes to the corporeality of an individual must unsettle any stable and fixed sense of self (Merleau-Ponty 1962). The coming together, then, of self and other in the material form of transplantation is no simple matter, but an enterprise of high affective significance. The dominant psycho-social imaginary of the Western world rests on the boundedness and singularity of each individual, so it is hardly surprising that the tangible experience of what is in effect a form of hybridity remains a largely alien perception. Going further, I suggest that considerations of microchimerism at the cellular level introduce new dimensions to the issue of identity, in that the continuing circulation and operation of 'alien' genetic material in the peripheral blood supply inevitably raises questions regarding the singularity of the self.

Before coming to the specific nature of microchimerism and its implications in transplantation, I want to look more generally at some of the other elements of stem cell donation that are not readily apparent to those involved on either side. What the PITH project has consistently shown (Abbey et al. 2009) – and we can reasonably speculate that similar forces are at work in stem cell transplants – is that the authorised discourse endlessly reiterated in the clinic and in the media acts to discredit or silence alternative narratives. Questions of hybridity, and the more so regarding chimerism, are clearly discouraged such that those involved may find little support or acknowledgment of the challenging concerns arising from their phenomenological experience post-transplant. As with organ transplantation, and prior to any clinical procedure, the focus for both those choosing to donate and those waiting to receive a stem cell donation, and for the wider families, is likely to be primarily on the prospective health benefits or risks. Yet at the same time, popular media representations of transplantation – though usually around more tangible elements such as heart, eyes or hands – abound with unsettling narratives that suggest an underlying fear that the personal characteristics of the donor might transfer to the recipient, or that s/he (the donor) might reappear as a spectral presence. It goes further than the phenomenological sense that corporeal changes – here the assimilation of donor material – may induce the emergence of a new embodied self, to speak instead of a self haunted as it were by traces of the other. For the majority of the recipients in the PITH study, whose biomedical recovery and well-being was expected to be coincident with a restored sense of singular selfhood, the path to the ontological state of well-Being was often challenging and sometimes impossible. The philosopher Jean-Luc Nancy (2002), who received a donor heart, speaks, for example, of becoming a stranger to himself, while Francisco Varela who had a liver transplant reflects:

> We are left to invent a new way of being human where bodily parts go into each other's bodies, redesigning the landscape of boundaries in the habit of what we are so definitively used to call distinct bodies (2001: 260).

Neither the trope of the spare part nor the expectation of gratitude for the putative gift of life can account for such experiences, and although they provide no direct template for understanding the familial context of sibling donation, there are clearly some similar existential disturbances at stake.

The expectation that SCT enhances health may, then, be somewhat offset by the intuition that there will be a change to the uncomplicated notion of an enduring sovereign self. Such a conception might well be experienced as intrinsically negative for those wedded to the Western logos, but it need not be so. The work of postconventional theorists, such as Jacques Derrida, takes a very different view as it moves away from the trope of singular personhood and individual identity. The insistence of the Western logos on self and other as separate and distinct entities is for Derrida an illusion. As he puts it, the arrival of otherness surprises the host,

> enough to call into question, to the point of annihilating or rendering indeterminate, all the distinctive signs of a prior identity, beginning with the very border that delineated a legitimate home and assured lineage (1993: 34),

but that arrival also marks the creative possibility of going beyond the metaphysics of the modernist concept of the self. For Derrida the coming of the other – and we can see it as both abstract and concrete – cannot be denied and it always speaks to a hauntological relationship not just between self and other, but also across past/present/future and between absence and presence, life and death (Derrida 1994). Existence, and that includes personal being-in-the-world, is always dependent on something else that is not present as such, something not graspable in the immediate moment. What matters is that the trace of the unknown other should be openly welcomed (and here we might think of the recipient's embrace of donor material), not in the expectation that we will benefit – for that can never be certain – but as a way of securing a future.

There is very little in Derrida's work that refers directly to transplantation but his largely theoretical 'logic of the supplement' is clearly of relevance. As with every form of augmentation or supplementation, the prosthetic nature of any transplant positions it as a vital element, not of a predetermined and settled being, but of a creative becoming. In letting go of the illusion of an unchanging, or at least restored, self, it becomes possible to accept the embodied hybridity that transplantation entails in a more welcoming and expansive way. The relation between self and other is no longer binary, still less antagonistic, but becomes entangled – "the guest becomes the host's host" as Derrida (2000: 125) puts it – and in the PITH project at least, the empirical material showed that those who comprehended the putative loss of corporeal singularity, who did not fetishize autonomy, were less unsettled by their unfamiliar experiences and affects. The recognition that transplantation – whether of a heart or bone marrow – promises restoration but more generally delivers unease speaks to a present reality for many recipients, and indeed the wider families, but, I would argue, a radical rethinking of the nature of embodiment could open up to more liveable alternatives. While the intimate encounters inherent in transplantation processes may provoke feelings of disturbance and anxiety, it is also the point at which we might rethink the temporal and spatial boundaries of all embodiment. I want, then, to explore another, related approach that brings together the philosophy of Gilles Deleuze and Félix Guattari – which pushes Derrida's insights further towards the existential state of becoming – with some contemporary developments in bioscience. It is here that the recent upsurge of biophilosophical interest in microchimerism becomes significant as that biomedical state plays into, and mirrors, on a very material biological basis, the central Deleuzian concept of assemblage.

Until the late twentieth century, the phenomenon of microchimerism was little known or researched, even in biological science. The term refers to a form of chimerism that operates specifically at the cellular level, unlike its broader meaning, which has its direct origins in Greek myth and figures a combination of body parts from two or more different animal species. Microchimerism denotes the existence – usually in very low concentrations – of what are identified as non-self cells with their own distinct sets of DNA and associated antigens, which arise from different individuals but are present in a single body. Although the terms hybridity and chimerism are often used interchangeably, there is a material difference in that the putatively non-self cells of microchimerism are not assimilated to achieve new uniformity across all cells, but remain distinct. Bioscientific understanding and explanations for the phenomena of both chimerism and microchimerism are uncertain, but the implication is that the conventional model of biologically distinct entities – whether as plants, invertebrates or mammals – where each individual organism is regulated by a single unvarying genome and displays genetic homogeneity across all cells of the body may be unfounded (Nelson 2012). The known circumstances of human microchimerism may indicate a natural state, as in the *in utero* fusion into a single body of dizygotic twins or the now widely acknowledged phenomenon of foetal cell engraftment into the maternal body, and *vice versa*. There are also many iatrogenic causes arising from biomedical interventions into the body, such as organ or stem cell transplantations. There are few observable morphological distinctions or evidence of external effects arising from the diverse DNA markers in natural microchimerism, so the actual extent of the condition is unknown. Nonetheless, microchimerism is now accepted – after decades of disparagement[6] – as a relatively common, and probably ubiquitous phenomenon, but one that is still largely unheeded in the absence of disease or ill-health.

Despite the low incidence of non-self cells, there are compelling reasons to believe that microchimerism is strongly enmeshed with the biomedical outcomes of many transplant procedures, and it is central for bone marrow transplants, where what might be more accurately called macrochimerism is the desired outcome. Most forms of transplant have yielded evidence that the donor DNA enters and circulates in the peripheral blood supply, thus maintaining a consistent presence of genetically divergent cells throughout the body. And occasionally microchimeric cells may accumulate at specific sites such as solid organs (other than the transplant organ itself), again resulting in distinctive instances of macrochimerism. Within immunology and transplant research there is an ongoing and highly oppositional debate with regard to the potential of beneficial or pathological outcomes in the presence of such chimerism, with much research investigating its possible, but as yet unrealised, therapeutic capacity as a counter to allorejection. What is striking, then, is that unlike the situation with solid organ transplants, where the authorised *clinical* narrative still insists that the DNA of the graft will remain *in situ* and play no part in recovery and future life (even though that claim is increasingly shown to

---

[6] See Martin's account (2010) of the difficulties faced by Diana Bianchi's lab.

be an illusion), the biomedical point of stem cell transplants is exactly the opposite. The explicit aim is to import active components that will both replace the originary stem cells, damaged, for example, by treatment for leukaemia, and boost the recipient's immunological responses. Where existing bone marrow has been fully or partially ablated, the primary intention is to stage a replacement with non-self cells.

In the biomedical context of transplantation, the concerns around microchimerism are less to do with 'alien' DNA than with its input to and effect on the immunological status of the recipient. Immediately following the transplant procedure, a regimen of immunosuppressant drugs is established, not just to aid short-term recovery, but sometimes over a lifetime to ensure continuing survival. Left to itself, the recipient's natural immune response to the unfamiliar donor cells – which carry their own distinctive Human Leucocyte Antigen (HLA) profile – would be an overwhelming onslaught on the putative intrusion, and rejection of the transplanted tissue, resulting in the recipient's further decline. Where it is possible, as in some kidney transplants and certainly in bone marrow transplantation, careful tissue matching between closely related donor and recipient can eliminate some of the problem. In the case of sibling donation, as in the present study, the parents and children involved express a strong psycho-social desire to keep the whole experience within the family, but that in any case is the preferred medical approach. Nonetheless, there is rarely a complete correspondence of HLA, which is highly specific to each individual, so the resulting histo-incompatibility that would prevent successful grafting is usually controlled by suppressing the recipient's own antigens. At the same time, a parallel problem arises as the donor cells mobilise a similar rejection response against the recipient. In what is called graft v. host disease, the functional immune markers of the transplant material recognise the non-self status of the recipient and attack the host who may have little defence, especially if already immunocompromised. The biomedical procedure of stem cell transplant is not especially risky in itself: the danger, as in all transplantation interventions, lies in effectively managing the incompatible HLA systems. Although post-transplant care and drug regimens may change over time, the underlying doxa remains the same – that the immune system of all animals naturally operates on the principle of self/non-self discrimination such that donor and recipient antigens are in an antagonistic relation. The success of transplantation procedures, including SCT, is therefore thought to devolve on a successful suppression of the otherwise inevitability of histo-incompatibility. In an interesting twist, peculiar to bone marrow infusions, that suppression may depend on promoting a complete engraftment of donor cells in order to directly counter certain existing conditions such as leukaemia. The graft versus leukaemia effect is a well-recognised benefit of SCT where the lesion is blood-borne and does not extend to subsequent cancers in other organs and tissues (Kolb 2008; Dickinson et al. 2017).

The militaristic metaphors with which immunology is commonly explained go back to the pioneering work of Frank Macfarlane Burnet and Peter Medawar in the mid twentieth century, which set out the seminal principles for most subsequent research. As they both understood it, the purpose of the immune system is to mobilise in response to the incursion of 'foreign' – non-self – antigens by releasing an abundance of biochemical agents that would eliminate the putative threat of otherness. They are credited for firmly establishing the apparently natural conflict of the self/non-self cellular relation,[7] but what is usually overlooked is that Medawar also identified the phenomenon of post-birth dizygotic twin chimerism in certain cattle known as freemartins, and even very rarely in humans. He recognised it as a form of *natural* immuno-tolerance, but was unable to move beyond calling such an occurrence a 'natural accident' and 'astonishing' (Medawar 1960). Instead, his legacy remains the conviction that the protection and maintenance of the boundaries between the supposedly normal self and the intrusive other is a natural function of the healthy body, and that in turn has been the dominant template for transplant medicine. It is only in relatively recent years that attempts to reconceptualise the nature and function of the immune system have emerged. Donna Haraway (1989), Polly Matzinger (2001) and more recently, Thomas Pradeu (2012) are notable here, but their influence is limited, albeit the very success of SCT must raise doubts about the viability of the standard model. The issue is that beyond bioscience itself, the socio-cultural imaginary, of which the biomedical imaginary is a subset, is no less committed to precisely the same core belief in the intrinsic nature of self/non-self conflict. The notion of the self embedded in the Western logos speaks to an atomistic, already complete and defensively bounded entity. Any suggestion, indeed any material research, that the immune systems of the self and its other(s) might ever be cooperative is an insult not just to the basic principles of immunology, but to the very understanding of what constitutes human being.

Once it is accepted that the immunological effects of transplantation extend throughout the body of the recipient, then we are obliged to reconsider the relation between self and other. Given that the DNA – and the associated HLA profile – of the donor circulate in the peripheral blood supply at very least, the issue of hybridity takes on a more radical significance. Even when the finer points of DNA coding are scarcely addressed by either clinicians or their patients, the recipient can no longer claim to be 'all me', and the intuition of hybridity is frequently an element in the post-transplantation context. Whatever the clinical narrative around SCT, both sides of the transaction display a feeling that the marrow graft signals that some aspects of a donor are incorporated. In a few cases there is a stronger sense that the particular essence of the donor is evident in the recipient. Hybridity is not a term commonly used in the interviews by either the siblings or their wider families; still less were respondents or donors aware of how circulating donor DNA in effect constitutes a microchimeric environment in the recipient body, yet there is surely a sense that the embodied self has changed. In biomedical terms, what may occur – and it is after all the intention of SCT – is that the donor cells may effect a complete engraftment of the bone marrow and peripheral blood supply, while coexisting with the recipient's own DNA still present in the epithelial cells, for example. It seems unlikely from the interview material that any of this was discussed as being of

---

[7] See Thomas Pradeu (2012) for a detailed exposition of the pioneering immunological work of Macfarlane Burnet and Medawar.

particular relevance with the families involved. As the father of family Rohde dis-
missively remarks, and his is the only direct reference: 'You know I find the concept
so crazy, the doctors are talking about chimerism (…), it's from //comes from the
Greek chimera' (Rohde, father, 106). For everyone concerned the cogent questions
are largely focused on the material consequences of SCT in terms of future health
and illness, but the philosophical implications of the coming together of self and
other should not be ignored. It is not a case of hybridity as such, which technically
indicates a form of assimilation, but precisely of chimerism where – at the cellular
level – the incoming components remain genetically distinct.

    In solid organ transplantation, the issue of chimerism was first recognised in
Edward Starzl's work in the early 1990s during a retrospective study of the outcome
of kidney transplants from almost 3 decades earlier. At that time, effective immunosuppressant drugs were unavailable, so mutual rejection processes between host and
donor were uncontrolled. Despite standard biomedical expectation, nonetheless,
several recipients had survived. In investigating this puzzling endurance, Starzl
showed that donor HLA was not just localised at the site of the transplant organ but
could be detected throughout the recipient body (Starzl et al. 1992). Other researchers then demonstrated that cell mobility was bidirectional, with the transplant organs
themselves showing evidence of incorporating the existing HLA typing of recipients (Quaini et al. 2002). In short, it was the first clear indication of extensive microchimerism. Starzl proposed that the problem of immunorejection might be countered
by keeping a balance between the immunogenetic effects of the two different populations of cells by means of recipients being given pre-treatment infusions of hematopoietic (stem) cells derived from the bone marrow of living donors. His underlying
aim was to find a way of minimising the need for highly toxic regimens of immunosuppressant drugs, which can generate a plethora of new morbidities. Because the
pre-treatment infusions did not prove reliably effective in solid organ procedures,
Starzl's insights were widely discounted, even though the whole enterprise of SCT
shows the potential of microchimerism in relation to immunotolerance. The contemporary absence of discussion about microchimerism among SCT clinicians[8] and
families is puzzling given that even the briefest online research makes clear that the
donor DNA and HLA takes over bone marrow function and circulates in the blood,
though on popular sites, there is little recognition that it may equally settle in solid
organs and other tissues. One might ask whether the omission of explanatory information about issues that may affect both future health and existential well-Being
raises the conventional question of what constitutes informed consent, especially
where children are the recipients and donors for whom proxy decisions are made.

    Where recognition of iatrogenic microchimerism is still relatively sparse in the
clinical discourse, the question of macrochimerism is all but absent. In one notable
case reported in 2008, initially in a professional journal and subsequently splashed

[8] I stress clinicians here in distinction to those doing SCT research. Talking to immunologists I
have been struck by the disjunct between the pragmatic treatments on offer and strictly research
findings – often in relation to murine models – that indicate more effective ways forward. Clinicians
cannot of course experiment on patients, but many seem unaware of alternative therapies.

by the media, the blood group of a 9-year-old female child switched from O-negative to O-positive following an emergency liver transplant, and her immunological profile realigned itself with that of the male deceased donor (Alexander 2008). The realisation that such unexpected and extensive chimerism had occurred resulted in all immunosuppressant medication being *withdrawn*, enabling the donor cells to rapidly effect a therapeutically beneficial engraftment and facilitating the patient's full recovery in the absence of drugs. Even though the *micro*chimeric process was relatively well known after liver transplantation, it was believed to be ephemeral and of little consequence; certainly it was not seen as a significant factor in graft acceptance. The case reported by Alexander, however, was not one of simple microchimerism – in which 'non-self' cells constitute no more than 1 in 1000 – but of enduring whole-body genetic translocation. The problematic of immuno(in)compatibility is not, however, limited to iatrogenic outcomes, and by exploring the wider context of cellular chimerism it becomes possible to trace its further significance. The incorporation of allogenetic material is one mode of inducing microchimerism but the phenomenon has many other grounds, many of them occurring naturally. Microchimerism in and after pregnancy is now well established and is believed to be frequent and possibly universal (Nelson 2012), and moreover, it may persist for decades, perhaps even indefinitely (Bianchi et al. 1996). A further shock was the discovery by Diana Bianchi's lab that women who have never been pregnant can also be carrying Y chromosomes, indicating the presence of non-self DNA (Khosrotehrani and Bianchi 2005), and it is now speculated that there are multiple reasons why non-self cells might circulate in the body.[9] Once microchimerism is established in the body of an individual, the bidirectional cellular traffic across the placental barrier indicates that whatever the initial cause, it will become intergenerational. The implication is that recipient and donor bodies may already be microchimeric, with the transplant material simply adding to the incidence of non-self cells. If indeed such populations of distinct DNA and HLA are durable over and beyond the normal life-course, it is not just our understanding of the immune system that requires revision. The projected ubiquity of such somatic multiplicity and intracorporeal malleability surely poses a fundamental challenge to the Western socio-cultural imaginary of singular selfhood that finds its biological justification in the individual uniqueness of DNA identity.

I turn, now, to a more detailed exploration of how bioscientific doxa around microchimerism could be opened up through a more philosophical critique of the relation between self and other, where the supposed boundaries of the one secure it against the intrusions of others. It is a surprise, as Cohen (2009) makes clear, to find that the original concept of immunity was confined to juridical and political discourse; it was not until the late 19th century that the more familiar biomedical

---

[9] There is little pressure to identify chimerism in healthy populations, but aside from its known incidence as a result of pregnancy, all types of tissue and organ transplant (Including SCT), non-irradiated blood transfusions, generational genetic transfer and human dizygotic fusion, there are also suggestions that lactation and the sexual exchange of fluids may be sources. More immediately accepted is the multitude of non-self cells that constitutes the human microbiome (Lloyd-Price et al. 2016), the majority of which have their own DNA and immune systems (Pradeu 2012).

understanding of immunity as a defence system for the body emerged. Contemporary philosophy is highly engaged with the notion and draws on both historical strands. Leaving aside for a moment Derrida's rethinking of hospitality as a mode that might speak to the nature of microchimerism (Shildrick 2019), the most cogent point of engagement is with philosopher Roberto Esposito's deconstructive analysis. The term 'immunity' may appear to be unrelated in meaning to 'community' – where community refers to a group linked together through conditions in common or indicates public ownership, and immunity is an insular attribute of the self – yet Esposito demonstrates that they are inextricably entangled. As he (2008) lays out, both words derive from the Latin term 'munus', which indicates an obligation of responsiveness to the other or a gift, such that the one who claims immunity is absolved from the self-abnegation inherent to community and eludes the reciprocity of gifting (Shildrick 2016). The trope of gift giving is ubiquitous in transplantation discourse, where the incorporation of donor material – which currently entails the deliberate suppression of the recipient's immune system – sets in place an enduring obligation of gratitude. For many that extends to a sense of mutual kinship between recipient and donor following transplant (Shildrick 2013a, b), or even shared identity as in the case of SCT between existing kin (d'Aurio 2015, current study).[10] Glossing Esposito's work, Timothy Campbell explains: 'Accepting the *munus* directly undermines the capacity of the individual to identify himself or herself as such and not part of the community' (Campbell 2010: x).[11] As Esposito recognises, conventional culture cannot tolerate the logic of the two-in-one or the one that becomes two (2008: 168) . Few recipients will think explicitly in such terms but they express precisely what may be disturbing about the transaction: prior to accepting the 'gift of life' they have lived as autonomous selves within the normative paradigms of Western modernism, with an unthinking, and probably unexpressed, belief in the corporeal distinction between one self and an other; afterwards the closure of individual identity is no longer possible. Small wonder then that so many of the families involved in the SCT study made a joke of such unsettling intuitions.[12]

Esposito's primary interest is in theorising biopolitics, but he draws on the materiality of biomedical immunity throughout. As Donna Haraway's prescient assertion reminds us, immunology is at the heart of biopolitics (Haraway 1989). Esposito also covers some of the same ground as Derrida, who has written extensively on the

---

[10] The issue of shared identity may be expressed in many ways with most donor-recipient dyads preferring to speak of heightened bonds rather than direct identity transfer.

[11] See also the take-up of Esposito in the work of Brown et al. (2011), Brown and Williams (2015) and Kent and Meachum (2019).

[12] It is noticeable that it is often fathers who carry the joke as in Diedrich (91) or Kunow (114). The comment offered by the Minz family recipient (98) is typical:

R: my Dad sometimes makes silly comments, if it's like (…) I dunno, if Malle [the donor], if there's some kind of opinion about Malle or Malle is supposed to make some kind of decision and isn't here, then he can – my Dad always says: yes, Marlena can do it, she has the same thoughts as he has, he has the same bone marrow or something like that, me and my brother, I mean we always think this is quite idiotic (laughs) or like that.

concept of autoimmunity and whose reworking of the gift and of absolute hospitality, as I briefly mentioned, brings new dimensions of understanding to the nature of transplantation (see Shildrick 2013a). By engaging with both the material and ontological transformations of embodiment, what concerns Esposito is the development of an *affirmative* biopolitics that goes beyond the neutral biomedical figure of tolerance. In place of a state marked in immunological terms by the absence of reaction to the other, effectively a form of *passive* coexistence, he wants to postulate a mode of positive relation between self and other. Where the microchimeric outcome of transplantation seems to stage a phenomenological insult to the notion of an individual life restored – given that the differential DNA of the donor cells resist assimilation and remain fundamentally other – Esposito offers instead a logic of dynamic multiplicity where dissimilarity itself is mutually productive. He writes:

> we need to find the mode, the forms, the conceptual language for converting the immunitary declension (…) into a singular and plural logic in which the differences become precisely that which keeps the world united. ('Immunization and Violence' (n.d.:13))

The notion of a radical hospitality proposed by Derrida (2000) has previously done some of that work in establishing the always/already interiority of otherness, but it is less directed towards an explicitly transformative and creative end. Esposito more clearly takes his lead from Deleuze, for whom the key purpose of philosophy is to enable new modes of thinking that will facilitate more adequate ways of conceptualising the events that transform life. Deleuze has little interest – even in a deconstructive mode – in modernist semantics that focus on individual and autonomous selfhood; rather he recognises not simply the one in the other, but the modality of an *im*personal vitalism that eschews the limitations of *being* and privileges instead the excessive potentiality of life's becoming. In conclusion, then, I offer some brief speculations on how the significance of chimerism might be read through a Deleuzian approach that takes for granted the illusory nature of self-other distinctions.

As with Derrida, Deleuze (both alone and in collaboration with Guattari) decisively breaks away from modernist thought, not only in contesting singular embodiment per se, but in opening up the disturbing ontological question 'Who am I?' that so clearly underlies the unease generated by the transplant exchange. It marks a fundamental challenge to the conventional paradigm of 'self versus other' that still – despite recent research discoveries around microchimerism – dominates the bioscientific discourse of immunology and the socio-cultural imaginary more widely, and an emerging theoretical shift to an understanding of the normal 'self' as constitutively chimeric. The Deleuzian rejection of the notion of an atomistic and sovereign subject of modernity, with an enduring sense of self, does not entirely deny the experience of individuality but sees it as at most provisional and always within a process of unravelling. In place of static 'being', the emphasis is on a state of becoming (Deleuze and Guattari 1987). The unique experiences and putatively contained embodiment of each person are enmeshed in what Deleuze calls assemblages, those multifarious and impermanent webs of interconnections that generate dynamic fields of energy. Life itself is an unlimited vitalist force that exceeds the individual life-span from birth to death (see Braidotti 2006; Shildrick 2013b). The concept of assemblages provides a convincing alternative to the logic of unity and wholeness, and a perspective from which to understand what is at stake in chimerism, which although not a term used by Deleuze has a similar import. To recap, chimerism – whether of whole parts or of cellular material – denotes not a simple assimilation that overrides the original differences, but a conjunction of disparate elements that both deform and reorganise each other, yet are still functional within a newly configured relationship. It is a way of thinking about human life as always and inextricably entangled not only with other organisms but with an assembly of technologies and processes, and that is precisely what transplantation exemplifies.

At a less rarefied level we might also think about the family itself as an assemblage – a coming together of individuals who in certain circumstances function as a conglomeration rather than as autonomous beings. Certainly the familial bodies at the focus of the SCT research project seem to take that view, and although they may be open to the changes wrought by events and processes and do not cleave to a static essence, there is still a strong commitment to an organised and organising intra-related entity. As the Bahr family mother commented: 'Something very special connects us, what we experienced together, what we endured and survived. That continues to connect us, you know' (89). It clearly matters to the members that they are seen as a family and that the fluid circumstances in which they find themselves can be managed within the unit. In that sense they satisfy the English language definition of assemblage as the fitting together of disparate parts to form a unified whole, but not the full Deleuzian sense in which the original word *agencement* indicates a loosely linked array of heterogeneous elements (Nail 2017).[13] Nonetheless, both the family as some kind of limited assemblage, and the nexus of chimerism, which they are implicitly obliged to accept, express the constructive power of interconnection and the ceaseless processes of transformation. The concepts of both assemblage and chimerism may help us to rethink transplantation, not as a singular and time-limited event leading ideally to restoration of the *status quo*, but as a continuing project for both the recipient and the donor. For Deleuze, human life is not limited to the temporal frame marked out by the conventional life-span of any individual, but rather persists as one variable element of the enveloping cycle of becoming that constitutes all types of living (and dead) organisms and machines. For all of us, the personal life course *is* undeniably marked by discrete episodes such as pregnancy, trauma, or transplantation itself, where there are tangible changes or transformations, yet in another dimension, events are also atemporal and intangible forces and points of intensity that are excessive to any singular or fixed form of embodiment. The science and politics of immunity that operate in terms of

---

[13] The supposed homogeneity and unity of family life following sibling donation – in other words, a coming together on characteristically parental terms – may indeed be the source of disquiet for the young people involved. Forinda and Posse found that the stress on families is high, and that a minority of recipients suffer significant psycho-social problems. As they put it: 'Their parents had already given so much of their time and they [the recipients] were afraid to "burden" them by talking about how they really felt inside' (2008: 307).

protection of singularity and the management of boundaries between self and other are superseded by the assemblage of communal becoming.

In the immediate and conventional context of SCT procedures – in which the individuality of each person is taken for granted – the point is to restore the prospective recipient to the self who preceded illness and the specific biomedical procedure. In contrast, Deleuzian philosophy contests any notion of the individual 'ownership' of embodied life and promotes instead an appreciation of the intensity of ongoing becoming in a process without beginning or end (Braidotti 2006). In any case, what matters for Deleuze is not whether the recipient re-establishes functional efficacy, the prospect of an extended life, or even ontological security, but what Rosi Braidotti calls 'sustainability':

> The sustainability of these futures consists in their being able to mobilize, actualize and deploy cognitive, affective and collective forces which had not so far been activated…These forces concretize in actual, material relations and can thus constitute a network, web or rhizome of interconnection with others. (Braidotti 2010: 413)

The science and politics of immunity that operate in terms of the protection of singularity and the management of boundaries between self and other is superseded by the assemblage of productive becoming. The recipient and donor in such an assemblage are no longer positioned as self and other, but are components of an apersonal correlation of elements that reflects the materiality of the unseen cellular chimerism that the biomedical procedures have mobilised. In addition to the predictable and desired changes that result from SCT, like the recovery of health, the overlooked transmutations effected by microchimerism must inevitably disorder existing corporeal boundaries. The authoritative discourse of conventional biomedicine that mirrors the modernist socio-political objective of maintaining the illusory singularity and integrity of the bounded self – a model that would thwart any move towards positive community – is contested in its very success. The transfer of bone marrow between siblings is at very least a step towards realising new potentials of becoming other than the separate and distinct self.

Research into the nature of microchimerism in organ and tissue transplantation – including bone marrow transplants and the projected use of stem cell transplants for neurological disorders – is driven by bioscience alone, but such procedures also constitute highly significant biopolitical objects. In effect, the *biological* ground that has reflected and sustained the biopolitical rhetoric of immunity, with its insistence on the distinct identities of self and other, is no longer viable. As both the postconventional humanities and bioscientific discourse increasingly acknowledge the plasticity of human embodiment, not simply in the context of established and future modifications of tissues or organs, but at the unseen cellular level, a new understanding of the inherent entanglement of corporeal materials is emerging. Multidisciplinary enquiry into transplantation suggests that rethinking the interweaving of chimerism and an immuno-politics could mobilise an ethical challenge to the damaging rigidities of the self/other model of modernity and insist instead on the fundamental diversity, mutability and connectivity of all corporeality. As it becomes increasingly clear that the incidence of chimerism and microchimerism is a ubiquitous facet of embodiment rather than a strange exception,[14] we should seek to find new models of thinking human life, not as a collection of time-bound individuals each defending the autonomous self, but through the fluid, interactive and communal dynamics of assemblage.

Literature

Abbey, Susan, Enza De Luca, et al. 2009. What they say versus what we see: Hidden distress and impaired quality of life in heart transplant recipients. *The Journal of Heart and Lung Transplantation* 28 (S2): 128.

Alexander, Stephen I. 2008. Chimerism and tolerance in a recipient of a deceased-donor liver transplant. *New England Journal of Medicine* 358: 369–374.

Bianchi, Diana W., Gretchen K. Zickwolf, et al. 1996. Male foetal progenitor cells persist in the maternal blood for as long as 27 years postpartum. *Proceedings of the National Academy of Science* 93 (2): 705–708.

Braidotti, Rosi. 2006. *Transpositions: On nomadic ethics*. Cambridge: Polity.

———. 2010. Nomadism: Against methodological nationalism. *Policy Futures in Education* 8 (3–4): 408–418.

Brown, Nik, and Rosalind Williams. 2015. Cord blood banking – Bio-objects at the borderlands between community and immunity. *Life, Science, Society, Policy* 11 (11): 1–18.

Brown, Nik, Laura Machin, and Danae McLeod. 2011. Immunitary bioeconomy: The economisation of life in the international cord blood market. *Social Science & Medicine* 72 (7): 1115–1122.

Campbell, Timothy. 2010. 'Bios,' immunity, life: The thought of Roberto Esposito. *Diacritics* 36 (2): 2–22.

Cohen, Ed. 2009. *A body worth defending: Immunity, biopolitics, and the apotheosis of the modern body*. Durham, NC: Duke University Press.

D'Auria, Jennifer P. 2015. Through the eyes of young sibling donors: The hematopoietic stem cell donation experience. *Journal of Pediatric Nursing* 30 (3): 447–453.

Deleuze, Gilles, and Félix Guattari. 1987. *A thousand plateaus: Capitalism and schizophrenia*. Trans. Brian Massumi. Minneapolis: Minnesota University Press.

Derrida, Jacques. 1993. *Aporias*. Trans. Thomas Dutoit. Stanford: Stanford University Press.

———. 1994. *Spectres of Marx: The state of the debt, the work of mourning and the new international*. Trans. Peggy Kamuf. London: Routledge.

———. 2000. *Of hospitality: Anne Dufourmantelle invites Jacques Derrida to respond*. Trans. Rachel Bowlby. Stanford, CA: Stanford University Press.

Dickinson, Anne M., Jean Norden, Shuang Li, et al. 2017. Graft-versus-Leukemia effect following hematopoietic stem cell transplantation for leukemia. *Frontiers in Immunology* 8. https://doi.org/10.3389/fimmu.2017.00496.

Esposito, Roberto. 2008. *Bios: Biopolitics and philosophy*. Minneapolis: University of Minnesota Press.

Esposito, Robertto. n.d. Immunization and violence, biopolitica.cl/docs/Esposito_Immunization_violence.pdf. Accessed 04 June 2018.

Forinder, Ulla, and Ebba Posse. 2008. A life on hold: adolescents' experiences of stem cell transplantation in a long-term perspective. *Journal of Child Health Care* 12 (4): 301–313.

---

[14]The growing literature on microchimerism makes clear that it is not simply the outcome of certain intercorporeal interventions but may be the condition of all human life. See Shildrick (2019).

Haraway, Donna. 1989. The biopolitics of postmodern bodies: Determinations of self in immune system discourse. differences. *Journal of Feminist Cultural Studies* 1 (1): 3–43.

Kaba, Evridiki, David R. Thompson, et al. 2005. Somebody Else's heart inside me: A descriptive study of psychological problems after a heart transplantation. *Issues in Mental Health Nursing* 26 (6): 611–625.

Kent, Julie, and Darian Meachum. 2019. 'Synthetic blood': Entangling politics and biology. *Body & Society* 25 (2): 28–55.

Khosrotehrani, Kiarash, and Diana W. Bianchi. 2005. Multi-lineage potential of fetal cells in maternal tissue: A legacy in reverse. *Journal of Cell Science* 118: 1559–1563.

Kolb, Hans-Jochem. 2008. Graft-versus-leukemia effects of transplantation and donor lymphocytes. *Blood* 112: 4371–4383.

Lloyd-Price, Jason, et al. 2016. The healthy human microbiome. *Genome Medicine* 8: 51. https://doi.org/10.1186/s13073-016-0307-y.

Matzinger, Polly. 2001. Essay 1: The danger model in its historical context. *Scandinavian Journal of Immunology* 54: 4–9.

Mauss, Marcel. 1990. The gift: The form and reason for exchange in archaic societies. Trans. W.D. Halls. New York: Routledge.

Medawar, Peter. 1960. Immunological tolerance. Nobel Lecture. 12 December 1960, http://www.nobelprize.org/nobel_prizes/medicine/laureates/1960/medawar-lecture.html Accessed 3 Jan 2015.

Merleau-Ponty, Maurice. 1962. *The phenomenology of perception*. London: Routledge and Kegan Paul.

Nail, Thomas. 2017. What is an assemblage? *SubStance* 46 (1): 21–37.

Nancy, Jean-Luc. 2002. L'Intrus, transl. Susan Hanson. *CR: The New Centennial Review* 2 (3): 1–14.

Nelson, J. Lee. 2012. The otherness of self: Microchimerism in heath and disease. *Trends in Immunology* 33 (8): 421–427.

Poole, Jennifer, Margrit Shildrick, et al. 2009. 'You might not feel like yourself': Heart transplants, identity and ethics. In *Critical interventions in the ethics of healthcare: Challenging the principle of autonomy in bioethics*, ed. Stuart J. Murray and Dave Holmes. London: Ashgate.

Pradeu, Thomas. 2012. *The limits of the self: Immunology and biological identity*. Trans. Elizabeth Vitanza. Oxford: Oxford University Press.

Quaini, Federico, Konrad Urbanek, Antonio Beltrami, et al. 2002. Chimerism of the transplanted heart. *New England Journal of Medicine* 346 (1): 5–15.

Shildrick, Margrit. 2013a. Hospitality and 'the gift of life': Reconfiguring the other in heart transplantation. In *Embodied selves*, ed. Kathleen Lennon. London: Palgrave Macmillan.

———. 2013b. Re-imagining embodiment: Prostheses, supplements and boundaries. *Somatechnics* 3 (2): 270–286.

———. 2016. Chimerism and *immunitas*: The emergence of a posthumanist biophilosophy. In *Resisting biopolitics: Philosophical, political and performative strategies*, ed. S. Wilmer and Audrone Zukauskaite. London: Routledge.

———. 2019. (Micro)chimerism, immunity and temporality: Rethinking the ecology of life and death. *Australian Feminist Studies* 34 (99): 10–24.

Shildrick, Margrit, et al. 2018. Messy Entanglements: Research assemblages in heart transplantation discourses and practices. *Journal of Medical Humanities* 44: 46–54.

Starzl, Thomas E., Anthony J. Demetris, Noriko Murase, et al. 1992. Cell migration, Chimerism, and graft acceptance. *Lancet* 339 (8809): 1579–1582.

Varela, Francisco J. 2001. Intimate distances. Fragments for a phenomenology of organ transplantation. *Journal of Consciousness Studies* 8 (5–7): 259–271.

Open Access This chapter is licensed under the terms of the Creative Commons Attribution 4.0 International License (http://creativecommons.org/licenses/by/4.0/), which permits use, sharing, adaptation, distribution and reproduction in any medium or format, as long as you give appropriate credit to the original author(s) and the source, provide a link to the Creative Commons license and indicate if changes were made.

The images or other third party material in this chapter are included in the chapter's Creative Commons license, unless indicated otherwise in a credit line to the material. If material is not included in the chapter's Creative Commons license and your intended use is not permitted by statutory regulation or exceeds the permitted use, you will need to obtain permission directly from the copyright holder.

Chapter 15
Intercorporeality: Giving Life from One Body to Another

Christina Schües

Abstract When a transplant is given to another person, the body material and its importance are at the centre of attention. Yet the meanings of the body, the body material, and the bodily relationship between the donor and recipient are unclear. This essay tackles the understanding of the body with regard to the practice of stem cell transplantation between siblings. The concept of intercorporeality embraces the "family body" and a singular body, the sense of bodily belonging and bodily ownership, and a relationship that inheres within a transplant. The intercorporeal relationship is basic and primary. Thematizing it may show a reality of body transformation that is more than just the distribution of body parts. It is a material approach to the human who has a body in the sense of a living substance that can be defined biotechnologically and made available. This essay shows that even though the transplant is body material, it is always more than that: a ground for personal traits, symbols, and a particular bond between the siblings.

Keywords Family · Body · Own body · Merleau-Ponty · Embodiment · Body sharing

The practice of stem cell transplantation (SCT) involves the body on a very material level: anaesthesia, immune suppression, taking and implanting the bone marrow, hoping that the bone marrow will do its work in the recipient, medical supervision to ensure that the "donor" body does not undergo further side effects. Such practice similarly includes concern for the patient and her illness, and issues of how well her body will respond to the treatment and how much she will suffer from possible side effects. There is also some concern about the donor, and both her physical well-being and psychological consequences after the treatment. The family will thus be confronted with many worries and concerns during the period of illness and the time

C. Schües (✉)
Institute for History of Medicine and Science Studies, University of Lübeck,
Lübeck, Schleswig-Holstein, Germany
e-mail: c.schuees@uni-luebeck.de

© The Author(s) 2022
C. Schües et al. (eds.), *Stem Cell Transplantations Between Siblings as Social Phenomena*, Philosophy and Medicine 144,
https://doi.org/10.1007/978-3-031-04166-2_15

thereafter: Will the stem cells do their work in the body of the sick child? Are the side effects tolerable? Can the donor child deal adequately with the situation and any possible physical or psychological consequences? My focus is not on these medical or psychological concerns but rather on the body concepts that may be involved in SCT practices and that emerge as themes in the interviews conducted in this study. The focus on the body and its meanings for SCT illuminates the way in which familial relationships are bodily embedded and how body images frame them.

The particular practice of SCT that we studied is carried out between siblings within the family. In normal circumstances, sharing is part of family life; members share their love and ideas, good and bad moods, bread and butter, or times of crisis or happiness. Physical and psychological care for each other involves the body as well, but – normally – the body itself, as material substance, is not shared, rather the body is a "medium" of caring through touch, presence or physical support. Even more so, the body, and particularly a child's body, is protected by the family, mostly the parents against injury or harm. In particular, on the level of care we may speak of an intercorporeal relation between the family members. Their care is not just practised by fulfilling duties, but is embodied in their daily shared life.

Interviews show that after SCT, even though the family survives, i.e. continues to exist, this does not mean it is still the "same family". The sickness and the transplant set off a family dynamic that provokes a questioning of the family body itself and of the bodily aspects of practices and family dynamics. In our study we analyze the structure and the experiences of the family, the specific relationships, and the role of the child's body. This last aspect is the specific focus of this chapter.

My basic concern is whether the passing on of body material could be understood simply as either an intervention in a physical body, or a matter for good decision-making and psychological care. I answer both these questions in the negative; instead, I am looking for a third position in the middle ground, involving the materiality of the body as well as the mental, emotional and social dimensions of the persons involved in these practices. This view of a middle ground involves the idea that the material and animated sides of the body merge in the concept of "corporeality"; an idea that also emerges in the concept of the family body vs. the singular body – here, the child's body. This involves the concept of *intercorporeality*.

15.1   The Family as a Body

We usually interviewed parents and their children, the siblings, in both family and individual interviews. Siblings naturally share the genetic heritage received from their parents; after a transplant they also share body material that they have not inherited. Sharing body material is done by transplantation; hence, on an intra-generational level. After a stem cell transplant, the siblings not only grow up together but they also share bone marrow; and this can result in new bodily features, such as having an allergy only the donor sibling had (Garzorz et al. 2016). In most cases the illness of one child and the treatment by stem cell transplantation will become part of the family narrative, and has the potential to change the relationships within the family body.

How can we understand the family as a body? The answer to this question will help to make sense of the experiences and mind-sets of the families who were seeking help and medical remedy from within the family by using the body material of their *own* child.

A family consists of intra- and inter-generational relationships that build a voluntary and involuntary community in which each member can expect help and care from the others. Family relationships are involuntary for some members because, for instance, children have not chosen to be born or to become a member of their specific family. Iris Marion Young understands family "as people who live together and/or share resources necessary to the means for life and comfort; who are committed to caring for one another's physical and emotional needs to the best of their ability" (Young 1997, 106). Whether a modern family definition requires members to be living together is not the issue here, and certainly children who are minors will not be living on their own. Depending on their age and capacities, acting to care for and show responsibility towards each other is also expected of them. This definition of family includes help and care for one another. In times of illness and when particular help and care are needed, or even bodily readiness is required, some families see themselves as *one body*.

Understanding the family as a body means seeing the family as *one* body in the sense of a unified system and, in a stronger version of bodily unity, expecting help in the form of bodily material as a remedy to come *from within* this unit.

As the mother puts it in the Lassen family interview:

> M: And at the end of the day you also know where the bone marrow comes from and I mean (..), like I say it simply feels good inside my head that we actually found it within the family at the end of the day. (Lassen, family interview)

The idea of having the resources within the family is important. These resources are certainly material ones, in this case the stem cells, but also the close relationship within the family that is strong enough to carry them through the crisis and to find remedies. By analogy with the words of sociologists Auguste Compte and Emile Durkheim, we can say that solidarity is their "cement". The rather romantic idea that family members are concerned for the well-being of the family as a structural unity is taken for granted, perhaps not factually, but ideologically at least, in some of the families interviewed.

When a child falls ill with a life-threatening or severe disease, the whole family is affected, often plunged into a state of crisis. A stem cell transplant affects not only the sick child but the whole family as well. The family members worry about the success of the transplant, the time before and after the stay in the hospital. But presuming that the remedy would best be found within the family body seems to be important for many families. It is a relief, and reinforces their unity.

> NDS: Well it was actually really a relief, when we heard that Kilian was a match. And otherwise in the search, if you have to somehow (.) search for something else, that really is even more difficult and takes longer. (.) And that's why it was really super like that. (Kötter, non-donor sister).

The relief at having "a match" within their own family implies that the child's body actually belongs to the family; it is a familial body.

15.2   What Is a Familial Body?

There are two dimensions at stake: the family is seen as a body, and the individual bodies are taken to be typical for the family. The family members see themselves, their family, as a kind of unity, a body system, in comparison with other families, and they understand the individual body as being part of the family unit. Just as with a body, they act on behalf of the well-being of the family, but they also distinguish different families on the basis of the individual body features and their similarities. To take care of the family's well-being also means caring for each person (and her body) who belongs to the family: the non-donor sibling of the Minz family emphasized a kind of "family body" whose basis was not just similarity of physical appearance but also the willingness to stand up for each other:

> NDS: it was also obvious, ALL OF US will do it, but (.) ALL OF US, really EVERYONE knew beforehand: it's Malle after all. (.) For some reason we all KNEW beforehand, we- both of them, like my sister already said, are so very LOHmann, that's my father and brother's side, er my big brother and me, we are so VERY on the Minz side, like my mum, in SO many ways and erm because of that it was all obvious and we all said it's Malle after all. (Minz, non-donor daughter)

A family body is bound together by a form of solidarity, help and being there for each other, and by a family resemblance that sorts the body features into specific bodies of the family. The familial body belongs to the family.

The interview study shows that during the illness crisis, families responded to two guiding threats:

First, they tried to find a way to act in concert and to fix the problem within the family. As far as possible, care for the sick child was provided within the family. Even further challenges for the parents, such as working for the family income or caring for other siblings and their problems, are met with the help of the core family. Second, therefore, stem cell transplantation between siblings is based on a narrow definition of family unit. Not only are kinship relationship and blood compatibility (HLA) necessary, but in addition most parents/families almost *naturally* approved of the therapeutic bone marrow being given from within the family by the healthy sibling. In fact, for many families it is *important* for the body material to come from within the family body: there should be no foreign material to interfere with their own. The family mentioned feeling uneasy about alien body parts interfering with the familial body. As mentioned above, the Minz family feels "good" about the idea that the bone marrow came from a family member whom they know, that – "at the end of the day" when all things are considered – they found the remedy within the family.

Holding on to a narrow definition of family, and worrying about getting the life-saving body material from within it, are both supported by the idea of the family's own body, the (imagined) similarities of body features, and established ways of how members within the family relate to one another. These relationships are strongly bodily; for infants especially, the "pre-semantic body language is vital" insofar as their "relationships are imbued with all their bodily needs, impulses, desires" (Stone

2019, 94). Families build their "typical" interactions in a highly bodily way, with members recognizing moods and feelings without much talking. The father's typical tone, the mother's way of moving, the children's responses, or the patterns of interaction, are all strongly bodily engraved and part of an imagined family resemblance that generates and reassures the family as a body. Members of the family are physically close, the family shares the "same blood", and the source of such blood, the bone marrow, is not strange but familiar, within reach, at their disposal.

Thus, on the basis of this formation of family, it seems to be easier for family members to accept their own familial body material for the reasons of similarity and closeness. This is not just because the child's body material is more easily at hand; the interviews also mention the idea that the body is somehow similar. As one donor says: "... so I simply had the hope, because we were so similar to each other, that Jennifer's body wouldn't even notice, (.) that- tha- that they are different cells or strange cells, that it wouldn't, like, twig" (Jaschke, donor). In this interview, similarity is clearly not part of a description of HLA compatibility, i.e. some kind of similarity that is medically important. Rather, similarity works on the level of personal body characteristics, or even emotional or mental likeness. In the following interview quotation the recipient reports that her father makes jokes about the similarity. These are jokes with some seriousness in them and they show that the presumed similarity is even detected in the mental life of the siblings.

> R: my Dad sometimes makes silly comments, if it's like (.) I dunno, if Malle, if there's some kind of opinion about Malle or Malle is supposed to make some kind of decision and isn't here, then he can- my Dad always says: yes, Marlena can do it, she has the same thoughts as he has, he has the same bone marrow or something like that, me and my brother, I mean we always think this is quite idiotic (laughs) or like that. (Minz, recipient)

The familial body as a system is not agonal but its unification rests on a strong notion of similarity, whether this be with regard to body features or to shared thoughts. In some families tattoos function as a "kind of bond that you can't just SEPARATE" (Molle, non donor). They "record" that the siblings had "grown together SO strongly" (Speidel, recipient). The tattoos symbolize the family as a body and the bodies that belong to the family. The belonging is realized by family themes, by particular styles and rituals, the idea of shared responsibilities and body parts, but it is also reinforced by markers such as tattoos that are more common today than they used to be decades ago. Each period has its own signs and rituals.

The idea of similarity between the family members and of sharing therapeutic body material within the family implies that the child's body is understood as belonging to the family. The next section therefore investigates the sense in which the child's body or parts of the body belong to a family.[1] The very fact that a donor child belongs to the same family as the sick child has the consequence that her body is taken for the practice of SCT. Some parents see it as a matter of luck, as unproblematic, or as justifiable that stem cells can be taken from the child's body if it is

---

[1] The question of whether the parent's body can be regarded in a similar way is still open to further discussion.

medically compatible. Theoretically, there are different models of ethical justification, such as the idea that donation of the body material (or accepting the medical
intervention) would be in the donor child's best interests, and that retrospectively
the child would be glad to have helped, or that actually the child *has* donated voluntarily.[2] With the diagnosis of the illness, knowing that the sick body could possibly
be cured by a SCT from the healthy and compatible sibling's body, there was no
dispute over whether the child's body material would be available as a remedy. In
most cases the family, and particularly the parents, acted on the basis of medical
self-evidence in following the therapeutic path of taking the healthy child's body as
a remedy for the sick child.

This self-evidence is based on a particular understanding of what it means to
belong to the family body. In order to clarify this thesis I will have to consider the
question of how to understand the idea of belonging. How does a child belong to her
family? With reference to the descriptions of the bodily relationships within the
family and family resemblance, the child's belonging is understood as a *bodily
belonging*. We can distinguish different senses of belonging and different aspects of
the child's body. First, I consider belonging in the sense of owning the body or the
child;[3] second, I spell out the reference to parts of the body.

15.2.1   Belonging in the Sense of Owning the Body or the Child

If belonging means parents own the body of the child, then it could imply that they
have the right and the power to simply decide over the body of the child.[4] Ownership
would indicate that family members may count upon the child's body to be used if
therapy is needed. According to this line of thinking, the availability of the child's
body to treat her sibling presupposes that her body is regarded as property. In his
essay, "The good that is interred in their bones", Barry Lyons asks: Are there
property rights in the child? He answers that yes, the children must be taken *implicitly* as property (Lyons 2011, 400). This is because, first, the parents have the power
in their relationship with the children; second, the concept of property implies a
right of disposal (*Verfügungsrecht*). Lyons argues, therefore, that "the property
model ...offers... the clearest mechanism to explain the parental right to authorize
the transfer of biological material from an unconsenting human to a third party"
(Lyons 2011, 400). There are legal constraints. Family law defines a limit: since the

---

[2] See Schües and Rehmann-Sutter 2015, Chap. 2 in this book. Ethical implications of donations by
children discusses Liebsch (2015).

[3] https://plato.stanford.edu/entries/property/
    See Gehring 2006, 44; Freeman 1997.

[4] Certainly, ownership does not always mean that the owner has the right to do anything she wishes
with what she owns. Ownership may also involve responsibility. To some extent this is seen in the
history of animal rights.

family belongs to the private realm and since the parents have the parental right, they have the freedom of decision (within limits) as to how to deal with their children. Despite this, Lyons laid out some lines of argument that question the implicit semantic shifts of the concept of property with regard to the body and transplantation practices.

Are children the property of their parents? Is their body the family's property? In what sense does a child and her body belong to the family? And if a child or someone belongs to the family, does this – the belonging – entail *giving* body parts?

The seventeenth-century philosopher and physician John Locke (1690) emphasized the relationship between labour and property: "Every man has a property in his own person" (Book II, Ch V, § 27). Through one's own physical and mental capacities we can turn things by way of bodily labour into our property, the fruits of our labour. But human beings are not allowed to put another's body at their disposal, not even after death. Children are not their parents' property, but are entrusted to them in the name of God, or put more secularly, parents have responsibility for them. Locke formulated defensive rights and, as Immanuel Kant later put it even more strongly, the right of integrity. Both lines of reasoning deny that someone has ownership rights to their own body, and even less to somebody else's.[5]

With new medical technologies, and particularly in reproductive medicine, the idea of property rights to the body have become more topical, especially with regard to ethical, social or juridical questions concerning abortion, surrogate motherhood, reproductive medicine, or tissue or organ transplantation. Property rights in the body concern, first, the issue of the body – both one's own and the body of another – and second, the difficult problem that in terms of these property rights the body is closely associated with the notion of commodity. The two aspects are intimately related because if someone considers a body to be property, the body has already been transformed into a commodity. "Commodity" refers historically to agricultural goods and raw materials: in the capitalist tradition, as described by Karl Marx, a commodity is a good that resulted from human labour and that can be sold on the general market. In any case, the term transforms a person and her body into a physical thing that has been introduced to the market circulation of medical remedies. The idea of the body being treated as a thing, an object, or even a commodity was of major concern to some interviewees.

For instance, there is the mother (Bahr) being afraid "that child just feels USED", and indeed the donor child is afraid she might be required to donate again in the future. Hence, imagining the child's body as a spare parts depot does not seem far-fetched. In reality, some of the donors were asked to donate more than once, giving tissues such as stem cells, blood, in one case even a salivary gland. The concern that the child's body or the child herself will be seen as a commodity that can be used is formulated in some interviews. For some donors, a SCT and having provided a body part as a remedy certainly triggers their imagination of themselves as a therapeutic tool.

---

[5] See different positions in Schües and Foth 2019.

The father in the Kunow family talks about the "sibling child who is ABLE to donate... due to compatibility" and he didn't want to put pressure on her, yet sees that it is impossible not to apply pressure and to see the child (not her body?) as a kind "of spare parts depot". Thus, in this context the reference is not made to the body part or to some liquid, but to the whole person, as if it were the child that was compatible (and not just the HLA marker). Since apparently the thought of being a spare parts depot (the depot being the whole of the body) was vividly present, one mother (Kunow) told the child: "You aren't a spare parts depot for your brother.... where did you get that from... I didn't have you so that you constantly have to keep donating something or other to your brother" (Wahl, donor). The mother wants to reassure her child that she – "as a person" – is not used *as* a spare parts depot even though bodily material had been taken from her. A consequential question arises: is the child or (just) the body being used as a commodity? In order to tackle this question, I shall turn to a phenomenological perspective on the body and on corporeality. The question is what it would mean to regard and treat someone or someone else's body as a spare parts depot. Here I am not just asking what it would mean for the person to be treated as a commodity. The above examples of the interview already show a concern, even a worry, that this would be the case. Rather, I want to thematize the body in its intertwinement with the person herself and her social context.

The phenomenologist Maurice Merleau-Ponty describes how a body is ambiguous, insofar as it is never just a physical object nor just a subject (self); I am my body and I have a body; and thereby I am related to and living in the world. The body is a lived body, and a person is embodied (Merleau-Ponty 2012, 431). If someone requires ownership of a body, then in this view the person herself would always be part of this property claim. One could argue that the parents claim to own the whole child. It is not only that we know, in the economic and social realm, about the history of colonialization and slavery, i.e. property on the basis of ratification, or about current situations of slave-like workers or housekeepers, but also that the question of ownership is equally debated in the medical sphere. However, reference to the ownership of one's own or another's body runs into metaphysical problems. With regard to being the owner of one's own body, the self would need to divide itself from the physical body in order to own it. In other words, ownership of the body presupposes a dualistic perception of human beings.

Claiming only to possess and to have the right of disposition (*Verfügungsrecht*) of the whole physical body does not make sense in the light of the body's complexity, embedded in a concrete situation and in between the self and the physical. Merleau-Ponty's concept of corporeality and intercorporeality demonstrates that the body is never *just and only* physical, that consciousness is corporeal and experience is embodied (Merleau-Ponty 2012, 265). The terms corporeality, intercorporeality or flesh indicate the ground from which phenomena may emerge, but they are not something to which we can point directly; rather, they are used as an adjective, for example in the sense of a corporeal experience. Corporeality as such remains anonymous. Intercorporeality underlies the relation between the self and the other, one's own body and that of the other. Intercorporeality is for Merleau-Ponty an anthropological condition of meaning constitution, which is bound to the body interaction. Being towards the world and being with others is always already bodily. "I am everything that I see and I am an intersubjective field, not in spite of my body and my historical situation, but rather by being this body and this situation and by being through them, everything else" (Merleau-Ponty 2012, 478). Phenomenologically, the body is made of a double structure because it is always sensitive in a double way which is most notable in self-touch (Husserl 1952, 164). In touching oneself, one is touching and being touched. Merleau-Ponty elaborates on this phenomenon with regard to the relationship with the Other, which is always bodily embedded, hence intercorporeal. Proposing the concept of a chiasmic structure, Merleau-Ponty differentiates three aspects that are important for understanding the concept of intercorporeality. The body is sensitive-sentient and as such displays an ontological intertwining between subject and object among sensitive things, physiological senses and linguistic expressions. Second, there is the lack of coincidence. As Edmund Husserl had already observed, we always perceive more than there is and there is always more than we perceive. It is neither entirely I nor the "body that perceives" (Merleau-Ponty 1968, 9). The sentient and sensitive are always distinguishable because of a divergence (*écart*) that suspends their coincidence. Third, intercorporeality nevertheless brings the Other into a co-presence with me. The example of the handshake allows Merleau-Ponty to discuss the phenomenon of my hand touching hers and being touched by her hand (Merleau-Ponty 1964). The concept of intercorporeality refers to this reversibility of being touched and touching, but also seeing and being seen; and therefore, it opens the space for the reversibility of perspectives by closing off the possibility of experiencing the Other just as a thing.[6] Likewise, we do know that people are able to treat – and have treated – other human being just as things, commodities or instruments.

To return to the worries expressed in the interview: owning the whole child is certainly thinkable; the commodification of the child may creep in through the back door. This much we can say: when the mother declares, "You aren't a spare parts depot for your brother..." she refers to her child (the donor) in the sense of a subject body and an embodied self. If indeed she had been used as a commodity, then it would not have been just her body but actually herself, her bodily self – she as a human being who had been turned into a spare parts depot. In other words, using someone else's body as a thing, as a commodity, disrupts the integrity of the person.

As researchers, it is not up to us to decide whether or not the parents simply saw and used their child as a commodity, but to consider what it means now to use parts of the body as treatment for someone else and as a matter of course (*Selbstverständlichkeit*). Even though there is an inseparable unity between the body and a person, we can certainly envision and use separable parts of the body.

---

[6] In his last and unfinished work, Merleau-Ponty uses the concepts of flesh and chiasm to allude to the described reversibility of sensing and sensed, but also to the intertwining of physiological and literary senses. In the following, intercorporeality is used only to refer to human relationships.

15.2.2 Body Parts Belonging to the Family?

Taking seriously the idea that parents do not own their children, one might still argue that by agreeing in all self-evidence to the stem cell transplant, they implicitly assume ownership of parts of their child's body and that they have them at their disposal. Even though some parents reported not feeling as if they had actively decided on the process, they certainly agreed to transfer body material from one child's body to the other. Thus, it seems that this discourse of agreement presupposes the division of a "physical body" into parts. However, this view needs to be questioned.

Theoretical or ethical approaches that understand the body *only* in terms of properties or physicality disturb an understanding of the integrity of the embodied self, the level of corporeality, bodily relationships, or intercorporeality among human beings.

The integrity of the embodied self, body, language and relationships is important for anchoring the child, or any person, in relation to herself and the world. The concept of integrity embraces the physical and psychological wholeness of the person in relation to herself and her world relationships, correlating psychologically with the person's resilience and morally with incorruptibility. Our intercorporeal and personal relationships are the basis on which we experience and they are the network in which we act and are treated. Therefore, integrity is a term that designates a normative as well as a relational state of affairs. Thus, any decision on the treatment of a child concerns not only her body but also her relationships in which she is bodily embedded as a person. It is therefore important to realize that the embodied self cannot be fully addressed in objective terms. We find our corporeality, and also our sociality, in "the thickness of the pre-objective present" that marks the personal existence in its entanglement and "communication with the world more ancient than thought" (Merleau-Ponty 2012, 457, 265).[7] Thus, the term "corporeality" stands for the pre-existence or pre-personal history that constitutes the core of the subject in its relationship with the other and the world. The in-betweenness among people is anonymous, because of the way that experiences with the Other in her cultural and social setting take place "under a veil of anonymity. *One* uses the pipe for smoking, the spoon for eating, or the bell for summoning, and the perception of a cultural world could be verified through the perception of a human act and of another man" (Merleau-Ponty 2012, 363, also 223).

A bodily disturbance in terms of objectivation, fragmentation, and naturalization captures the experience of a person who feels ill. The sick body gives the feeling of falling apart. The body that one *is* becomes the body that one *has*. Perceiving someone with regard to her bodily material parts, taking her parts and thereby giving her the experience of illness and injury is an affront to the whole body subject. The

---

[7]Merleau-Ponty uses the term "corporeality" cautiously in *Phenomenology of Perception*, and he unfolds it with some variations in his later work including his 1954–55 lecture *Institution and Passivity* and his final uncompleted manuscript, *The Visible and Invisible*.

integrity of the embodied subject is fragmented by being forced to feel injured and by being discussed in terms of pure material, the level of corporeality is reduced to the biomedical substance, the ambiguity of in-betweenness is forced into determining one feature, namely the HLA compatibility of body material.

By feeling into oneself, and within the phenomenological tradition of the twentieth century, authors like Husserl, Merleau-Ponty, Heidegger, Sartre and Simone de Beauvoir do not comprehend the body as a thing but as "a situation: it is our grasp on the world" or even our outline for the future (Beauvoir 2009, 68). The body is not just a thing with a context, but is bodily lived; not simply a biological object, but a subject of experience.

Since the body is a subject of experience and is situated in a situation, intercorporeality has a context of praxis that, in our study, is the praxis of medicine, the family and society. Practice includes particular ways of perceiving and sense-making, structures of behaviour and acting, and dimensions of moral responsibilities and values. Each of the fields concerned has its own paths, structures and dimensions. The concept of intercorporeality emphasizes four central aspects that are not thought of when talking about a close relationship or social bond.[8] Intercorporeality indicates, first, the material side and, hence, that it is part of a common symbolic-material structure; second, that this structure is bound to a concrete praxis that is not actor-centred but corporeally transmitted; third, the structure does not have a beginning or end in the sense of a positivism; and finally, therefore, the bodily relationship and its further dimensions have an openness that may generate a tendency to enable or disable in the further praxis of the family and its social context. Distinguishing these different sides of intercorporeality can be helpful for interpreting the interviews and understanding the body relation in SCT praxis.

With reference to these aspects, approaching the body in terms of its corporeality and its subjectivity enables us to address how the bodily relationships between the siblings are lived following the transplant. In the case of SCT it is not just a relationship based on familial interaction, biological kinship, or a shared daily life and beliefs, feelings or narratives. More than that, it is a relationship based on a shared materiality, i.e. the same type of stem cells that grow in both bodies. It is an intercorporeal relationship. The meaning of this particular type of sharing is grounded in the participation in a common materiality and an intersubjective field.

The transplantation of body parts may lead to an imaginary that transforms the body parts into character traits. This transformation accommodates the lived corporeality and relationality of the embodied self.

---

[8] My thinking about intercorporeality with regard to transplantation praxis has also been influenced by Gail Weiss (1999) and a description in the final pages of *Korporalität und Praxis* by Selin Gerlek (2020, 254).

15.3 Body Material Lives in Personal Traits and Characteristics

After the transplant, the physical material, the transplanted bone marrow, still plays a role for some families, donors and recipients. Family members are amazed, and observe new physical attributes and psychological characteristics in the recipient. The transplant is not just a remedy that might heal the body of the ill child. The body transplant becomes part of the inter-corporeality and relationality, for the recipient and within the family. Furthermore, and perhaps even most important, the donated body material becomes the metaphor for a saviour, and stands for a new life, a rebirth.

The observing non-donor sister acknowledged the whole procedure: "... that was kind of funny, to know that the cells are taken out of one of them and PLANTED in the other..." (Rohde, non-donor sister). Generally, family members used many metaphors to describe the transformative act of the bone marrow transplant: the notions of rebirth and new life often recurred. These metaphorical uses of "birth" (Wahl donor), as well as the very concrete reference of having helped with a "healthy bit of me now inside her" (Rohde, donor), indicate the relational aspect of transplantation. Thus, the donor Wahl said: "Life... comes from me."

A "birth" always takes place in relationship; a rebirth or a new beginning takes place when there had been "something" – life – before; and the metaphor of a rebirth or a new life is not expressed with the end directly in sight. I think, therefore, that if a donor uses the word "birth", she expresses a particular optimism. The mother refers, laughing slightly, to a "spiritual... moment" (Molle, mother) that is involved in such a body-relation and personal relation of helping. The dimensions of the concept of life are different when the bone marrow itself is seen as "a life-saver" (Jaschke, mother).[9]

> M: I said to Janine, I er (.) I'd like to be there at the time because (.) I know it's actually just a bag just like BLOOD, but it's (.) a bit different, it's bone marrow, it's a life-saver (.) and it's just going to go in. It's not a big deal but I've simply got to to be there, it's simply the MOMENT, now the bone marrow is going in. (Jaschke, mother)

Thus, the understanding of the body and the value-laden interpretation of the body material are put forward by some interviewees, and not by others. Some donors understand their body material as having the potential to be good or bad, helpful or not. Some of them therefore reported feelings of responsibility for their sibling's health and for the outcome of the bone marrow transplant (both survival and after effects). Even though parents in the study told us they reassured the donating child that she was NOT responsible for the outcome, their feelings remained, sometimes many years after the transplant.

---

[9] Bone marrow is also understood as merely a medication, a remedy, some liquid. Some interviewees thought that an organ, like a lung, is a more special thing.

M: the child who donates feels responsible for it not working, and for us that really did almost happen and it WAS like that, that Zorro doubted himself and Zorro really did look for blame in himself or his bone marrow

F: Which is nonsense of course

M: Which is OF COURSE nonsense, which I also tried to explain to Zorro, that it's nonsense (Zucker, family interview)

I: So how was it actually for you, when you found out that (..) Zedrick became ill again even after the first donation?

D: Erm I blamed myself, because my bone marrow, or I thought, my bone marrow must be bad.

I: Did your parents say anything about this?

D: No. (Zucker, donor)

Another way the merely medical discourse of stem cells is symbolically transformed is the observation by some family members that they recognized new body traits in the recipient. They formulate this in the following ways:

After the interviewer remarks that there may be "really a part of the body (.) in the other body and it lives on //and works there too//", a non-donor sister says:

> NDS: //Yes exactly and lives and // WORKS and also obviously works on her appearance and and on erm, oh, what else was there? (.) Karolin told us that she got implausibly hard fingernails, such UNBELIEVABLY hard fingernails so that you almost can't cut them and that she still has now. I mean particular attributes, I think yes, they're (.) actually appropriate for Karsten, you know, like these (.) yes. (Kirstein, non-donor sister)

The donor in the Bahr family was looking for a change of character but actually found physical things, such as hair, that had changed after the transplant.

> D: I mean whether his character has (…) has adjusted more to mine or (.) there are things of mine in him, I can't put it like that at all. (.) I have noticed physical things though. My brother (.) when he was erm (.) little, he had straw-blond hair (..), completely smooth and erm (..) yes, suddenly after the transplant, when his hair grew back, (.) it had got substantially darker, it had got curly, and those are things that were really obvious to me, because (.) it wasn't like that before and erm (.) was when- (.) as a child I was terribly enthusiastic about it, yes, but that's (.) in inverted commas a detail, (.) he's actually still the person he was before, but for him to change physically over such a detail, how can that be, it it can overturn everything like that? (.) Erm (..) but in terms of character I can't say that, it's too long ago or perhaps I was too little as well. I can't say that precisely. (Bahr, donor)

There was an attention to bodily traits and the physical and hormonal changes, as well as to emotional ones, that were observed. Family members wondered, or even worried, that the transplant had changed the recipient because of the donor's body substance.

D: Well I NEVER thought like that (.), erm, now my sister is (laughs), yes, the same as me, how stupid, now I'm no longer unique or something. (Rohde, donor)

F: What we asked ourselves as well, by the way, at that time for example they, it was this thing, well yes, after they'd explained it: it's now MALE blood that Marlena will be developing, not female any more. What does that mean actually, later on for SPORT, if they really get the idea to do a blood test and erm and so on and so forth. We asked ourselves that at that time and erm I don't even remember which doctor we talked to about it and then he said: yes but (.) you can explain it like this and it's nothing that enhances performance or similar, it's just disconcerting. (Minz, father)

Even gender aspects came up when the donor and receiver were of the opposite sex. The gender aspect was formulated in a very stereotypical way, such as the "soft, feminine.... Perhaps it affects the hormone system a bit" (Wahl, mother). On this level of character traits, family members (and actually there was no noticeable difference between parents, donor or recipient) were unsure but wondered whether a change of character would be noticeable.

D: even if you think it maybe sounds a bit odd but I KNOW who that person is, a BIT of whom my brother is carrying around in him (.) and (…) I don't know. Maybe that might have (.) changed more of his character of it if you knew that it was (.) a stranger (.) like in- in the place of my brother, so that it was a stranger- (.) or an unconnected part (.) and whether that maybe would have changed something for him or for someone in the family. (Bahr, donor)

Some people imagine the body parts – the stem cells, the bone marrow – as being character laden, but at the same time they also feel that it is *"nonsense of course"*. The medical discourse of transplantation seems to guide their thinking, that in fact the body material is just physical and has no influence on bodily traits, and certainly not on the psychological level. Yet family members – people in general – do not relate and are not bound to one another in terms of what medical vocabulary phrases as real. They need signs and imaginaries of relationship and family narrative. Perception and imagination are intertwined. The phenomenon of what is seen as change or a new characteristic is intersected by a real imaginary, formed by the discourse of the already embodied past and anticipated future. Following Jean-Paul Sartre, Merleau-Ponty explains that attention to or expectation of something will allow oneself to be affected by what had already been on the horizon of the expected and pre-known. "Imagination is without depth; it does not respond to our attempts to vary our points of view; it does not lend itself to our observation. We are never geared into imagination" (Merleau-Ponty 2012, 338). Observing such described changes in the recipient and her body seems to trouble people to a degree. Their abstract judgement allows them to "know" that it is "nonsense", but their perception lets them see that the stem cells have changed the body of the recipient. For these observers it is conceivable, certainly in the realm of the imagination, that along with new stem cells new character traits have also been introduced into the recipient. And if body material had been taken from a stranger and introduced into the family, then new characteristics would also have been introduced into the family. The family resemblance, which supports the idea of the family as a body, would have been threatened. If all of this is true, and in view of the description of the family body, for those who worry about the unity of the family it is better to have a donor from within the family, and not some stranger.

However, not all interviewees shared this view; others understood stem cells as merely physical things, as nothing special. A bit provocatively, the interviewer asks the recipient Preuss whether it would be an issue for her to have a "piece of Pascal in you". But actually her response was that she would not think "much about it" (Preuss, recipient).

In fact, many family members say that they don't think much about it.

F: Like it's (..) it's exactly like if you, you know? receive donated BLOOD or something (.) after some sort of accident you know, it- it's actually nothing really strange (.), that I've now got (.) a stranger's blood in me, I dunno. So me- like for ME personally (.) it's not. That moment when- when- when she- when she received it from him, that was (.), like. That was a really big moment, like, but right now, that bit of Pascal that's (.) in Pia, that's (.), I dunno, like for me personally (.) not (.), not anything special (laughs). (Preuss, father)

Although some might feel that having received body material from a sibling is nothing special, it still opens up space for new imaginations, perceptions and family narratives. The sense of the corporeal and the novel relationship are taken into a new realm of meaning constitution.

The imaginaries include issues of responsibility and the metaphor of "birth", bodily and psychological character traits, and rather impressively, the distinction between one's own self and the strange. The idea of distinguishing between the family's own traits and a possible new character that belongs to a stranger presupposes that the body sharing takes place within the core family.

15.4   Intercorporeality and Body Sharing

Children are generally supposed to share all sorts of things. Immanuel Kant considered that a child should learn to share her bread. The requirement to share alludes to a fundamentally civilizing task of solidarity. Sharing a piece of bread means that, once given to and eaten by someone, it will be gone and digested by the person to whom she gave it. When she shares a toy, she might get it back; and sharing a music file means that one doesn't really give away anything, because sharing means copying it. Again unlike a slice of bread, if bone marrow is given then – if all goes well – it will be reproduced in a functionally identical manner; but it does not stop there, because it continues to grow, and to be incorporated into the new body. It becomes a narrative part of the life story of both donor and recipient. For sandwiches, on the other hand, incorporation means their destruction; but they would go mouldy if they were not incorporated.

When sharing blood stem cells the donor gives away body material (by way of a medical intervention), she experiences side effects, and in the end her body replaces what has been taken. She gives life without losing life. For the recipient it is important for her body to accept the given material; the bone marrow must become part of her body in order for her to survive. In the interviews, the mode of sharing a bodily part came up as something very special.

D: I'm really and 'cos we were als- also so SIMILAR, I can only EMPHASIZE that we really (.), I don't know if the DNA is so similar or whatever is so exactly alike, (.) that tha- it was just relatively rare for siblings to match so perfectly (.) and I thought that was somehow cool. I thought it was REALLY cool, as our characters are basically different (.), but inside (.) we were kind of THE SAME (..). I thought it was so fascinating that you can be so different on the outside yet be so much the same on the inside. (Jaschke, donor)

NDS: well (..) he saved her life and [there's] so much (.) similarity and [they're] so much the same that they now also share through the shared bone marrow, that is (.) something very special. (Minz, non-donor sister)

One mother reports that she sees sharing bone marrow as creating a very special bodily bond, "a tighter bond to one another" (Zucker, mother). A bodily similarity is imagined because of the transplantation. The aspects of saving life and similarity create a bodily relationship between the siblings of a form that is usually not imagined. A bodily relationship seems different to an emotional closeness because the former stresses the *material* side of *inter-corporeality* that interacts between the body subjects.

Similarly, a mother would say the siblings had already had a *close* relationship, but this had become even deeper *because* of the transplant and *because* of sharing the "same thing".

I: did it feel strange that somehow left behind in Klaas (.) was a piece of Kira? M: No. (..) no. (.) through it all, 'cos, 'cos they were SO (..) so CLOSE to each other, erm it wasn't an UNRELATED body (.), you know. (Kunow, mother)

- siblings were "closed", "it (singular) wasn't an unrelated body". (Kunow, mother)
The mother reports that non-donor daughter believes that because of the "same thing" ... "flowing through them" the siblings are bound a bit "closer together". (Kunow, mother)

I: Also in their relationship, well not right now...
M: Exactly.
I: ... only through their actions, more like
M: yes.
I: ... that they are otherwise connected than they were beforehand?
M: Exactly. (Preuss, mother)

These two mothers talk about the closeness of the relationship based on the siblings sharing the "same thing", that is, the blood created from the same stem cells. The idea that, by transplanting the stem cells and having them grow in the body of the recipient, they would perhaps change and become less like the previous body, does not occur to them. The material side of an intercorporeal relation is thematized and evaluated.

But reality and its observation may be manifold, and for some interviewees the transplant does not change the relationship much.

M: Well, the relationship is exactly like it was before (.), oh, sometimes I think: rather more distanced perhaps because of the age difference or something, I don't know, perhaps [when they're] doing gymnastics, they've got their (.) similarities, but otherwise no. (.) NO like I said the doctor asked as well, that MUST make such a bond between the two of them, (.) I say: no, I don't notice anything of that, I mean outwardly you don't see anything. Mhm (negative) (Kötter, mother)

In this quote, the mother reports two observations: the relationship between the siblings seems not much different, perhaps even more distant; and she also refers to the problem of not being able to see anything from the outside. What could she possibly see? Behaviour that shows closeness by common social standards, a similarity in opinion, emotions or character traits. In this article, I have discussed some of these aspects, with the concept of intercorporeality placed quite centrally. This, however, is something one cannot see from the outside or report on. The atmosphere of intercorporeal closeness can be felt in a horizon of practice, yet as soon as it is reported about, its pre-conscious horizon is transferred to the level of recognition and expressed imagination.

Interestingly, most parents actually observed a close tie between the siblings: but this bodily relatedness is not something that is always consciously formulated or thought of. The interviews also show a whole set of imaginaries that may ground or simply add to the family and sibling's intercorporeal relationship. Certain imaginaries may be necessary to pursue a practice of transplantation at all, and the practice may give rise to others. The intercorporeal relationship is basic and primary. Thematizing it may show the attitude of body transformation behind the distribution of body parts. It is a material approach to the human who has a body in the sense of a living substance. This substance can be bio-technically defined and made available. Availability implies rights of ownership and access.

On the basis of medical progress and medical-ethical understanding, the body or body parts imply a reinforcement of the Cartesian dualism of substances: namely as raw material ("nature"), as productive and reproductive substance ("life"), as a means to produce other body substances (resource, "instrument"), as a useful thing, commodity, donation or remedy. Thinking in terms of the history of ideas, it is not self-evident that an internal, life-supporting body part is *donable* at all. If is understood as a material substance, the body is easily divisible. Thus a body substance can be distributed like a "useful thing", a piece of bread. After a transplant, such distribution is re-transformed in a family narrative and in corporeal relationships. Considering the work of Merleau-Ponty in reference to SCT practices, the idea of intersubjective relationships becomes one of intercorporeal relationships that much better illustrates the pre-objective ability to encounter the other and to feel close to her. The family members reported on their relationships, but whether these reports actually have access to the understanding of the intercorporeal dimension is left to the reader to decide.

Literature

Beauvoir, Simone de. 2009. *The second sex*. Trans. Constance Borde and Sheila Malovany-Chevallier. New York: Random House.

Freeman, Michael. 1997. Taking the body seriously. In *Property rights in the human body*, ed. Kristina Stern and Pat Walsh, 13–18. London: Centre of Medical Ethics.

Garzorz, Natalie, Thomas J, Eberlein B, Haferlach C, Ring J, Biedermann T, Schmidt-Weber C, Eyerich K, Seifert F, Eyerich S. 2016. Newly acquired kiwi fruit allergy after bone marrow transplantation from a kiwi-allergic donor. *JEADV*, 1136–1138. First published: 16 March 2016. https://doi.org/10.1111/jdv.13617

Gehring, Petra. 2006. Kann es ein Eigentum am menschlichen Körper geben? In *Was ist Biomacht?* 35–54. Frankfurt/New York: Campus Verlag.

Gerlek, Selin. 2020. *Korporalität und Praxis*. Paderborn: Fink.

Husserl, Edmund. 1952. *Ideas pertaining to a pure phenomenology and to a phenomenological philosophy, second book*. Trans. by R. Rojcewicz and A. Schuwer 1989. Dordrecht/Boston/London: Kluwer Academic Publishers.

Liebsch, Burkhard. 2015. Gewebespende als 'Gabe'. Ethische Implikationen von Gewebespenden an Geschwisterkinder. In *Rettende Geschwister*, ed. Christina Schües and Christoph Rehmann-Sutter, 259–279. Munich: Mentis.

Locke, John. 1690. An essay concerning the true original, extent and end of civil government (book II). In *Two Treatise of Government*. Berlin: De Gruyter.

Lyons, Barry. 2011. 'The good that is interred in their bones': Are there property rights in the child? *Medical Law Review* 19 (Summer): 372–400.

Merleau-Ponty, Maurice. 1964. The philosopher and his shadow. In *Signs*. Ed. and trans. by Richard McCleary, 159–181. Evanston: Northwestern University Press.

———. 1968. *The visible and the invisible*. Trans. by H. E. Barnes. Evanston: Northwestern University Press.

———. 2012. *Phenomenology of Perception*. Trans. by D. A. Landes. London/New York: Routledge.

Schües, Christina. 2015. Dem Willen des Kindes folgen? – Das Kindeswohl zwischen Gegenwart und Zukunft. In Rettende Geschwister, ed. Christina Schües and Christoph Rehmann-Sutter, 215–239. Münster: Mentis.

Schües, Christina, and Hannes Foth. 2019. Elternschaft. In *Handbuch Philosophie der Kindheit*, ed. Gottfried Schweiger and Johannes Drerup, 90–98. Stuttgart: J.B. Metzler Verlag.

Stone, Alison. 2019. *Being born. Birth and philosophy*. Oxford: Oxford University Press.

Weiss, Gail. 1999. *Body images. Embodiment and intercorporeality*. London: Routledge.

Young, Iris M. 1997. *Intersecting voices. Dilemmas of gender, political philosophy, and policy*. Princeton: Princeton University Press.

Open Access This chapter is licensed under the terms of the Creative Commons Attribution 4.0 International License (http://creativecommons.org/licenses/by/4.0/), which permits use, sharing, adaptation, distribution and reproduction in any medium or format, as long as you give appropriate credit to the original author(s) and the source, provide a link to the Creative Commons license and indicate if changes were made.

The images or other third party material in this chapter are included in the chapter's Creative Commons license, unless indicated otherwise in a credit line to the material. If material is not included in the chapter's Creative Commons license and your intended use is not permitted by statutory regulation or exceeds the permitted use, you will need to obtain permission directly from the copyright holder.

Chapter 16
Open Questions

Christoph Rehmann-Sutter, Martina Jürgensen, Madeleine Herzog, and Christina Schües

Abstract The families we approached have two exceptional things in common: they all experienced the dramatic event of a life-threatening disease such as leukaemia affecting one of their children; and, in all of these families, that child was treated with a stem cell transplant taken from a sibling's body. In this last chapter of the book we reflect very briefly on our interview experiences, analysis, and discussions. In the end, we identify open questions and further areas which may invite further research.

Keywords Family narratives · Interview experiences · Responsibility · Care · Decision-making · Family body · Healing

The families we approached have two exceptional things in common: they all experienced the dramatic event of a life-threatening disease such as leukaemia affecting one of their children; and, in all of these families, that child was treated with a stem cell transplant taken from a sibling's body.

In richly informative interviews they showed us what they had experienced, how they remembered the events, and how they narrated them – in a great many different ways, and at various time points afterwards. Beyond the transplant itself, some of the families and family members encountered entirely unforeseen challenges and obstacles, and despite their efforts often found themselves able to solve the problems that confronted them. We felt welcomed and accepted as empathic observers. We heard from families who experienced the interviews as an occasion to reflect on that time in the past, and also to exchange views with us and with each other. We are extremely grateful to the families and all interviewees for being so open and sharing their perspectives with us. On these occasions we heard explicit accounts and also

C. Rehmann-Sutter · M. Jürgensen (✉) · M. Herzog · C. Schües
Institute for History of Medicine and Science Studies, University of Lübeck,
Lübeck, Schleswig-Holstein, Germany
e-mail: christoph.rehmannsutter@uni-luebeck.de; martina.juergensen@uni-luebeck.de;
c.schuees@uni-luebeck.de

© The Author(s) 2022

C. Schües et al. (eds.), *Stem Cell Transplantations Between Siblings as Social Phenomena*, Philosophy and Medicine 144,
https://doi.org/10.1007/978-3-031-04166-2_16

recognised more implicit, but nevertheless vital, overarching family narratives. Complex issues were explained to us and detailed memories shared.

After analysing the collected materials, we discussed our main findings and sketched out preliminary conclusions. We invited a number of colleagues to join us in this process: they contributed commentaries, which have grown into the chapters of this book. We are very grateful for the inspiration and insights that originated in them. As summarised in the opening chapters to the four sections of this book, what we have seen has shown that the theme of 'transplantation between siblings' goes well beyond straightforward moral considerations. In order to grasp the issue, we needed to address not just the ethical complexity, but also familial and psychosocial considerations, ontological and existential aspects, and even the interrelation between the donor and recipient bodies.

The ethical question is not solely about weighing advantages against disadvantages of the transplantation – but nevertheless our study gave us a more comprehensive understanding of the issues around utility as well. While confirming some of the medical and psychological benefits for recipients and donors, the study might add some weight to the other side of the balance – the disadvantages and burdens of the procedure of sibling donation, compared to unrelated donors or haploidentical transplants from parents. Besides the weighing of advantages against disadvantages, the ethical issues of transplantation also include the possibilities of an emotional transformation of family relationships as well as of the quality of family life itself.

Overall, we do not want to conclude that sibling donation should not take place, but we still want to raise awareness of the long-term implications, downsides and psychosocial difficulties of the procedure in the context of whole families, difficulties which are perhaps less clearly visible from a purely medical, outcome-oriented perspective.

Ultimately, we certainly have more questions than we did when we started. Some of them may lead to further discussion beyond this book. We want to mention five areas where we think that there remain open questions, and invite readers to give them more attention.

1. Action and outcomes

The situation of a child's severe illness, together with the option of treating her with a stem cell transplant taken from her sibling, is one that is utterly exceptional and beyond everyday care. Such a situation and its consequences are difficult to understand, yet understanding seems important in order to make decisions under considerable stress and urgency. Understanding the meanings connected to the option of 'donation' by the sibling is also important for family bonding and for the narratives that evolve, after either consenting to this option or rejecting it. Physicians have clearly described the action of extracting stem cells from one body and infusion into another. It entails a small risk and some burden on the side of the donor but is a tremendous chance for the sick child. Physicians present the whole procedure as being manageable.

However, a closer look reveals that the issue of stem cell transplantation is actually far more complicated. There may be unsuccessful outcomes, there is a risk that re-transplantation will be needed, or that there will be other potential complications, and much more. Thus, it must be clear to the parents that the decision taken *now* will matter in the future and will be an exceptional experience for the family. In conditions of such overwhelming complexity there is a need to simplify, to see the basic structure of the situation, to distinguish the essential from the peripheral.

From a theoretical perspective, other questions arise. What is, in fact, 'the action' under scrutiny? What is the 'choice', what is the 'outcome' of this action? Amartya Sen has written extensively about this. While criticising utilitarianism and thinking more fundamentally about social choice, in particular about what counts as the 'outcome' of a choice to be ethically evaluated, he calls our attention to the danger of reductionism in some of the dominant streams in the consequentialist literature (Sen 2000). This is relevant to our context as well. Outcomes are plural and cannot be reduced to one or more measurable results ('outcome parameters'), such as life years or contribution to happiness and welfare. Two aspects would be lost: There is first the act of choice, and then the processes and events that lead to certain results, and that continue to have repercussions in the lives of the families. Sen writes: "A person's preferences over *comprehensive* outcomes (including the choice process) have to be distinguished from the conditional preferences over *culmination* outcomes *given* the acts of choice" (Sen 1997, p. 745). Comprehensive outcomes include the essential question of *who does the choosing*, i.e. who are the agents in the choice process. And they include all other relevant aspects of the choice process as well. For some of our respondents in the study, the processes of choice and of coming to terms with it retrospectively were more burdensome and complicated than the act of the transplant itself.

One important aspect of the outcomes of the decision, which many of our respondents emphasised, is the fact that the primary responsible decision-makers are the parents. As a consequence of their (and ultimately no one else's) decision, they treat one of their children in an instrumental way that is at least partly in conflict with their parental obligations to care for the child who is used as a stem cell donor. Parents apply what Sen calls 'agent-sensitive' responsibility and evaluation (Sen 2000, p. 488). They are aware of their obligations to each of their children. The situation is seen by moral philosophers, and some parents, as a conflict. The impact and the aftershocks of the decision on the family system are related to what the parents (and physicians) have inflicted on a child, who may have experienced a psychosocial benefit but certainly not a medical one, and these choices are attributable to them as parents.

The question of the inclusiveness of the concept of outcomes also extends over time. In the history and narratives of the family space, where are the limits to the consequences that must be attributed to 'the action'? Both the actions involved in transplantation and the outcomes of the actions are far more complex and extensive than parent and child decision-makers could reasonably *foresee* at the point of decision-making. Even years after, the transplant is still alive in their memories and is recognised to have changed many things in the family. In some families it remains an ever-present feature of their family history and is surrounded by family narratives.

From these observations and reflections a set of questions follows: What can be learned from this for our ideas about action and outcomes of action, and about foreseeability more generally? What are the implications for medical ethics and beyond? The 'action' at the centre of stem cell transplantation is clearly much more complex than only a transfer of tissue and the medical primary and secondary outcomes.

2. Ethics in care practices

Apart from its consequences, moral questions also circulate around the transplant itself. When we reflect ethically on the key decision in the stem cell transplantation context, we have good reasons to argue that a consequence-independent, duty-only moral perspective is as inadequate as a consequentialist one. The injunction of a child's 'duty to donate' seems rather misplaced. For similar reasons an outcomes-only perspective (such as the utilitarian) is inadequate in that it does not do justice to the moral perceptions of the people who are actually the responsible decision-makers. A consequences-only perspective would not properly address the questions that are raised by the initial act of making one child a donor, such as the legitimacy of conferring the donor role on the child.

A consequence-sensitive relational assessment of care as practice seems more appropriate. However, it also needs to include a critical reflection on the virtue-related offers to the donor child (to become a saviour, a hero, or even to have made a sacrifice). This assessment should be based on an ethics of care (Barnes et al. 2015; Vosman et al. 2020), which allows us to understand the conflicts and relational intertwinement of responsibilities (Walker 2007) that arise in caring for one child, for the other children, for the parents caring for each other and for themselves, and even for the children caring for each other.

Care and responsibility are terms that capture the essence of the ethical concerns moving the actors in these dramas. A key question raised for the further development of an ethics of care is therefore: In what sense did the attention and responsiveness of family members towards each other change as a result of their different experiences during the time of illness and transplantation? How can we understand and evaluate the *conflicts* of responsibilities that arise in the practices of care relationships during and after such difficult situations?

3. Framing the situation of decision-making

In the standard view, the key ethical question in stem cell transplantation between minor siblings is whether it is permissible to use tissue from the body of a healthy child who is too young to consent in order to help another person. We have heard families narrating that they felt they had no alternative in that situation, and were unable to take a different decision, or that they did not even see the decision as 'a decision' to be taken but as a matter of course.

How far is this situation constructed by the medical professionals who present it to the parents in a certain way? Recent developments in the registry of unrelated donors and also in transplantation of partially mismatched, haploidentical parents (*haploHSCT*; Berger et al. 2016) suggest that the situation for the parents would be significantly different if they had to think first about an unrelated donation, then about themselves donating as parents and, only if neither strategy worked out, about asking another child to be tested and if possible to be a tissue donor. The two scenarios A and B (A the standard view; B the view of transplantation using children as a last resort) clearly have different implications.

Clinical routines need to be more reflective about framing the situation of decision-making as scenario A or B, i.e. about how to present it to the parents, rather than concerned only with the justification of stem cell donation per se. This is of course a topic for medical ethics and law. The German Transplantation Law § 8a stipulates that before a minor sibling can be considered as a donor, an adult donor should be sought. In *practice*, however, this is usually not done if there is a family with two or more children. Thus, the relationship between the law, medical ethics, and practice needs to be investigated more thoroughly.

4. Healing of a family

Families are involved both in caring practically for a child and in the worry about the child's illness. We encountered many different examples and were able to study them to a certain extent. When a child becomes seriously ill, the rest of the family, while physically unaffected by the disease, is very often affected emotionally and morally, both individually and on the level of organisation of family life. Sometimes (but not always) family life had to be reorganised in order to cope with the new circumstances. Illness is therefore more than just the disease of one individual child. It is a family issue, sometimes a family crisis. Understanding this affects our understanding of a disease and also our concepts of treatment and healing.

What is transplantation as a treatment? Sibling donation contributes to making this disease a family affair: in some ways a dangerous adventure, in others a difficult experience, and sometimes a tragedy. Nevertheless, for some families the transplantation also became an experience of pride, agency and strength because they were able to regain control and influence over a situation of serious illness. Such an experience may also strengthen family ties. Hence, the topic of family transformation within a medical context raises many questions for further study by a sociologically and philosophically informed child psychology, psychology of the family, and medical ethics.

5. Familial bodies as a remedy

The development of new successful treatments and emergent styles of clinical research, for example in 'precision' or 'personalised' medicine, brings the physical body into the realm of family debates and, in new ways, into negotiations of responsibility as well. To our families it became quite normal to consider having a family member's body at their disposal when transplantation had to take place, or when information for 'multi-omics' medicine together with certain kinds of surveillance were needed.

Do we therefore need to think about new social-ontological concepts of the body? Will these medical options transform our family relations, or at the very least introduce a substantial new dimension? The bodies of the family members become a resource for healing purposes. Once the data, for instance about HLA compatibility, are collected they remain potentially useful in future.

Our research into this rather specific situation of stem cell transplantation between minor siblings has revealed rich realms of questions and themes that will be fruitful for further debates extending beyond the concrete scenarios discussed in this book.

Literature

Barnes, Marian, Tula Brannelly, Lizzie Ward, and Nicki Ward, eds. 2015. *Ethics of care: Critical advances in international perspective*. Bristol: Policy Press.

Berger, Massimo, Edoardo Lanino, Simone Cesaro, et al. 2016. Feasibility and outcome of haploidentical hematopoietic stem cell transplantation with post-transplant high-dose cyclophosphamide for children and adolescents with hematologic malignancies: An AIEOP-GITMO Retrospective Multicenter Study. *Biology of Blood and Marrow Transplantation* 22 (5): 902–909. https://doi.org/10.1016/j.bbmt.2016.02.002.

Sen, Amartya. 1997. Maximization and the act of choice. *Econometrica* 65 (4): 745–779.

———. 2000. Consequential evaluation and practical reason. *The Journal of Philosophy* 97 (9): 477–502.

Vosman, Frans, Andries Baart, and Jaco Hoffmann, eds. 2020. *The ethics of care: The state of the art*. Leuven: Peeters.

Walker, Margaret Urban. 2007. *Moral understandings: A feminist study in ethics*. 2nd ed. Oxford: Oxford University Press.

Open Access This chapter is licensed under the terms of the Creative Commons Attribution 4.0 International License (http://creativecommons.org/licenses/by/4.0/), which permits use, sharing, adaptation, distribution and reproduction in any medium or format, as long as you give appropriate credit to the original author(s) and the source, provide a link to the Creative Commons license and indicate if changes were made.

The images or other third party material in this chapter are included in the chapter's Creative Commons license, unless indicated otherwise in a credit line to the material. If material is not included in the chapter's Creative Commons license and your intended use is not permitted by statutory regulation or exceeds the permitted use, you will need to obtain permission directly from the copyright holder.

Appendix: Study Description and Additional Quotes

Study Description and Sample

Research Questions/Aims of the Study

The aim of our retrospective qualitative study was to investigate the short-, medium- and long-term family and psychosocial effects of blood stem cell transplantation between siblings of minor age. Our interest focused on whether and in what way the sibling donation changed family relationships and dynamics from the viewpoint of each individual family member and of the family as a whole, and how family members judged and interpreted these changes in retrospect. For example, did new patterns of responsibility and dependency arise? Are there family discourses of guilt or gratitude? What impacts and implications does the experience of sibling donation have for the personal development of individual family members? How are ideas about the integrity of the body and individual bodily uniqueness affected by the transfer of body material from one family member to another? And what enables families to cope positively with their experience of a radical crisis: a child's critical illness?

The research questions of our project were complex, and address several topics at different levels:

- Blood stem cell transplantation takes place against a backdrop of a serious, generally life-threatening illness (such as leukaemia). There is ample literature confirming that both the threat posed by the illness to the life of a child, and the possible consequences for the family as a whole and its individual members, place a major burden on the *whole* family (e.g. Hendrischke 2010; Schoors et al. 2018; Alderfelder and Kazak 2006; Alderfer and Stanley 2012; Björk et al. 2011).
- The practice of paediatric stem cell transplantation touches on central ethical questions, such as the basic legitimacy of an intervention into the life of the donor that only benefits someone else, especially since a child – and often a very

© The Author(s) 2022

C. Schües et al. (eds.), *Stem Cell Transplantations Between Siblings as Social Phenomena*, Philosophy and Medicine 144,
https://doi.org/10.1007/978-3-031-04166-2

young one – cannot legally give informed consent. Questions arise as to changing duties within the family, with dependency relationships as a background (see American Academy of Pediatrics 2010; Beverley and Beebe 2018; Rehmann-Sutter et al. 2013; Schües and Rehmann-Sutter 2013, 2014).
- The time perspective presumably influences the interpretation and evaluation of individual and family experiences – not least since children develop new perspectives in the course of their maturation and development.

Study Design

Addressing the research questions of the study needed a multi-dimensional approach (to data collection and analysis). First, the experiences, perceptions and interpretations of the individual family members (parents, donor children, recipient children, other siblings, possibly other persons the family considers relevant) are central, and must be lifted out of individuals' own subjective perspectives for analysis. In addition, families are also specific entities: they produce shared "stories" and experiences, they refer back to their own horizons of knowledge and values, they demonstrate family-specific dynamics and have family-specific resources (e.g. their social setting, communication within the family and with the outside world, financial resources).

We decided to use qualitative interviews with a strong narrative focus, combining family interviews and subsequent individual interviews with family members who were more than 4 years of age and were prepared to take part. The family could decide for themselves who counted as a relevant family member. The experience, advantages and disadvantages of this methodological approach have been summarised in two publications (Herzog et al. 2019; Herzog et al. submitted).

Questions targeted to the particular interviewees were formulated to stimulate narratives, differentiated by family or individual interview, and phrased age-appropriately. An (optional) set of follow-up questions was also developed to generate the narrative.

Recruitment

To recruit study participants, all the clinics on the German Society for Paediatric Oncology and Haematology's list (a total of 60) received information flyers and other material about our study, and were asked to help us with recruitment by passing on leaflets to suitable families. Clinics were also offered a personal presentation on the study by one of our researchers for further information. The DKMS (German bone marrow donor register) and children's hospices were also contacted.

Further, approaches were also made to the four German aftercare clinics for children/families, and to 25 regional and supra-regional self-help groups, parents' initiatives, and associations to support sibling children. A total of approx. 1500 study leaflets were disseminated, either displayed or passed directly to the families, via these routes. Regular follow-up and personal contact-making (e.g. at conferences, and working meetings of the Deutsche Krebsstiftung – German cancer foundation) were used to win stakeholders on the ground for long-term support in recruiting study participants.

To inform families directly about our study, and also to reach those who were no longer under medical supervision, study information leaflets were sent out via various mailing lists in the researchers' professional and social fields, and flyers were distributed at central public places (e.g. libraries, cultural institutions and cinemas) in 10 large cities in Germany.

The study participants were recruited from across Germany. They comprised families in which a minor child "donated" blood stem cells to a sibling. In order to gain the most comprehensive insight into the subject and to cover the whole bandwidth of possible experiences, we tried to involve as many different families as possible. They differed in various ways, including

- the age of the child receiving the transplant
- the age of the donor child at the time of the transplant
- the time since the transplant
- the family's social and cultural background (educational level, home, religion etc.)
- the sick child's diagnosis
- the result of the illness / transplant: cure, mitigation, serious complications or sequelae, relapse, death.

Families with inadequate German were excluded.

Sample

A total of 73 persons from 17 families took part in our study. We carried out 16 family interviews and 66 individual interviews. This allowed us to achieve a high degree of heterogeneity of the sample in terms of the aspects mentioned above (children's age etc.).

At the time of study participation the transplant had taken place 0–5 years previously for 5 families, 6–10 years for 6 families, and 11–20 years for 5 families. In one family the interview took was conducted 2 weeks before the transplantation. The donor children were aged between 2¾ and 20 years at the time of the transplant, and between 3¾ and 35 years at the time of the interview. Those receiving the transplant were aged between 2 and 23 years at the time of the transplant and between 3 and 32 years at the time of the interview.

In two of the 17 families, the transplant did not stabilise the sick child's health longterm and the children had died after years of treatment. At the time of the interview some of the recipient children were still suffering from the longterm effects of the illness and the transplant; others had recovered completely and were living without any constraints.

In four families more than one blood stem cell transplant had been carried out; in two of these, the second donation had come from the same sibling, and in one the first donation from a sibling was followed by one from the mother and then a further one from an unrelated donor. In the fourth family, the sibling donating bone marrow had then also donated further body material (salivary gland).

Most commonly, the illness that had led to the need for a blood stem cell transplant was leukaemia (different forms). This diagnosis was present in a total of 10 families, while a diagnosis of myelodysplastic syndrome was present in two families, and of adrenoleukodystrophy (ALD), metachromatic leukodystrophy (MLD), aplastic anaemia, Fanconi anaemia, and haemophagocytic lymphohistiocytosis (HLH) in one family each.

A detailed description of the participating families and family members is given in Part C of the Appendix.

Study Procedure

An initial telephone conversation informed the family about the purpose and procedures of the study. Family members had the opportunity to ask questions and to choose the time and location for the interview. All the families chose to have interviews in the family home or that of a family member. The definition of which persons were family members, and who should take part in the interviews, was left to the families themselves.

All the interviews were carried out by the authors (MH and MJ), in most cases jointly. The study day began with introductions (see below) followed by the family interview, and continuing with the individual interviews. This order was chosen for the following reasons:

- At the start of the visit there was an initial go-round in which all participants introduced themselves briefly and got to know each other, the timetable for the day was discussed, and the formalities (informed consent) completed. This shared round with all those involved led on logically to the shared family interview. This procedure proved its value particularly with younger children, who in this way could get to know the interviewers and become familiar with the situation, in the presence of their family. We believe it also raised the quality of the subsequent individual interviews.
- The family interview was designed primarily to make visible the dynamics, interactions, distribution of roles, communication structures, shared meaning-making and joint "stories" of those involved. The content of this family interview (see above) offered the interviewers a good general overview to which they could link the individual interviews.

The interviews were an hour long on average, although they were significantly shorter for smaller children.

Audio recordings were made of all the interviews, with the participants' permission, and were then transcribed verbatim. The transcripts pseudonymised names, places, dates and other facts that might allow the interviewees to be identified.

Analysis

Interviews were analysed according to the typical iterative approach of qualitative research in parallel with data collection. This approach ensures constant linkage of data acquisition and evaluation, and that the narrative-generating follow-up questions and clarifications were continuously updated.

The data were analysed using a process based on the documentary method. This aims to reconstruct and interpret both implicit meanings and the interviewees' empirical knowledge (in this study, knowledge of family rules, norms, behaviour patterns, things the family finds relevant or takes for granted. The method is characterised by constant within-case or cross-case contrasts, through which commonalities or particularities of the cases (and their underlying structures and behaviour patterns) could be mapped out. For a more precise analysis of the family dynamics, communication patterns, resources and resilience, a detailed structured case analysis was drawn up.

The data were analysed by two interviewers jointly and discussed at regular meetings of the whole interdisciplinary team. In addition, the analytical approach and the (interim) results were discussed with an external expert (Nicoletta Eunicke, Johannes Gutenberg-Universität Mainz) at a two-day workshop. Further discussion and interdisciplinary working through of the study materials and results took place as part of the project's final conference on "Care, responsibilities and integrity", on 14 and 15 February 2019 in Lübeck, out of which this book project arose.

Additional Quotes

Topic I: Mapping Responsibilities

Donation as a Family Responsibility: A Matter of Course
(*"Selbstverständlichkeit"*)?

> Father: that what's nice about the whole thing, that a family like that can solve something like this, these problems. (Kötter)
> Mother: because it's not a matter of course, is it, even though Zorro was then under 18 and I took the decision for him, but erm despite that it shouldn't be taken for granted and they should also get it across to the child that it wasn't taken for granted but it was something special and a BIG achievement. (Zucker)
> Non-donor sister: that she has to have bone marrow and that we all need to get ourselves tested or whether we wanted to get ourselves tested and I think, that's actually not something to question. (Kirstein)

Father: I don't know, he always took it for granted. There wasn't anyone else who put him under pressure or anything, there there WAS no discussion at all. "I'll do that for my brother" and erm like like like they also got everything started, I mean somehow (.) not that you'd say, that's somehow been forced on him by his parents or something. It was his voluntary decision. (Kötter)

Non-donating brother: Well (..) er, it came up that Marlena needed a bone marrow transplant and they would have to [tissue] type for this. I can't now remember the moment when my parents asked me, Manuel, would you like to get typed? It was a sort of thing, that you, like it SHOULD be like this in the family or as I understood it, you want to get TYPED, you HAVE YOURSELF typed. (Minz)

Non-donating sister: and Maximilian and I wouldn't have thought about it for a moment and Marlena too, if she had NOT been in this situation, but had been the DONOR, she'd had done exactly the same thing. And I think that's why this she won't have this feeling, no way do I have to do a good thing, because Malle and Lena both know, the other way round she'd have done exactly the same, yes. (Minz)

Donor: And so it was LITERALLY a matter of life and death. Of course it was clear that (.), I mean that I was now saving his life. Y'know. (Wahl)

Donor: so I was then asked if I wanted to do it, but there was never ever any question, I mean it just fitted and then (laughs) it somehow simply had to get done. (Grohmann)

Non-donor sister: Then she explained shortly beforehand that it wasn't working with the chemo, that she just needed to have bone marrow and that we should all get ourselves tested or whether we wanted to get ourselves tested, and I mean, there's no question actually. Yeah, and then we all got ourselves tested. (Kirstein)

Donation as a Family Duty?

Mother: it was also clear to me, without us having a massive discussion with Zorro, that Zorro WILL donate whether he wants to or not. And as a result this matter was, er, initially not debated with Zorro much at all, rather, like, it was ACTUALLY already CLEAR for us, whatever Zorro wanted. (Zucker)

Donor: Yes, but then for me as a child that was, you also asked me if I would like to do that, I still think it was right, but for me as a child I was still aware: if I don't do this, I'm to blame

Mother:/Exactly, if Björn dies, exactly

Donor: if Björn is dead.

Mother: That's what I mean. Yes, that was the quandary and you were very frightened, weren't you?

Donor: Yes.

Mother: Yes. (Bahr)

Donor: because then I got so much PRESSURE from my parents: come on, and you have to do this, he's your brother after all and erm, if you don't do this, then erm (..), yes, then- you you won't forgive yourself for the rest of your LIFE and come on, just do it. And then at some point I'd been put under such emotional pressure that I just said: OK, you know what, you're not going to give up anyway and I don't want afterwards to have to take responsibility, I didn't donate bone marrow to my brother. (Kunow)

Father: Right now, when I heard about your study, it went through my head again: what would you actually have done, if she had refused. (..) Quite frankly, I don't know, I'd like to

Interviewer: Difficult to say, isn't it?

Father: Yes, well I'd probably erm of course first have pleaded with her, we've got – well we did say in the first conversation, Ronja, it's your decision, erm but quite frankly it would probably (laughs) not have been Ronja's decision alone, would it, I mean as an adult you're, that you think, well if necessary I'll persuade her or somehow or I'll somehow put the pressure about feeling guilty or what do I know. Well I think, we would have pulled out all the stops, erm (sighs) erm I am glad that it didn't work out like that, I'd really have to say. (Rohde)

Mother: I said at once we'll check it out, if she's a match then she'll have to do it. Of course that was selfish, sure, we should perhaps have talked to her before: WOULD you? But we'll just do it. That's then, if she's a match, it is well, our hope MUST we do this, we don't have any other alternative. No no, that was actually clear from the outset. (Jaschke)

Donor: I still remember how that often, it SOUNDED like I'd done something good, all in all though it's just chance and genetics, that I was able to donate and it was sometimes, not EMBARRASSING, but in the sense of, well yeah, what you just said, taking credit for OTHERS' achievements, but in the sense of well, it was chance and I did it. Well, I don't need to talk about it much now. [...] It was presented at that time as though I'd done something fantastic, but I think to myself (..), but what have I got to do with it? Now I've, I was just compatible and I did it. (Minz)

Father: [Thinking about it] right now, when I heard about your study, it went through my head again: what would you actually have done if she'd refused. (..) Hand on heart, I just don't know, I'd like

Interviewer: Difficult to say, isn't it?

Father: Yes, well I'd probably have, erm, tried talking her into it of course, we said, then- in the first conversation we did say, Ronja, it's your decision, erm, but to be honest it would probably (laughs) not have been just Ronja's decision, would it, if you're the adult then it's like, you think, well if it comes to it, I'll somehow persuade her or put her under some sort of pressure with a guilty conscience, or I dunno. Anyway I reckon we'd have pulled out all the stops, uh (sighs), uhhh I do have to say I'm pleased that didn't happen. (Rohde)

Differentiated Responsibilities/Obligations

Parental duty: Caring for (all!) the children? Conflict of care (in relation to the donation and transplantation)? Do the parents feel "guilty"? Do the family members identify a dilemma?

Interviewer: it was DESPITE that for you somehow, how it feels, I mean, that's basically a healthy child

Father: THAT was never an issue. Absolutely never an issue. Of course we (laughs) asked Pascal, you know, but he also, well, saying no was never an op- OPTION for him. So none of us thought about NOT doing it, you know that was absolutely never an option for us, you know. (Preuss)

Mother: for us it was always that if Greta was a MATCH, then, um, Greta would obviously be a donor. We never gave it a second thought because it was, yeah, that's what everyone SAYS and you just don't think about it and, er, later on I was asked by friends years later, 'did you actually ask Greta if that was what she wanted?" and I said: "it never, it never occurred to us, for us it was actually ALWAYS going to be the case, like, if Greta was a match then that's what would happen (swallows), you know?" Like, you know (..) ultimately it's also a risk for Greta (..), we were actually NEVER a hundred percent I wouldn't say aware, but you put it to one side a bit, you know, that you think that, like, something might also happen to her. (Grohmann)

Non-donor sister: it did feel like they were worried about Ronja and then they discussed it with Ronja really often, whether she would really like to to do this, whether she was totally sure about it, and everyone was just a bit unsure about the whole thing, how it was going to turn out, no-one was certain, it will be JUST GREAT, we're definitely doing it, but all of us hesitated a bit had and our doubts about it and Mummy and Daddy were scared, we had a sense of that, beforehand. (Rohde)

Dilemma

Mother: Speaking for myself I always thought, it's a- it's not such a major intervention. OF COURSE, you're interfering with a perfectly healthy child, Zorro is basically healthy, erm but when you look at the BENEFIT of it, then that is NOTHING. For me it was like having an ultrasound scan during pregnancy, it wasn't any MORE than that for me. And because of that it was clear to me, without us having a massive discussion with Zorro, that Zorro WILL donate whether he wants to or not. And as a result this matter was, er, initially not debated with Zorro much at all, rather, like, it was ACTUALLY already CLEAR for us, whatever Zorro wanted. (Zucker)

Interviewer: Do you know how it was for your two OTHER children, that time, how they experienced it, have you talked about it or what?

Mother: YES (wearily), not that well (laughs), yes. I know that, looking back now, er, at the time we didn't think too much about it, things just had to work. I mean, they got their food, they got their their their clothes washed, stepmum sorted everything out and so on (.), but, er, they were just going through puberty, like. Mmm (positive), (…) they actually needed me TOO, but it just didn't happen, you know. (Kirstein)

Non-donor sister: I didn't know how I could have done things better and of course I also at some point, like much later realised that if I'd imagined myself in my mother's position I COULDN'T have DEALT with things any other way, because if you believe you're losing a child then it's- then this child has a different status in the family. And after all I was ALL RIGHT, wasn't I? So I didn't have a problem with it, I was OK, despite everything it was really hard somehow. (Minz)

Father: First of all you see the child who's lying there, and secondly, (..) erm, sounds stupid, you you see, er, er, first of all you can see: you're healthy after all, you can surely do without something. Like a ki- kind of spare parts- yeah, spare parts depot, kind of. But, erm, that shouldn't be a problem now and then, but as to what happens in the end regarding not only psychological but also physical limitations, that that is actually TODAY's problem for her. That's, erm, not what you consider and er (..) like I said, it's wrong to keep piling on the pressure. But that's not what you know in advance, we know that NOW. That you try to lead your child gently through this whole business (..), this erm, like I said, that's, that is a a serious intervention. In principle it's an intervention for the parents AND the donor. (Kunow)

Mother: Now this really is always an issue: here we have a healthy PATIENT, and to do the bone marrow donation, they administer a general anaesthetic, when they put the central line in (..) they also administered a general anaesthetic, it always involves some sort of risk, which probably might also put some other families off, but what that means right now, that we need to administer something to a healthy human being, not for their own benefit, rather so that they have to, so to speak, help someone else. (Preuss)

Father: of course I was able to put myself into Greta's situation but all I could think of was oh God, oh God, oh God, the poor girl. (Grohmann)

Mother: like with Maria we FORGOT her that whole- during those three wee- three months, that is, end of Mar- end of March, end of April, end of May, for those two months we totally overlooked Maria. (Minz)

Donor: then if a child in your family gets ill, then everything centres around them […] and yes, for my sister it was REALLY bad of course. But (..) I remember, I think it was every year after that when we er whenever we went on holiday we always talked about it, OH YES, because- whenever I had anything wrong with me it immediately put my mother in a PANIC and then er (.) my sister or my siblings would then always said something like: OH YES, it's Marlena, the favourite child, that sort of thing. (..) (sighs) HMM even if I probably wasn't- like erm who knows, no idea if if you are or not, but whenever something is wrong with one child and you're more concerned of course if one child has such an extreme history and so of course the others feel disadvantaged if I say something like: OH my toe's hurting and my mum immediately says: OH NO, I say it's OK, but we still need to look at it and if my sister has anything wrong with her then it's just YES, it's, that's how it is. (Minz)

Non-donor sister: I was somehow like the er the BYSTANDER. I had, yeah, I had nothing to DO, I wasn't a donor, I wasn't a donor match, so I was in a way, spare, and so could only observe from the outside. That's how it was, somehow: HMM, yeah, and what about me? (laughs) At the time er (.) SPARE. And that continued in the months afterwards and even when things were better for her, whenever Lena said, I NEED something, I've got a runny nose or a tummy ache, then it would have completely different status than if I'd said: I've got a tummy ache, because it was just, as far as my mother was concerned, ALARM bells would suddenly start ringing and that's how it was for me, yeah definitely! you know? And so I felt I'd been somehow left on my own, but (.) hm (..) at the time it was very hard to comprehend. In the meantime I think, that- I wouldn't have known how else they should have done it, if you have a sibling who is so unconnected how do you really INVOLVE them? Because like I said, I had to go to school, I had to get on with things so that I could somehow get my life on track. I took my- my interests kind of elsewhere, yeah, like (..) hmm (sighs) I (.) I didn't know how I could have done things better and erm (.) of course I also (.) at some point, like much later realised that if I'd imagined myself in my mother's position I COULDN'T have DEALT with things any other way, because if you believe you're losing a child then it's- then this child has a different status in the family. And after all I was ALL RIGHT, wasn't I? So I didn't have a problem with it, I was OK, despite everything it was really hard somehow. (Minz)

Mother: the other siblings realise, you know, what's being done for the poorly ones and what's not being done for those, who are just there you know, the so-called shadow kids and that's ACTUALLY true, that they are just sitting in the shadows and erm because everyone is just focusing only on the ill (.) on the ill child and erm the other child doesn't completely disappear into oblivion, I wouldn't say that, but no-one has a MIND to bother with the HEALTHY child in inverted commas, because they are simply just occupied with the ill child. And it's not only the parents, it's actually the whole family who does it, you know. And if phone calls come in then first of all they ask about the ill child and only later about the other child, and of course they get that. (Zucker)

Mother: there were rounds and rounds of family conversations that (…) siblings, it has nothing to do with donating, but at the moment we've got a child who's got cancer or is seriously ill so that it really often was the case that the siblings were somehow ignored based on: (.) do you want to swap places with your ill sibling or something like that? And I tried to avoid that if possible because I think that it's bad for the healthy child AS WELL. For example I'd rather have done it the other way round. It was in city A that it happened, I'm pretty sure, when she was really unwell (..) or during the transp- transplant period when we were alternately sleeping with her, but during the whole preparation stage, whilst she was on the ward, students who were looking after the children came at 5 o'clock in the afternoon. [...] I then drove home late in the afternoon and when they were getting clingy I said: look, Pascal ALSO needs his parents for a few hours each day at least, I said to them, you've got your own things to get on with. [...] And it was also important for me that I had some time with him too. (Preuss)

Mother: I didn't spare a thought as to how Zorro felt at the time. As far as I was concerned it was quite bad enough, the way things were, so at that time I didn't have a SINGLE thought at all for Zorro, like that. (Zucker)

Mother: We were not there AT ALL for him, we weren't able to help him at- at all or to supp- support him. (Zucker)

Mother: I think that Kaila, she also wanted to get part of me back with stuff like: "Kina's allowed to be with Mummy the whole time, but not me". So she didn't say that, but (..) she started to self-harm. (Kelling)

Donor: for me and Stina it was clear that Sven basically had priority and that our parents would primarily look after Sven and as for our own needs we, yeah, postponed them. Now I don't want to say we were neglected, I wouldn't want to say that under any circumstances, rather it was simply, it was clear to us, one of them is with Sven and we're looking on. So that was, mind you, completely OK that way. (Speidel)

Donors' Responsibilities Before Donation: The Chance for a "Rescue Attempt"

Donor: that I now [have] like this this feeling of responsibility, I'm responsible now that it – that that the cells are OK now, that I don't somehow, no idea, that I erm like I said, don't smoke and don't drink or something, al- although there I think isn't a connection like that not directly, but you don't want that either (..) erm (..) not afterwards be left with the feeling, OH I didn't like live healthily enough or something (laughs) before it. (Wahl)

Donor: in any case before, I broke my arm when doing gym and my first question was straight away, that I asked the trainer , who's also a bit of a medic and also works here with the St John Ambulance, I ask straight away whether I could still donate. Well (swallows) you already have that in the back of your mind, that everything should go well. (Kötter)

Mother: She wasn't allowed to get an infection either, you know, she had to- you- wasn't allowed to go out so much either and then you have to explain to a child who's 12, yes explain to them that she's not allowed to GO OUT, why she can't go out and then all those Harry Potter films came out, Greta really wanted to go to the cinema, her friends all went to the cinema and Greta wasn't allowed to go WITH them, because she

Interviewer: All before the transplant?

Mother: It was all before the transplant, wasn't it, because these crowds of people, you know, they told us, she was supposed to avoid them. (Grohmann)

Donor: Well, I still remember that erm at that time, when I got that medication to induce these stem cells, OH I WAS EIGHTEEN or seventeen, well I mean then – of course I thought, can I go to a festival or not, can I go to a concert, CAN I like SMOKE or DRINK or do I have to always go home by taxi because I, it was clear to me, if I, for whatever reason if I DIE, then they'll die too, I mean so that- that's a feeling of responsibility at that age, then- where you actually erm think, you're only responsible for yourself, so then somehow not like that (..) (swallows) or that afterwards I also take stock of the situation again, that I then sometimes (takes a breath) OH, what do I know, one night at a swimming pool like (laughs)) erm er with friends I like brok- BROKE IN and then it was like, I don't know, it was like in, where was that, I was like such a such a erm (..), in any case it was a tricky situation, because like young people attacked each other and with knives and so on, you know, and we also ran away at once and we then made sure that we got away, but afterwards I also thought, if I know – if something had happened to me THERE, that I like, everything that I'd experienced beforehand, where I'd sometimes been in a TRICKY situation, erm (..) I didn't regret it, but I though OH MAN, I can NEVER do that again or something, you know and that really is a strange feeling I mean at that age, if you (.) like deny yourself THINGS, not because you're like scared or something, but because you think, I have to (..) erm because for that I- because I'm not just responsible for MY body but also for another body, erm like and act like that. (..) I mean I feel like that now I'm pregnant as well (laughs). (Wahl)

Responsibility for the "Success" of the Transplantation?

Mother: the child who donates feels responsible for it not working, and for us that really did almost happen and it WAS like that, that Zorro doubted himself and Zorro really did look for blame in himself or his bone marrow

Father: Which is nonsense of course

Mother: Which is OF COURSE nonsense, which I also tried to explain to Zorro, that it's nonsense [children very loud in the background], but erm (..) YES, that- there was that situation as well. (Zucker)

Donor: and it's also important to know that, if something goes wrong, that you yourself are not to blame. I mean (..) THAT could always happen and then you should- I mean, and then you really have to see that you somehow get rid of these feelings of guilt or whatever. (Rohde)

Interviewer: So how was it actually for you, when you found out that (..) Zedrick became ill again even after the first donation?

Donor: Erm I blamed myself, (4) because my bone marrow, or I thought, my bone marrow must be bad. (6)

Interviewer: Did your parents say anything about this?

Donor: No. (Zucker)

Interviewer: she did respond, definitely, she had side effects and complications. That was NOT what you thought: oh, that could somehow [happen]?

Donor: Not at all, yes. And no one made me feel like that either, (..). And I didn't think about it either, to be honest, but no, I have felt [...] that- sure, for me all that with the BMT was done and dusted. Because ultimately the BMT itself was successful. Then at some point Marlena started producing new blood and then for me the thing really was done and dusted. And everything that was connected to the long-term effects, and for one thing the MG [myasthenia gravis], for another the whole thing with the warts. She has a lot of things, she'll tell you about them too, erm (..) I didn't feel responsible at all. I was sympathetic, but feeling responsible? (Minz)

Interview: At first it worked very well with the with the transplant and then there were problems in the end. How was THAT for you?

Donor: That was (..) um, if I put it in plainly: it was SHIT, (..) because erm, well for me it really wasn't good, because I then partly blamed myself, that I'M to blame because in the end it was MY bone marrow that then erm worked against his cells and destroyed them. (Kunow)

Donor: of course that was another strange feeling, that I first thought like this: now everyone is blaming me a bit (..), I'm to blame that my cells didn't manage it, but I really couldn't influence that. (Jaschke)

Mother: she partly erm, blamed herself, erm partly they also eh from outside suggested it like this. Along the lines of, erm so brother got got ill, your bone marrow wasn't good enough. (Kunow)

Donor: I also erm (.) dumped a lot on my friends and then specially on my best friends. There was one I had who always- she always said: no, you're not to BLAME, YOU CAN'T do anything about it, but you (.) you don't realise that at once, that you're not to blame. It's just like, pfff that was YOUR product and you're responsible for it, (..) but you actually can't do anything about it, that erm it takes a long time until you understand that. And I really only started to understand it, erm, when my brother wasn't there any more, that erm (.) I'm not to blame at all for the whole thing, but it was a MEDICAL MISTAKE, because they only saw too late that these medications aren't compatible and that then everything else was built on this and that does take an awfully long time until you understand it. (Kunow)

Long-Term or Life-Long Duty for Further Donations/"Gifts"

> Mother: one time she came erm (..) from somewhere and erm she said, erm they'd um told her, um she'd already donated bone marrow, so she could also donate half her lung to Klaas.
>
> Interviewer: That was a doctor, or what?
>
> Mother: No, that was someone here from the village and I said: you aren't a spare parts depot for your brother, I said, where did you get that from, I didn't have you so that you er constantly have to keep donating something or other to your brother. I mean, apart from the fact that it wouldn't have worked anyway. But I thought was really quite hard, that people just say, yes, she can do that again, isn't it.
>
> Interviewer: And what did Kira say about it?
>
> Mother: Kira was devastated, she was crying her eyes out, (…) you know. [...] I mean um not just that Kira had gone through through a very hard um thing because of the bone marrow transplant, but afterwards it wasn't good either. (..) Where (.) where would it have stopped? (..) Well, that the people were certainly (..) very hard. (Kunow)
>
> Mother: So he assumed that he's actually already in the donation database and but then I told him, that he's (..) only sort of been tested for his sister, and isn't in the file and in his case I advised him to leave it at that, because you've seen it now, he would always be considered for her again in the future. (Preuss)

Does the Recipient Owe Something (to the Donor)? Gratitude?

> Mother: Melissa was also TOTALLY cool, yeah? and Mighel had just been um discharged from the BMT and the two fought again for the first time (.). "oh," Melissa says to me, (loudly), "YEAH YOU KNOW WHAT AND NEXT TIME YOU WON'T GET ANY MORE BONE MARROW FROM ME" (laughs), I thought that was so cool. I had to LAUGH so much, because it was so cool, so childish, so normal you know, yeah. (Molle)
>
> Recipient: well [I was] also very depressed and then I tried to kill myself and um my brother could never approve of that like, because he said: I SAVED your life and now you just want to throw it away! (Kirstein)
>
> Recipient: what worried me a bit for quite some time, was that I felt I OWED him something, on the principle of: "Yes, you saved my life and I owe you something". But erm for one thing I can't owe him erm my whole life long erm- I mean that he like, I mean that I have a DEBT towards him or something. That can't be the case, can it, and it can't be the case either that erm he makes some kind of statements and I just HAVE TO listen to them and be sad. That can't be the case either, you know? Because he doesn't have a RIGHT either to say, no way: you don't have the right to KILL YOURSELF, because um I donated bone marrow to you or whatever, yeah? So he got in a huff and when I say: why don't you just ask me WHY I tried to kill myself anyway, you know? (Kirstein)
>
> Donor: like for everyone else, if somewhere it, let's say I'd donated in city A and the recipient was in Munich, then you wouldn't have seen, it would have been like, you wouldn't have noticed at all, but then in the immediate family and then, YES (swallows) and then you're also like, YES, you you yourself have a life, you see how erm the person whose life you've well indirectly perhaps you've saved, erm throws away their life, or tries again DELIBERATELY to destroy it, and you want to prevent that. (Kirstein)
>
> Mother: Kira said now and then: I donated bone marrow to you as well, didn't I, and now you have to be grateful to me (laughs) (..) but

Interviewer: But that kind of thing did happen?

Mother: YE-ES, well there were normal jealousies. I mean I wouldn't wouldn't, who knows how to gauge that. (Kunow)

Donor: I know- well occasionally there was a bit of that as well, he's in my DEBT because of this donation and so on [...], that he somehow a bit. I don't want that of course and I NEVER wanted it either or that- like, but that can't, I think, perhaps be avoided, that he feels, I- I owe Wilke like SO MUCH and so on and that because of that he of course I don't want to like DENY myself of some things or somehow want to be- begrudge or something. (Wahl)

Interviewer: But you don't somehow feel, I mean I'm now asking quite directly, because I've often read that it does arise that you somehow have to for ever your whole life be unbelievably grateful for or how how is it?

Recipient: Nooo (quietly), mhm (negatively). No, well that erm that's what, I think, the doctor said as well, that it's erm like siblings or something, that you then become like siblings, but I don't think that and I don't think either that you should then feel you would be in debt or something. I think that would be wrong somehow. And why? (Kötter)

Mother: Yes, but like I said not for Kilian, okay, it may well be, if Kai is being bitchy to him, listen, think about it, what I did for you, no, that's NEVER happened, and I think that's good. If you always kept bringing that to the table, I think, that wouldn't be helpful either somehow. I think everyone has like, I think Kai knows exactly, what he owes to Kilian and Kilian also knows, what he DID. (Kötter)

Topic II: Experiences in Times of Illness

Shock and Denial: "We Don't Belong Here!"

Father: well, there was stuff where I realised: OK, well and my wife also said later on, we didn't WANT to belong there. I mean it was an internal barrier like, I don't want to have anything to do with these people here, to get involved, you know, I mean, to say, yes, I'm here too, I'm one of them or something, erm it was a big effort to overcome that. (Rohde)

Father: then the transfer happened erm quite quickly, to the university hospital. And I can remember very well that I was stressed OUT, as my wife also said, about the situation with the BUILDing. About what we had seen there. There was stuff that you'd seen previously on television and you'd turned off because you didn't want to see this wretchedness. And erm it was also the same for me, I, we, we arrived at the ward and then I-I wasn't able to realise that AT all, what it, I mean that were affected by this as well now. That WASN'T us [...] That WASN'T us. That was OTHER people. (Speidel)

Mother: Well that was erm (..), I mean that moment, yes it was as though you were somehow being catapulted from from ONE galaxy into another. It's (..) well really like a sort of high-speed [ejector] seat from one world into another. It's (.) there's nothing the same as before and well, I mean it's really crazy, I mean just this diagnosis itself, hearing that, it's (..), you can't imagine it at all. [...] Well I'm glad that my husband was there, that we weren't alone, that I wasn't sitting there on my own, I always had a bit of support, but in the end (sighs) yes, yes, it's, you're just searching somehow, for how you (.) how you can stop this (laughs) high-speed train that's just setting off, I mean it's CRAZY and then of course another world begins. I mean (..) sure, then came the move to the Onco ward and then, yeah, then then EVERYTHING is new, everything different and erm then you first have to get used to it, that you're surrounded by all those (laughs) "Oncos", onco patients, and you've always been certain that it won't hit you, I mean for children especially it's SO rare that even, if you've heard that somewhere in your wider circle of friends or or relatives, where you could always say (very quietly) well yeah, that's so rare, that won't affect you erm and erm (.) and then suddenly there you are in the midst of this world and (..) and it's somehow, I dunno, you poor little sausage (laughs) first of all because the others already live in this world and know their way round, you yourself are completely completely disorientated (..), well, how was that before and then it only begins then (…) YES, it takes a very long time till you, or WE took a very long time till we found our feet there I mean at all, at all with the DIAGNOSIS, being able to take it in, that it's like with this life situation, the new one. I mean I didn't want ANYTHING AT ALL to do with any of it, I didn't want to talk to anyone, the doctors also said, yes, you'll get to know (laughs) other parents, what a thought mhm (negatively) (laughs), no way no thanks. (Rohde)

Loss of Control, Being at the Mercy of Something

Mother: I mean you sort of entrust your whole- I mean, it's my life, they're my children, it's everything for me and you're entrusting them to some people and they can do things [to them.] (Kelling)

Mother: it was terrible, always standing on the sidelines and erm, watching how they fed some kind of remedy into your child and erm TORTURED them, yes really, yeah, and you always just stand to one side and say, oh come on, it's not bad or something and comfort them and give them support. (Schubert)

Mother: and then access was established and I just DIDN'T know. The doctor just said "OK, do you need anything else or shall we just get straight on with it". Like, oh God. And they hadn't prepared her for it, not properly I felt, that now she- and that was really bad for her, so she was afraid of falling asleep and it hurt and actually there was nothing in there but she's a child and there was still that feeling there was a needle in her. (Kelling)

Mother: then no more [information] came and at some point I asked the doctor, "well, erm is it going to happen now and is Lena a donor or what"? Yeah, he didn't know anything different. So I say, "ok, well I haven't heard anything either, and just now, we'll drive over there and we'll assume and afterwards they'll say, erm-

Interviewer: That isn't right or what.

Mother: AFTERWARDS I'LL HAVE TO whatever, but then I would like to have known in advance." Then he said, yeah erm pf- "it's okay like that." […] I mean you sort of entrust your whole- I mean, it's my life, they're my children, it's everything for me and you're entrusting them to some people and they can do things [to them]. (Kelling)

Who Is Ill? For How Long?

Non-donor sister: Well, I believe that she is still not quite free of [it], that she still has psychological problems because she's well been at death's door twice. She did have a chance, but she doesn't USE it, she doesn't perceive it and then sometimes I have the impression she'd rather have died, or I don't know at all how I should put it. Well I think sometimes like, she should actually be glad and and happy that she's still alive and that she has a family and that she's ACTUALLY healthy, with limitations, but there are also quite different cases, where their legs, arms, they've had to have something amputated, you know, and then, well yeah. But that's what it is. (Kirstein)

Mother: well, my mother is simply, let's say, at an age, for her Sven is still not well and never will be. She always says, "oh God, the boy shouldn't do so much sport, what's he doing again?" Recently he did a 24-hour table tennis tournament, played really round the clock, day and night. "But he can't do this, he really can't cope with this." I say, "sure, why shouldn't he do this, of course he can cope with it, he's young, of course he can play table tennis for 24 hours" (laughs), that, like, my mother is always just afraid, like. He's still the poor little tender boy, who's ill, and that won't change either. I think she's at an age where she just worries too much, like, and erm, but the relationship hasn't changed, no, it's, otherwise not, not much has happened, no. (Speidel)

Recipient: Exactly, trying somehow not to focus on it, but really to focus on other things. Like, I dunno, sport, which I do now, my hobbies, my friends, somehow I'd rather concentrate on that than to know, like, let's say, I'm still very thin, very small, I still have the consequences of all the chemotherapies, THAT's what people could look at of course, like, that's still present. But that, I don't WANT that. (Speidel)

Mother: It's everything, doesn't matter what, I still look at her skin ten times a day, [to see] whether there's anything there, well I don't know, if you can someday find- I said after two years perhaps I'll be able to a bit

Interviewer: But for that this experience is I think too drastic, that suddenly like "bam" that you can-

Mother: Yes the counselling service in city B also said that you'll still get frightened in ten years' time if she has a temperature. It's just like that, you can't, I think, ever get out of it. (Kelling)

Donor: after the next one (laughs) that he the body (.) erm can't be returned to the level of- that was there before the illness. Like, and that was I think simply a- the feeling that he can't trust his body any more or he has- he can't any longer no longer to some extent rely on it or have a goal in mind, which had previously been (takes a breath) determining himself, so that erm (.), it did I believe, erm yes, das that was in the end. (Wahl)

What Does It Mean to Be Ill?

Recipient: Well you also notice it in sport for example, that you're not quite as fit as the others, because you've spent a year just lying around in bed and yeah, among friends, because if- if you just blurt it out, then, um I think, then they're gone so quickly, because then they- then to begin with they're all really afraid that they'll get it TOO. (Diedrich)

Mother: but that he doesn't want to talk about it, I think, he doesn't want to talk about it, because he wants to be like other children. And he is too, isn't he, and he doesn't want to stick out on any account. (Diedrich)

Recipient: so you get packed straight into a crate: CANCER KID. (Minz)

Recipient: but otherwise I really do try to avoid the subject, as far as I can. Because it's a subject, I think, that for one thing generates a very bad mood. Somehow that's always immediately a depressive, "everything's stupid" mood, if you even just mention the word cancer, [...] it's always a part of me, or of all of us. (Speidel)

Non-donor sister: Yes, it's always so uncomfortable when they find out about it and then they spread it and

Non-donor brother: And then the whole world finds out.

Non-donor sister: (laughs) Not really. I mean, even if it isn't bad, but it's

Non-donor brother: We just don't LIKE it.

Non-donor sister: Then some say: hey, look, Mads and Macy are contagious or whatever from cancer and isn't at all TRUE, but

Non-donor brother: Cancer isn't catching. (Molle)

Interviewer: IS it like that or- or do you already feel able to talk about it?

Recipient: yes but, it really has to be someone who trusts me, because I don't want it to GO somehow halfway round the world, afterwards, no idea, on Instagram or Facebook. (Diedrich)

Interviewer: How is- how was that for you?

Recipient: I never wanted to be [that child]! I also had, I had, I wore a wig, many people thought it was my real hair or at least that's what (laughs) I imagined they believed. Because I just wanted, YES, I didn't want to be the cancer- I mean the sick child for everyone. Of course I was at school, because I walked around and they all knew, because I had three older brothers and sisters and in all the classes you explain that to your friends and it gets around. And a lot of people talked about it. (Minz)

Recipient: Now that I think about it, or if it happened to me NOW, I would, I think, I mean I'd walk around without hair, I mean without a wig, because now you have a bit of a different VIEW of it and that, well, it's not cool, but I would stand by it. Because, no idea. But at that time I wanted to hide behind it a bit and wanted at least for people in the town to say: OK, you're just a normal young girl and quite pretty, nice and tall. But: there's nothing in it. And that was also a bit of a protection for me, of course, if someone looked twice, he'd have seen that it was a wig, but (Minz)

Dealing with Illness (Coping Strategies)

Recipient: Exactly, yes, I'm not just the one, exactly not just the one who, like was ill and did well despite that, but I also have a lot of other things that I CAN do, rather than just being ill (laughs), that sounds stupid, but that's what it is. (Minz)

Toughening Up

Mother: and in my DEEPEST insides I'd had the feeling the whole time: THIS is what you were expecting. Everything was going too well for the past t- fourteen, twelve years, everything was going way too well. I was always very preoccupied with the topic of DYING, I read a lot of books about children who have to die

Interviewer: How come?

Mother: Because I always- I'm made like this, that I believe I can tou- I can toughen up. If I've already thought stuff through twenty times, I can deal with it better. I mean, I can't read crime novels, I can't stand anything exciting. When I was a child I could only watch Daktari from behind a chair, like, well I was always unbelievably fearful, but things like this I DID stand up to them in the HOPE: if something really does happen, you're completely hardboiled, then you're better able to withstand it. (Minz)

Resignation

Father: My sister died of cancer in 2011 and then you just, I mean I, when the woman told me, I just drew a line under it.

Interviewer: Because: no point, or what?

Father: Well, I was completely convinced, OK, if there's a diagnosis of cancer, then that's that. Well, I didn't reckon on ANYTHING. (Kelling)

Father: normally I wouldn't say this out loud, but sometimes erm I, I I was still saying a year ago, if I had the money for my funeral, I I'd put an end to it. But then you think: "Bloody hell, you can't do that to your family," and my wife, I know I, how my wife reacts, she'd probably [do it] as well (..). Because, at that time she, on several occasions she said, "Hey, I've already chosen the tree" [inaudible]. I already HAD one! (Kunow)

Ignoring/Having Done with It

Mother: Well, now we're, lots of people are like, that they live so much in this illness, or with it, they NEED it, this exchange of experiences. For me (..), Pia actually thinks just like this, I mean because these illnesses are so individual that I (…) actually don't want to engage with it all the time. Pia also says: I don't fancy one of those circles of chairs, where the Kleenex box is on the table and this bloke tells this story and. I mean, she actually feels WELL and not like a sick person, I mean and then she doesn't want to be in a group like that (takes a breath) where she's kind of viewed as sick. That is so not her thing. (Preuss)

Interviewer: just a question for you, how was it at that time, what happened, how did things proceed?

Donor: Well I NEVER thought much about it, I have to be honest. (Minz)

Mother: Well I blotted out the subject of cancer, I said, well everything is possible, but it's definitely not CANCER, because they hadn't found any stuff either. (Minz)

Father: at some point they told us, hm just BURY the old photos (..), because I still have a lot on my mobile and we still have old photos from that time. Just bury them and just LET the past be the past, but I I still think, that's part of it, of OUR life it's just part of it, why should I BURY it? Why should I FORGET it? (..) I mean for ME I decided: no, I'll leave it on my mobile, I'll leave the photos on my phone, I- we'll leave the photos, I decided that for myself. What they decided I don't know, but it's but it's not not a subject for discussion between us. (Grohmann)

Acceptance

Mother: not perhaps thinking too much about things you can't influence, and just letting things run their course. (Bahr)

Non-donor sister: it will never be completely done and dusted, it's always like [just putting] a plaster on it. (Minz)

Mother: Well you just get to GRIPS with the situation, that's now a FACT and like I said, close your eyes and hope for the best, so that you can get your child through it OK, and the family doesn't somehow get NEGLECTED, that you scrape everything together, yeah. (Preuss)

Recipient: so this whole subject of cancer was dumb of course, but ultimately I also thought, yeah OK, it's also just a bloody awful illness, there's no great difference. (Minz)

Keeping Control/Regaining Control

Mother: I am someone who has to know everything precisely, I read everything I can find, I ask everyone I know. Sometimes I felt I understood the illness better than those who were involved. Yes, but because I well, I SOLVE it for myself analytically, I consider it controllable. (Minz)

What Is Helpful in Dealing with the Situation?

Maintaining Everyday Life/Structure and Functioning

> Mother: but basically: It's no longer living, it's actually only really, you're functioning, you know. It's (.), you also try to think ab- as little as possible about it, simply only to do what you have to do and everything else just really doesn't matter. (Jaschke)
>
> Mother: Everything has to be arranged, everything has to and stuff and you still have a daughter and this and that and how is everything supposed to function and ggrrr and then it comes to mind, you know and actually you just want to fall on your knees and scream and (laughs) like, shout at almighty God. (Bahr)
>
> Mother: The benefit to ME, in that sense I did have a benefit to me, because I HAD to be there. So that was how I benefitted. I couldn't just collapse as well. (Jaschke)

Hope/Belief that Everything Will Be All Right

> Father: What was on the horizon was: "Sven will get well". That was our starting position and we pushed it through rigorously. (Speidel)
>
> Father: we didn't allow for any alternatives either. We had an unspoken resolve that, for us "things are only going to get better", right. And that- then, then it also makes it easier for you, right. So for us it was clear. Er, even although we never spoke of it somehow "isn't that what we're hoping for?" and so on. No question. NO QUESTION, right, you know. (Speidel)
>
> Mother: I don't know, I somehow always assumed the best. I actually spent most of the time totally convinced that everything was all right, and actually also- always, 'cos wh- I don't know why, because he also had this kind of leukaemia, which is the at best or at least the one which lots of others get and they have a good chance of recovery, no idea. From the start I was actually hardly ever er, that I was somehow really afr- afraid that David would die. That was actually (.) actually never really the issue. (Diedrich)

Making the Best of It

> Father: when I also thought: my God, that is really crap for this little one, but compared to so many others he's actually doing all right. And er I often had this feeling as well, heading towards the transplant, this feeling: oh man, we should be so bloody glad that we are HERE in this situation, suppose Marlena hadn't been at home at that time. We wouldn't have had the chance to go to the doctor's if she'd been away on a school trip or been somewhere else like: WHICH child who doesn't just live in an industrialised developed country like we do, they would have been dead a long time ago, they would never have had this opportunity. What actually is all right for us, even in this situation, when you (laughs) when you've constantly had your feelings reflected back to you from your surroundings: oh man, it's hard for them, they've got it really tough now, they've got it, you know. (..) LIKE, (.) THESE thoughts, they actually determined those months for me. (Minz)

Sense-Making of the Illness

> Father: for me it was always the thought, we have to remember, OK, if this thing is so massive, then there will be some time BEFORE, some time DURING and some time AFTER. (Schubert)
>
> Mother: Basically I'd always imagined it like, oh man- it's like a station where only one train (..) arrives and stops and then- and you don't know where it's going to (.) and either you get in or you stay where you are. Yes and if you (.), if you stay there at the station,

you don't know when the next train will come, so you get in, (..) you don't know where this journey is going. And no one can take that away from you, the decision doesn't go [away]. (Kunow)

Mother: So I called the GIRLS again and then we sat down together again and I said: Girls, what's going on now, we're in God's hands. We are in God's hands and somehow we will get through this thing. Based on this attitude we then did it and then everything actually went like in a film. (Minz)

Mother: and in my DEEPEST insides I'd had the feeling the whole time: THIS is what you were expecting. Everything was going too well for the past t- fourteen, twelve years, everything was going way too well. (Minz)

Interviewer: And you couldn't do anything ABOUT IT, that you're ill. Like, it wasn't your FAULT.

Recipient: It's always just me.

Interviewer: It's always just you? really?

Recipient: I can't do anything about it. (Dietrich)

Father: YES, how was it? (sighs) (..) I reckon everyone would say first of all: shocked, bewildered and then they let's say they TRIED somehow, yeah to FIND OUT something so they simply say: where has this come from? (..), why us? So actually, I think, these- these questions are asked by everyone who is in such- such a situation and that's actually what- what was crucial or what- what questions which which I was presented with, why US and yeah, where did that come from. (..) Yes and the SEARCH, the search which which is, you know, yes ultimately what what what for me at least, I'm telling you, mostly took up my time, when I tried to understand how an immune system can suddenly stop working. And so I spent loads and loads of my time on internet forums. […] yes, doing THAT I really spent MANY MANY hours, in order to SOMEHOW find out, I'm saying, WHY the immune system stops working, why why this lifeblood-producing system simply gives up (..), yeah and I never got an answer, ever. Yeah, that's actually how it it is, that that how, shocking it was, that you, like, actually ever got hardly any answers. Yes, it could have been due to some illness, it could be down to some chemical product, it could have been cau- caused by some some kind of NATURAL causes, but as for answers (..), we never got any. (Grohmann)

Father: this discussion, from the start I refused to tolerate it. I mean I refused to let myself talk about GUILT or WHY, I mean it's fine for folks to speculate how how these disorders come about and so erm it's OK, but erm that's how I felt, this discussion, it doesn't lead anywhere. (Schubert)

Retrospective

"A Part of My Life"

Father: I tell myself clearly, it's part of my life and why should I forget it, why should I REALLY make an EFFORT to forget it. I don't want that at all, because it's all part of it. (Grohmann)

With Hindsight, It Benefited the Family and Changed Attitudes

Donor: Yes I'm also THANKFUL for it, that we could witness it so CLOSELY like that, you know, and that erm (..), of course I'd have experienced other things instead, but it was or I had such a BEAUTIFUL experience because it was- because I was so sad and then like also (takes a breath) erm THANKFUL or- soaked up like a kind of SPONGE, like everything, like everything that was beautiful, I soaked it up (laughs) and made it even more beautiful internally. It could also be that- like it was, but despite that (...), yes, there were really beautiful moments there. (...) Yes. (Wahl)

Father: I look at a lot of things with different eyes today (swallows) (...) and so I say to myself, you have- you DO things a bit differently today and I don't get obsessed about it like, you (.) and you shouldn't get obsessed about the problems of tomorrow or the day after or whatever, you should also just enjoy [things] a bit more (.) and I have to say, for me personally I have ALREADY (..) changed my attitudes a bit. I just don't want to miss it any more. [...] (..) I don't want to be sitting in front of the TV at eight, quarter past eight, I mean on Saturday evening at eight (.) I went cycling through the field, whatever, at quarter past eight or something, that you're watching something, you don't have to [watch] everything at all (..) and for me personally I find that, I feel a bit like this is the biggest change I mean in the whole subject. (Kötter)

Mother: they hold really, really fast together as siblings. I think it's great, I like watching it, to be honest, I think it's great, I mean I really like seeing it, hm. And if that's the effect of the illness, then we always say, that's great, I mean, the illness has also done great things. (Speidel)

Donor: yes, I [changed] my attitude towards life, that everything that happens to us, doesn't matter whether it's good or bad, has in the end made us into the people we are and I'm actually content with what I AM and who I am. (Bahr)

Interviewer: Do you feel that these experiences CHANGED your family, the family?

Recipient: Certainly. I mean even if it sounds silly, erm above all because now, in the years when it happened like that, it sort of surfaced, that you should live EVERY day like it's well, like it's your last one. (Minz)

Mother: Other things are more important for us and erm, it's a pity that you have to learn something like that, but I think I can say that, since that first day of being ill, we as a family really have lived every day as if it were our last, every day. It IS like that. And they say it so lightly, but EVERY day we go as a family, we do lots and lots of things, we are conscious every day that we are together as a family, that Sven is here, that the world is beautiful. Money is money, well okay. COMPLETELY unimportant! There are so many things that are important, erm, and we live like THAT, and that, well it's a pity, but as I said, the illness also brings a lot that is good. Like Sebastian said, it, we also see a lot of positives in it, that your viewpoint is set differently, yes it really is like that. (Speidel)

Mother: The whole thing did weld us together as a family, you know, because we all pulled together and not one of us like this and the other like that. (Lassen)

Mother: It also welded us together very strongly in a way, you know. Something very special connects us, what we experienced together, what we endured and survived. That continues to connect us, you know. (Bahr)

Non-donor sister: Well I think we have grown a bit closer together through this and we know how to value the little things, eating together sometimes and so on, yes, well I do think so, yes, such a positive outcome, I mean somehow that does weld you together. (Kötter)

Topic III: Processes of Decision-Making

Decision-Making About Therapy

Mother: the likes of us really had to put up with everything that they chucked at us.
Interviewer: Yes, of course, yes.
Mother: Yes. I have to swallow the bitter pill again
Interviewer: Yes, you simply can't judge it for yourself, can you.

Mother: No, I CAN'T judge it, I can't say, is this (..). Of course I think it's all stupid, what they're doing, everything that harms her, of course I think it's STUPID. I don't think it's good that my child is harmed like this, even just this pathetic (.) chemo, eight days long, I think is totally dumb. Surely that doesn't have to be the case. Yes, of course it does have to, it couldn't work another way. I don't have another choice, I mean, I can always only be grateful for what they're doing for my child, at least trying to keep her alive. It doesn't work any other way and not everyone succeeds either, I know that too. (Jaschke)

Decisions Under Time Pressure

Father: we were sitting, we all listened carefully, without

Mother: [imitates doctor's voice] "Do you actually understand why we're TALKING or (laughs) what we're talking about?"

Father: And th-th-th-th- then it was like, the doctor says this and erm, I could basically say it like that as well, I said, YES, we are listening to you carefully, we UNDERSTAND it like this, but we can't ALLOW ourselves, shall we say, to sit here in dismay or burst into TEARS. I have to UNDERSTAND what you say so that I can make a DECISION AT ONCE, because from the first day on we knew, erm, we're racing against TIME. Every day, every week, every month just brings us a CHANCE to stop this disease earlier and then he told us that and it was actually also relatively short, I mean very dramatic that that, I mean, he showed us, this and that and that and that can happen. (Schubert)

Interviewer: And did you have a sense before the transplant, of having enough time to reflect on how everything- what sort of consequences there were for the family, how it would pan out psychologically, did- were you aware of what the extent would be?

Mother: No, I didn't think about it either. The- erm my sole concern was to save my child. No, everything else comes much later. (..) No, no, it's just tunnel vision, like, just tunnel vision. The next blood test, the next, this test, that test (sigh), from one test to the next, thank God, like, thank God, it's all OK, everything's working, everything OK. (..) It's crazy (laughs). (Bahr)

Decision-Making About the Transplant

Interviewer: I mean, was this transplant an option straight away or (.) or (..) how was it, that this subject came up?

Father: It was, to use the words of Mrs Merkel, there was no alternative. (Wahl)

Interviewer: Was that a question somehow, I mean (..) whether a a erm a bone marrow transplant should be done or not, was evidently no question

Father: No.

Interviewer: it was simply medically necessary.

Mother: Yes.

Father: Well, we did question it, but we questioned the medical medication, not the therapy itself. (Lassen)

Mother: Right, we were always weighing up between QUALITY of life

Father: Yes.

Mother: and lifeTIME, so OK, how much quality of life will she still have if we do this now

Father: It's no use, let's say, keeping a child that needs to be permanently ventilated alive. Of course we're in a discussion, we evaluate what's worth living. But who's going to do it apart from us and it makes the decision so difficult as well, eh, the two of us

Mother: Yes, we agreed on a common denominator, it was

Father :We always agreed on a common denominator like

Mother: Neither of us said, okay, we have to do it in any case, you know, keep the body, like.
     If I say okay, if nothing else is there any more, then perhaps better a terrible ending than
     unending terror, and life has to go on for everyone as well. I mean the boys wouldn't
     have a normal family life either, if someone was still lying somewhere attached to tubes.
     (Schubert)
Father: we were away over Easter and we were already saying, well this is the last holiday
     together, because once the bone marrow transplant erm has been carried out, that was
     our way of thinking, it's not only the the underlying disease, but (.) with just the bone
     marrow transplant itself we are DESTROYING quality of life. I don't think we have
     anything- I mean that like a
Mother: No, (are they hitting [each other]? [inaudible] the first time, I mean they are
     KILLING the first time, at the moment when the chemo runs in, life for HER is finished
Father: For other people you'd say, even just (.) yes, exactly.
Mother: And then it's up to her, whether she surfaces again or not. I mean I mean (.) I mean
     we are to BLAME, that it's finished. (Schubert)
Father: And that that is our fear, that makes this bone marrow transplant all the more
     FRIGHTENING for us because erm (..) this medical treatment has an influence on
     which ABILITIES she has and clobbering her again and then, YES, well- erm normally
     I'd expect, now we're having a treatment and then it'll be GOOD, yes or not good and
     we just don't KNOW after all. And that means we are confronted with: this treatment is
     terrible, erm we don't know what'll happen, it could go in any direction. The underlying
     disease can go in any direction, yeah, organised chaos actually. (Schubert)
Donor: then at some point they said, there is no other option, we now have to erm talk about
     a transplant like this and consider it as a possibility. And (..) they didn't actually ask us
     much, WHETHER we really wanted to. It was like, pfff, yeah, this is a done deal and
     then erm you have to, like, comply. And with hindsight I have to say, I didn't think it was
     so bad that it worked like that, how it worked. (Kunow)
Father: we have one train of thought, where we deCIDED about it, it was like this: what
     would we do if we ourselves were ill, erm how would we ourselves decide, I'd want that
     or I WOULDN'T want that. (Schubert)
Mother: we have a chance now, your son has to have a transplant, we're going to do it like
     for leukaemia, there isn't another chance, otherwise Björn will have a miserable
     death. (Bahr)

The Decision About Siblings' Donation

Mother: But also as part of the testing. It was just like, now the family will [go] first.
Interviewer: Yes.
Mother: You weren't asked. They just said, "Who wants to go first?" like. (laughs)
Interviewer: Everyone form a queue.
Mother: Yes, basically. (Kelling)
Interviewer: Your wife and your son were considered as donors, did you think about an
     unrelated donor or was it clear, that it'll just…?
Father: Then of course we DIDN'T at first think about an unrelated donor. No, it was actu-
     ally clear, one of the two would have to do it. (Kirstein)
Interviewer: Do you remember, was there the question: donation from a sibling, donation
     from a stranger, or what?
Recipient: Erm yes, as far as I can remember, of course I first asked how that would pro-
     ceed, because sure, you want to know how it works, after they tell you chemo won't
     achieve anything, or hasn't achieved anything. And then the doctor tried to explain to me

that they would now try to carry out a blood transplant and erm, there are two possibilities, either erm from the family or from a stranger. And they would test the blood from the family of course, because that would be BETTER or, yeah (.) it would be very good if someone from the family was a match erm but if it didn't work, you could fall back on a stranger and ask them for blood, if that would be ok, if it would match. Erm and then they did this blood test relatively quickly and it came out that Sebastian was a 100% match and from then on there was no question any more, of whether there would be a donation from a stranger or not, because it was clear, we'll take the blood from Sebastian. So, exactly. From then on it was actually clear from the outset and I hadn't reckoned with anything else either and I knew, it would match 100%, I mean, I assumed that it would work. (Speidel)

Father: YES, well there was no discussion in any case that I can remember, but it was just clear that you have to do something for your little sister and for your daughter. (Minz)

Interviewer: And you decided for a sibling donation and against an unrelated donor, because?

Mother: Well that was of course ultimately on the DOCTORS' recommendation, they did say that you can't say at this point that the surviv- survival rate is necessarily HIGHER, if you take a sibling donation, but the well the SIDE effects are often less and it's better tolerated overall in the long run. (Rohde)

Interviewer: Ah, well the question about an unrelated donor wasn't for you such

Mother: Not like, no, we would have gone there if neither of us had been a match. Then we'd have shed new light on the subject, but yes, then it was clear for us that it would take some time until the results were in, when- they took swabs from us. (Molle)

Donor: I did hope secretly, that it would be me. I don't know why, but I just wanted, I I just wanted to be it and erm when it really was the case, that was really erm how- I can't describe it now, the feeling, it really was so RAD. (Jaschke)

Donor: for ME myself of course it was also very positive, I mean I did erm, I also think it's GOOD to be a donor and so in retrospect, if I look back, independently of the fact that it was my brother, being able to help someone in THAT way, is of course also very, very beautiful. (Speidel)

Donor: I am by now extremely glad that I was the one, because it's my brother, I was able to help him. (Bahr)

Mother: and then I thought, WELL, if it goes wrong, also if Melissa donates at eight years old and Mighel doesn't survive, then we would have mourned a lot of course, but we had Melissa as well and if Melissa, this always brings TEARS to my eyes, if she then feels guilty (cries) and thinks, he died because I wasn't good ENOUGH. OH I thought, I can't do this, at that moment. Should I lose my child and then have another child who is tortured by issues of GUILT. THEN rather Merik who was two and a half, then WE would at least have time to grieve, I mean yeah, I wasn't thinking so negatively, but just realistically, yeah? Hm and we could then still explain to Merik [...] later on with help from outside somehow. Yes, I also told Melissa all that honestly, at eight years old, which was of course a lot, but I WAS like that, it all had to be honest (..) but then it was like that, that the (.) doctors talked to us all together

Interviewer: As a family?

Mother: No, first just with Maurice and me, just with my husband and me and they told us: it's just like this, that ERM, that the chromosomes of the opposite sex are identified better and are able to adapt better. I mean, that erm Melissa would have a bit of an advantage, but Merik would be just as good a match, it's just this minimal ADVANTAGE, erm (.) but that would be a LUXURY decision, well then we thought, no, now talk to Melissa again, SHE has to decide, even if she's eight, she just has to decide now, what she wants. And then she did do that. Then it was clear for her, NO, I mean every little thing that makes it better, I'll do it!

(Molle)

The Rationale: The Advantage of Sibling's Donation

Mother: because Zorro was the donor, that was the advantage, we were flexible. With an unrelated donor that wouldn't have been so simple. (Zucker)

Father: There were I think five- five people who were eligible and one was like in in I think in Africa or something and then there was the question of whether erm erm erm unrelated donors across the continent were erm AFFORDABLE. (Wahl)

Mother: And you know in the end as well, where the bone marrow is coming from and I think that (..), but it's, let's say off the top of my head, simply a good feeling that you do find someone from the family after all. (Lassen)

Donor: and then the chance was of course, that we were so similar, (..) so there was a greater chance of the body saying: "HEY I KNOW THAT, I'VE ALREADY SEEN THAT. (Jaschke)

Father: Actually we were even, I mean not just actually, we were even really glad that she was allowed to do it, you know, because erm and they told us, it's better tolerated, yeah, she will tolerate it better, she needs one one drug less and it's precisely this drug that is really difficult to tolerate or not not very well tolerated for children and erm (..) yes, that's why we were actually really glad and then we could also, after it was clear that we had them, straight away we could plan everything else and start it, without being afraid that it'll get pushed back and anything else, we could just (.) well, go ahead with the treatment, you know. (Lassen)

Mother: let's say, an unrelated donor is again (..) well, something QUITE different, because you don't know the person [...]. We have also experience of other cases, where the unrelated donor said: no, I'm going on holiday first, I don't have any time now. Or: no, I'm not going to do it any more. And I thought- was really totally grateful to the woman for doing it, but it's- it feels like something else again, it's a stranger. She's saving my child's life or she's at least trying to do so, but she really is a bit further away, if you like, either your daughter does it or you do it yourself. (Jaschke)

Non-donor sister: Well it was actually really a relief, when we heard that Kilian was a match. And otherwise in the search, if you have to somehow search for something else, that really is even more difficult and takes longer. And that's why it was really super like that. (Kötter)

Children and Adolescents Involved in Decision Making Process?

Mother: So we'd already made the decision for Dorothea, but we made the decision as if it were for ourselves, I mean as if we'd been a match, as we would have done. (Dietrich)

Mother: For me it was like having an ultrasound scan during pregnancy, it wasn't any MORE than that for me. And because of that it was clear to me, without us having a massive discussion with Zorro, that Zorro WILL donate whether he wants to or not. And as a result this matter was, er, initially not debated with Zorro much at all, rather, like, it was ACTUALLY already CLEAR for us, whatever Zorro wanted. (Zucker)

Mother: I've- I know- I can remember one scene, when Kira and I were upstairs, standing outside the bathroom and KIRA somehow came out with: "I REALLY DON'T WANT TO DO THIS"-

Donor: No, I didn't want to either

Mother: "I DON'T want to donate any bone marrow" and I was weeping, totally devastated: "and er then then Klaas will die"

Donor: as bonkers as it looks

Mother: "And is- is that what you want?" and that's how it is with our family. You build up such an insane pressure, you don't want this to happen to one of them at all, you know you're also basically afraid for both children, but that's after all the only chance you can see at that moment, that (..) the sibling can donate to the one who's ill.

Father: yes.

Mother: And (..) no child should have to go through that, no-one. (Kunow)

Mother: And so I wished it could be an adult and then it was like that for my daughter, yeah (laughs) what a stroke of luck THANK GOD, OH NO, ironically our little Berit who PANICS in front of doctors, she panics over every injection, every visit to the doctor's she screamed and screamed, cried, raged and then [she was] just a child you just can't believe what it was like. (..) She was beside herself (..), so that was, for the child that was hell. As she says, I knew, I had to do it, I (.) she sensed the PRESSURE, she HAD TO- she didn't have a choice. We asked her and explained it to her, said to her, ARE you going to do this, do you want to do this, but actually everything was really obvious, she's got to do this, even if we ask her, it was a charade, you see. It was clear to all of us and SHE sensed the pressure, yeah (.) great, I am terribly scared. No way could I dare say- I can't say no, like. (Bahr)

Father: 'cos I'd also explained it to her. I'd- I'd told her, yeah it just doesn't work without TALKING, you know, so we talked for ever and ever and why we are doing this, also why we're doing it this way. Of course you've got to talk about these things. Also this whole bone marrow transplant thing, we asked Greta, do you really want this, is this REALLY the way? (Grohmann)

Donor: YES, so the first time, like I didn't know at that time what I was supposed to donate or what a transplant was. I didn't know what bone marrow was etc. etc. All I knew was that if they ask me if I'd like to donate and I say yes, that I would be saving my sister's life, so to speak, by doing that. So that was actually (.) so it was all er (.) I had of an impression and for me it was completely obvious. I just didn't know why they had to ask me at all (..) and I also didn't know why anyone at all would refuse, yeah and as far as I was concerned I was right there I tell them straight that I will do it, yes. (Preuss)

Donor: Then my parents also asked me, erm (..) I have to say I really don't know what might have happened, if I'd said no, whether my parents would have in any case decided or not for my brother, but erm that was important at the time, to get my opinion on it and not simply to take decisions completely over my head. I'm still OK with that. (Bahr)

Non-donor brother: We already had the feeling that they were concerned about Ronja and then they talked to Ronja really often, whether she would really like to do this now, whether she is really certain about this and everyone was actually a bit unsure about the whole thing, how it would turn out; no-one was now completely sure that that will be JUST GREAT, we're definitely doing this now, but we all hesitated a bit and had our doubts about it and Mummy and Daddy were worried, we just had that feeling about it, before. (Rohde)

Father: So this was never a solo decision, it really was a family decision. (Grohmann)

Evaluation of Decision-Making Options and the Decision Made, in Retrospect

Donor: only in retrospect we're now actually just happy that everything went so well and that we were somehow able to help and yeah. (Grohmann)

Mother: (sighs) that's how it was ,a burden of choices (...). YES and then we did it and it was OK that we did it and I believe, yes.

Interviewer: You'd do the same thing again?

Mother: Definitely, I'd do the same thing again, of course, yeah yeah. So (.) definitely. (Bahr)

Topic IV: Familial Bodies

Bodily Substances/a Change of Nature

>   Father: It was rather well a bit, this is how I feel about it, that the body fights against it.
>   Actually it's something good, the transplant, but I mix in a bit this uniqueness somehow,
>   it it that's how I feel about it. It's not necessarily something that God wants and that's
>   why I call it something dangerous, as far as you can- get mixed up in it as a human,
>   yeah, is- that's a bit what I think I wanted to say. You have to be hellishly careful I think,
>   that there are also medical boundaries that you're not allowed to overstep. (Kötter)
>   Donor: Well I NEVER thought like that, erm, now my sister is (laughs), yes, the same as
>   me, how stupid, now I'm no longer unique or something. (Rohde)
>   Mother: we didn't think about it that much, that's it's now erm (.) a piece of Manuel or
>   something. It wasn't like that. (..) Sometimes I think it's like this: if someone donates
>   a- an organ, you know, this organ has already done something somewhere else and is
>   now supposed to do something in another person. But bone marrow is something that
>   continuously re-forms itself, erm although you call it an organ it's like skin, which has
>   to, if it TAKES ROOT in Lena, in that it's- at that moment it's her own, because some-
>   thing new is growing up there, which then makes this blood, YES: The trigger certainly
>   came from Manuel, but what's HAPPENING with it in Marlena's body, that's Marlena's
>   thing, isn't it? I mean it didn't bother us, didn't bother us, wasn't a topic of conversa-
>   tion. (Minz)
>   Father: What we asked ourselves as well, by the way, at that time for example they, it was
>   this thing, well yes, after they'd explained it: it's now MALE blood that Marlena will be
>   developing, not female any more. What does that mean actually, later on for SPORT, if
>   they really get the idea to do a blood test and erm and so on and so forth. We asked
>   ourselves that at that time and erm I don't even remember which doctor we talked to
>   about it and then he said: yes but you can explain it like this and it's nothing that
>   enhances performance or similar, it's just disconcerting. (Minz)
>   Donor: that's it's somehow like this and that, BECAUSE, I dunno, and that we speculate
>   like this sometimes, yeah, I dunn- that I'm a GIRL and I've donated my stem cells to
>   him, you sometimes say [turns towards her mother; MJ] you know, that erm (..) (swal-
>   lows) that he now has female (laughs) stem cells or something, and now because of that
>   some ways of behaving are eh erm DIFFERENT or something or (..) in that direction,
>   you know. (Wahl)
>   Mother: that something like something soft, female, is ticking inside him somehow. I don't
>   remember any more what it was about, but (.) erm (…) yes I can't- don't REMEMBER
>   any more. Well he reacted very, so very sensitively and soft, like he perhaps wouldn't
>   have done before, but I don't remember any more what that was about. Mhm
>   (affirmatively).
>   Interviewer: And you're linking that a bit?
>   Mother: That is MY, I don't know, that I think like this, perhaps erm (.) the BLOOD in him
>   is talking (laughs), you can also be determined by something like that. It's nonsense of
>   course, but erm (..) yes, really like like one of those (..) (sighs) yes, that perhaps it affects
>   his hormone system a bit. (Wahl)
>   Non-donor sister: well (..) he saved her life and [there's] so much similarity and [they're] so
>   much the same that they now also share through the shared bone marrow, that is some-
>   thing very special. (Minz)
>   Recipient: my Dad sometimes makes silly comments, if it's like (.) I dunno, if Malle, if
>   there's some kind of opinion about Malle or Malle is supposed to make some kind of
>   decision and isn't here, then he can- my Dad always says: yes, Marlena can do it, she
>   has the same thoughts as he has, he has the same bone marrow or something like that,

me and my brother, I mean we always think this is quite idiotic (laughs) or like that. (Minz)

Donor: I mean whether his character has (…) has adjusted more to mine or (.) there are things of mine in him, I can't put it like that at all. I have noticed physical things though. My brother when he was erm (.) little, he had straw-blond hair (..), completely smooth and erm (..) yes, suddenly after the transplant, when his hair grew back, (.) it had got substantially darker, it had got curly, and those are things that were really obvious to me, because it wasn't like that before and was when- (.) as a child I was terribly enthusiastic about it, yes, but that's in inverted commas a detail, he's actually still the person he was before, but for him to change physically over such a detail, how can that be, it it can overturn everything like that? Erm (..) but in terms of character I can't say that, it's too long ago or perhaps I was too little as well. I can't say that precisely. (Bahr)

Interviewer: but despite that like this idea that, there's really a part of the body in the other body and it lives on and works there too

Non-donor sister: Yes exactly and lives and WORKS and also obviously works on her appearance and and on erm, oh, what else was there? Karolin told us that she got implausibly hard fingernails, such UNBELIEVABLY hard fingernails so that you almost can't cut them and that she still has now. I mean particular attributes, I think yes, they're actually appropriate for Karsten, you know, like these (.) yes. (Kirstein)

Mother: for him it was like this, he gets his brother's blood, so he BECOMES his brother. That means he started to do sport, the same sport as Sebastian and he always says: yes, it's quite clear, I've now got it in me, that I'll become a good table-tennis player. Sebastian plays table-tennis, quite well, and for Sven it was clear, yes, I'll also become a great table-tennis player (laughs). (Speidel)

Interviewer: Mh, how does it feel, that you now have something of Sebastian in you?

Recipient: Well, it's it's funny, yes. I mean I think if you see Sebastian and me now you notice how similar we are. Whether that really has something to do with it, I don't know. But I have to say, since that point (..) it has felt like I was CLOSER to Sebastian than to Stina. Without being mean, judgemental, to think something, you know. I mean, I dunno, it's just a feeling, you've got your brother's blood actually IN you. Like and, mh, yes, it's FUNNY to describe. It's as if you were linked even more closely than you would be anyway, like and yes, somehow the development or how I have developed is very similar, really to Sebastian, w-w-we have the same hobby. (Speidel)

Interviewer: does that exist, like, in your head, that you now have a piece of Pascal in you too, is that an issue for you or what?

Recipient: Well I do know that but (laughs) (….) no it's just, (..) I don't actually think that much about it. (Preuss)

Mother: apart from that we always just made jokes, you know like, that Gino was, you know, if there was something up, OH, you're like Greta, you know like, you've got like her blood or I dunno, if we were watching a crime drama like, yeah, if you leave your blood at the scene, they'll say afterwards that it was Greta, you know like. That kind of thing, you know. (Grohmann)

Interviewer: how was it for you, the idea that, like, there will be bone marrow like from my daughter in my- I mean was there somehow also this idea like, there- there will be really a sort of life

Mother: Yes, totally, I saw it like a union (laughs), that Melissa is in him like that. (Molle)

Father: I should say, if David's blood were tested now, then it's, let's say, yes, you'd think, yes, it's a woman, you know, that's, exactly, from the from the from the DNA, yes, I thought, I wasn't so aware of it at first, but I do also find it somehow (laughs) interesting, that it's like that, but good, it's like that. Somehow there's also a crime scene where erm (laughs) I mean with the culprit like that, they looked for a guy and afterwards it was a woman or the other way round, I can't remember, I saw it a couple of years later, I thought it was really interesting (laughs). (Dietrich)

"Spare Parts Depot" ("Ersatzteillager") - Lasting Responsibility, Including Keeping One's Body Available for Future "Donations"

> Father: and, erm, like I said, you, you put this outside pressure on someone, you actually keep piling it on and somewhere in this is the, the sibling child who is actually ABLE to donate, due to com- you know this, like really good compatibility (.) erm, the pressure, you keep piling it on, even if you don't want to, you do it unconsciously. First of all you see the child who's lying there, and secondly, (..) erm, sounds stupid, you you see, er, er, first of all you can see: you're healthy after all, you can surely do without something. Like a ki- kind of spare parts- yeah, spare parts depot, kind of. (Kunow)
>
> Mother: then we had some DEEP conversations and such (..) terrible things came out, like I already said, you know: I was so afraid and you just USED me. (Bahr)
>
> Donor: then (.) erm Wido asked erm (swallows), how is it then, can you like register it, that the organs are for ONE PERSON only or just erm and I reckon he somehow even used the term RESERVED IN ADVANCE, (laughs) somehow, like, that's not what he MEANT and it also wasn't er like, I didn't get it wrong, but it simply SOUNDED like (.) a bit like that, you know, STRANGE, you know, at that moment (.) and basically I th- think it's OK- thought it was (laughs) totally all right. Like I mean, if something happens to me and somehow he suddenly needs a lung or something, that's somehow completely er er yeah I'd want that, that HE got it and not (draws breath) er, because it's my brother after all, you know, but th- th- there WERE a few times when that thought somehow came to me, mmm, what is that actually? Like if if now this (..), like what what actually is the point of my body erm (.) regarding our relationship with each other too, like how important erm (..), I'm important to him as a person, that I know, but how important am I to him, given that, that I simply (.) now, that he's got my stem cells as well, you know. Yes. I had those kind of thoughts somehow, but that was more like somehow a few years on. (Wahl)
>
> Mother: and I said: you aren't a spare parts depot for your brother, I said, where did you get that from, I didn't have you so that you er (.) constantly have to keep donating something or other to your brother. (Kunow)

Transplantation: Concepts/Metaphors/Ideas

> Donor: yes, I always thought that was somehow nice, that erm that (..) that somehow even now (..), that I could help her in this way and that it (..), that- like the healthy bit of me is now inside her and (.) (laughs) in a manner of speaking driven out the bad bits. You know I think that's actually somehow a really lovely concept (..), yeah. (Rohde)
>
> Mother: well, (..) I know that I, when I was sitting there with Melissa (swallows) and that, when that, when it had been EXTRACTED from her and I knew it's being delivered right now and stuff. That was a kind of (..) spiritual (laughs) moment, really, yeah, that I thought- like I'd really imagined that Melissa's production of life has now docked with him and somehow new production does that, yeah. (Molle)
>
> Mother: I said to Janine, I (.) I'd like to be there at the time because I know it's actually just a bag just like BLOOD, but it's a bit different, it's bone marrow, it's a life-saver and it's just going to go in. It's not a big deal but I've simply go to to be there, it's simply the MOMENT, now the bone marrow is going in. (Jaschke)
>
> Mother: for Rebecca it's a major issue, having Ronja's warrior cells in her blood. I mean that is for- like for REBECCA much more an issue I reckon than for Ronja, that she's

got Ronja's warriors and that her own warriors weren't that good, but Ronja's warriors are great. (Rohde)

Donor: it's like a birth or like a (..), like a sort of transfer of now- now- as if life is somehow flowing in right now or something and that COMES from ME and like (laughs) somehow, you know. It was, yeah. It really was... (Wahl)

Non-donor brother: well it's of course it's like another a different kind of bond, you know? I mean if I had for example donated bone marrow to my brother, I think then the bond for example between my big sister and my brother, I mean not dramatically, but like DIFFERENT, because it really is something that connects you. (Molle)

Mother: I know that I, when I sat down with Melissa (swallows) and her, when her, when they had REMOVED it from her and I knew, so it's being transferred right now, you know. That was like a (..) spiritual (laughs) moment, really, yeah, that I thought- like I'd properly imagined that what Melissa had produced from one life becomes docked onto him like that and goes on to produce something new, like, yeah. (Molle)

Using Your Own Body Material as a Medicine?

Father: for me it's just an integral part of modern medicine, like transplanting organs etc.

Interviewer: so it's like a kind of medication

Father: like, exactly that, yes// may- maybe not comparable to a pill that you take, like me, I'm diabetic and I've got everything you can think of to swallow or inject. No, it is actually different, how something like an organ er or a bone marrow donation functions. But that's, yeah, something that happens at every street corner, I mean nothing that really occupies, yeah, totally occupies my mind, that's for sure, mmm (affirmative). (Minz)

Mother: as I said, that is a piece of KILIAN and I'll always think that, AAH Kilian is a healthy boy and I always think, now Kai is too. I always think, if Kilian's well, GREAT, then everything's fine with his bone marrow and I tell myself that it's now working just as well for Kai, that's how I imagine it, yeah that's right, I watch Kilian, and think: aah, he's FIT, Kai is just as fit, great. (Kötter)

Recipient: it wasn't such a strange feeling that I had at the time: like, bah, I'm getting a new organ or stuff, 'cos I had somehow at the time the bone marrow too, like no idea, that's just it, but I somehow didn't know much about it at all. So no idea, something like a lung transp- a lung transplant, yeah, you hear more about one of those

Interviewer: Yes, then you can picture it in your mind //somehow, like

Donor: Exactly and like AH, they're putting something new into her, like a heart or something I dunno, but bone marrow I always thought it's a liquid, isn't it? (Minz)

Mother: it could be a kind of medicine as well. Like as far as I'm concerned it's actually IRRELEVANT, I mean whether they now say OK, we've got this packet here erm, it's a medicine, we'll inject it, or that's come out of another person. So I'm not sensitive about that. (Schubert)

Father: Like it's (..) it's exactly like if you, you know? receive donated BLOOD or something after some sort of accident you know, it- it's actually nothing really strange, that I've now got (.) a stranger's blood in me, I dunno. So me- like for ME personally it's not. That moment when- when- when she- when she received it from him, that was, like. That was a really big moment, like, but right now, that bit of Pascal that's in Pia, that's, I dunno, like for me personally not, not anything special (laughs). (Preuss)

Family as a Body/as a System

Interviewer: did it feel strange that somehow left behind in Klaas was a piece of Kira?

M: No. (..) no. Through it all, 'cos, 'cos they were SO (..) so CLOSE to each other, erm it wasn't an UNRELATED body, you know. (Kunow)

Donor: so I simply had the hope, because we were so similar to each other, that Jennifer's body wouldn't even notice, that- tha- that they are different cells or strange cells, that it wouldn't, like, twig. (Jaschke)

Donor: I'm really and 'cos we were als- also so SIMILAR, I can only EMPHASIZE that we really, I don't know if the DNA is so similar or whatever is so exactly alike, that tha- it was just relatively rare for siblings to match so perfectly and I thought that was somehow cool. I thought it was REALLY cool, as our characters are basically different, but inside we were kind of THE SAME (..). I thought it was so fascinating that you can be so different on the outside yet be so much the same on the inside. (Jaschke)

Non-donor sister: it was also obvious, ALL OF US will do it, but ALL OF US, really EVERYONE knew beforehand: it's Malle after all. For some reason we all KNEW beforehand, we- both of them, like my sister already said, are so very LOHmann, that's my father and brother's side, my big brother and me, we are so VERY on the Minz-side, like my mum, in SO many ways and because of that it was all obvious and we all said it's Malle after all. (Minz)

Inscribing Family History in the Body: Tattoos

Father: my daughter, she had a tattoo on her arm. I'll just put it like this, erm, it's a tree with words, with the date of the transplant and she wasn't even 18, I had to sign, the tattoo, that was her wish, it's like a new life. Like the words and so on, for his brother and his brother had also already had a tattoo [...] Without, without my saying anything. (Molle)

Mother: Kira had a TATTOO done (.) 9 February, which erm I mean it'll always remind her of it. (Kunow)

Donor: I mean, I think tattoos are actually THERE for something like this, I mean (.) I mean of course it can also be an art, but for me it's very clear that I'd actually like to have SOMETHING LIKE THIS, that's very important for me [...] But for me. For me it's like, I (.) I forget it sometimes as well, that I have the tattoo, because I don't FEEL it, let's say, but more often I think about it again and erm it's something very POSITIVE as well actually and yes. I think it's somehow very good as a companion (laughs), yes. Exactly and erm for example Merik ALSO wants to get a tattoo (laughs).

Interviewer: The same one?

Donor: Yes (.) I mean like here in this shape or form, let's put it like that. I don't know if he still wants it and I think it's actually very nice and it shows again that, I mean for me it's like this, yes: OF COURSE he should also have it (.) like, because he could just as well have donated and Mighel can also get a tattoo and Mum and Dad too, if they want, I mean if they want! It's all the SAME to me because it's actually so beautiful, because (.) yes, because everyone carried it and yes, of course, everyone as he pleases, but like I said, especially for Merik. I think it's somehow, I thought it was really good that he thought: yes, I'll get a tattoo of it as well! Because I was thinking that maybe he thinks that he's not allowed to do it or something, because I was the donor.

Interviewer: Because he didn't do anything, aha

Donor: Exactly and it's still- for me it was again like, YES, he sees himself equally as a part and it's, yes it's also like, because we all worked together like a cogwheel (laughs) I should say, yes. (Molle)

Non-donor brother: that is something that connects you. Hm (.) I don't know if you've also seen this: I mean my big sister also has a tattoo here on her arm

Interviewer: No.

Non-donor brother: of a TREE erm and here in the roots is the date of the bone marrow transplant, something like that and my brother now wants to do the same thing AS WELL. And that does somehow connect you. It's like (..), it's a kind of bond that you can't just SEPARATE like. (Molle)

Interviewer: I think your father did, your father talked about it, that you had one of those TATTOOs

Donor: (laughs) yes.

Interviewer: done.

Donor: Yes, here, I mean it's a tree […] with the date (.) yes. (laughs) Exactly. Like one of those trees of life.

Interviewer: Are these stars down here?

Donor: (laughs) Yes like, yes.

Interviewer: GREAT, that- did you design that yourself or what?

Donor: No, a friend of mine did it and it's really not the per- perfect TATTOO, I should say, but's it's like perfect for this whole situation, I should say. I mean here as well, that the roots are so open. Actually the date was supposed to go in there, but it didn't FIT and then I just- just […] left it open, like and yes, exactly.

Interviewer: And then- and you now think it's quite good that it's so open, you just said, the roots?

Donor: Yes because, I mean // actually it would, I mean it would have been MORE PERFECT (laughs), if it had been filled in, but everything ISN'T perfect at all and it WASN'T either and I think it's as good as it is just I mean

Interviewer: So this openness sort of this, this

Donor: Yes and that, yes.

Interviewer: Ambivalence as well, put a bit like that?

Donor: Yes yes, well for ME simply that it (.) well it grew like that as well (laughs), yes. (Molle)

Interviewer: And you really thought of the tattoo together?

Recipient: Exactly, then there was the idea that in the meantime we had grown together SO strongly as siblings that we would like to record that in some way and a tattoo offers that, because it lasts a lifetime. Erm, then we thought about, yes, a sibling tattoo is simple, I think, it's something very good, that would connect us even, even more closely and then we thought of what motif we could have, something that all three of us like very much erm the three of us like so much that we want to have it. That somehow [connects] us to one another or that marks us out, that connects us to one another and without necessarily [focussing] on this story erm of the illness erm, yes without putting the focus on that, we nevertheless came up with this date and then we jointly decided that that was simply THE most important, or one of the most important things that determined our life and that we wanted to record, exactly. (Speidel)

Detailed Sample Description

Family (members)	Role/function	Diagnosis	Number of transplants	Kind of transplant	Time since transplant/donation	Age at transplant/donation (children)	Age at interview (children)	Notes
Bahr		**Adrenoleuko-dystrophy (ALD)**	1	**BMT (donor sibling)**	**18 yrs**			Recipient: Progression of disease was stopped by BMT but he has physical and mental impairments (severe disability). Parents separated and divorced approx. 10 yrs after diagnosis/BMT
Barbara	Mother							
Bernd	Father							
Björn	Recipient					$9^4/_{12}$ yrs	27 yrs	
Berit	Donor					$5^9/_{12}$ yrs	23 yrs	
Dietrich		ALL	1	**BMT (donor sibling)**	**7.5 yrs**			
Doris	Mother							
Dieter	Father							
David	Recipient					$5^1/_{12}$ yrs	$12^7/_{12}$ yrs	
Dorothea	Donor					$2^5/_{12}$ yrs	$9^{11}/_{12}$ yrs	
Detje	Non-donor					2 months	Did not participate	
Dana	Non-donor					Unborn	participate	
Grohmann		**Aplastic anaemia**	1	**BMT (donor sibling)**	**8 yrs**			

Name	Role		Diagnosis	No.	Transplant	Age at transplant			Notes
Gabriele	Mother								
Gerd	Father								
Gino	Recipient						10⁷/₁₂ yrs	18 yrs	
Greta	Donor						12²/₁₂ yrs	20 yrs	
Jaschke			AML	3	1. BMT (donor sibling) 2. PBSCT (donor mother) 3. PBSCT (unknown donor)	1. 12 yrs 2. 10 yrs 3. 7 yrs			Father refused to take part in interviews Recipient died 7 years ago after several complications, at age 17.
Jutta	Mother								
Jennifer	Recipient						1. 12⁷/₁₂ yrs	Did not participate (see notes)	
Janine	Donor						2. 15⁷/₁₂	28 yrs	
Kelling			AML	1	BMT (donor sibling)	1 year			Recipient: GvHD (skin, liver, heart)
Kristin	Mother								
Kristian	Father								
Kina	Recipient						2¹/₁₂ yrs	Did not participate	
Kaila	Donor						7³/₁₂ yrs	8³/₁₂ yrs	
Kirstein			ALL	1	BMT (donor sibling)	16 yrs			

(continued)

Family (members)	Role/function	Diagnosis	Number of transplants	Kind of transplant	Time since transplant/donation	Age at transplant/donation (children)	Age at interview (children)	Notes
Karin	Mother							Both Karsten and Karin (mother) were possible donors. Recipient: GvHD (arthritis esp. knee joint, intestinal problems), psychosocial problems: depression, substance abuse Donor: long-lasting back pain
Karlheinz	Father							
Karolin	Recipient					$13^3/_{12}$ yrs	29 yrs	
Karsten	Donor					19 yrs	35 yrs	
Kerstin	Non-donor					$17^5/_{12}$ yrs	33 yrs	
Kötter		**Myelodysplastic syndrome (MDS)**	**1**	**BMT (donor sibling)**	**$2^3/_{12}$ yrs**			
Karen	Mother							Kilian and Kaja are twins.
Klaus	Father							
Kai	Recipient					$16^4/_{12}$ yrs	19 yrs	
Kilian	Donor					$13^4/_{12}$ yrs	$16^1/_{12}$ yrs	
Kora	Non-donor					19 yrs	22 yrs	
Kaja	Non-donor					$13^4/_{12}$ yrs	$16^1/_{12}$ yrs	
Kunow		**AML & ALL**	**1**	**BMT (donor sibling)**	**7 yrs**			
Kirsten	Mother							
Kurt	Father							
Klaas	Recipient					$10^4/_{12}$ yrs	Did not participate (see notes)	Recipient: GvHD (especially pulmonary disease). Donor: long-lasting back pain
Kira	Donor					$15^6/_{12}$ yrs	22 yrs	Recipient died after several complications 3.5 years ago at age 14.

Family	Name	Role	Diagnosis	N	Treatment	Time			Notes
Lassen			ALL	1	BMT (donor sibling)	11 months			Only family interview
	Linda	Mother							
	Lars	Father							
	Lene	Recipient					4⁹/₁₂ yrs	9 months	
	Louise	Donor					2⁴/₁₂ yrs	3¹⁰/₁₂ yrs	
Minz			Myelodysplastic syndrome (MDS)	1	BMT (donor sibling)	7 yrs			Recipient: GvHD (skin & joints), myasthenia gravis
	Martina	Mother							
	Michael	Father							
	Marlena	Recipient					12¹⁰/₁₂ yrs	19 yrs	
	Manuel	Donor					18 yrs	25 yrs	
	Maximilian	Non-donor					20 yrs	27 yrs	
	Maria	Non-donor					14¹⁰/₁₂ yrs	22 yrs	
Molle			ALL	1	BMT (donor sibling)	12 yrs			Both Melissa and Merik were possible donors. Mads and Macy are twins.
	Michaela	Mother							
	Maurice	Father							
	Mighel	Recipient					5¹⁰/₁₂ yrs	17⁸/₁₂ yrs	
	Melissa	Donor					8²/₁₂ yrs	20 yrs	
	Merik	Non-donor					2¹⁰/₁₂ yrs	14¹⁰/₁₂ yrs	
	Mads	Non-donor					Unborn	8⁸/₁₂ yrs	
	Macy	Non-donor					Unborn	8⁸/₁₂	
Preuss			Fanconi anaemia	3	1. BMT (donor sibling) 2. PBSCT (donor sibling) 3. Lymphocytes (donor sibling)	1. 16 yrs 2. 9 yrs 3. 9 months			

(continued)

Family (members)	Role/function	Diagnosis	Number of transplants	Kind of transplant	Time since transplant/donation	Age at transplant/donation (children)	Age at interview (children)	Notes
Petra	Mother							Recipient: severe infections after transplants
Peter	Father							
Pia	Recipient					1. 11 yrs 2. 18 yrs 3. 27 yrs	27 yrs	
Pascal	Donor					1. 8 yrs 2. 15 yrs 3. 24 yrs	24 yrs	
Rohde		**AML**	**1**	**BMT¹ (donor sibling)**	**$3^{6}/_{12}$ yrs**			Recipient: mild GvHD symptoms
Rita	Mother							
Ralf	Father							
Rebecca	Recipient					$2^{1}/_{12}$ yrs	$5^{8}/_{12}$ yrs	
Ronja	Donor					$12^{10}/_{12}$ yrs	$16^{4}/_{12}$ yrs	
Raphael	Non-donor					9 yrs	$12^{6}/_{12}$ yrs	
Roberta	Non-donor					$6^{2}/_{12}$ yrs	$9^{8}/_{12}$ yrs	
Scholz		**Metachromatic leukodystrophy**		**BMT (unknown donor)**	**Prospective! (2 weeks before BMT)**			
Sabine	Mother							
Stefan	Father							
Saskia	Recipient					$5^{8}/_{12}$ yrs	Did not participate in interview	
Two older brothers						Approx. 7 and 9 yrs		

		Diagnosis		Treatment	Years	Age at transplant	Age at interview	Notes
Speidel		ALL	1	**BMT (sibling donor)**	10 yrs			
Silke	Mother							
Sascha	Father							
Sven	Recipient					$8^{1}/_{12}$ yrs	$17^{5}/_{12}$ yrs	Recipient: GvHD (arthritis fingers, dwarfism)
Sebastian	Donor					$13^{8}/_{12}$ yrs	24 yrs	
Stina	Non-donor					$15^{5}/_{12}$	Did not participate in interview (see notes)	Stina did not refuse to participate but was unable to attend due to a stay abroad.
Wahl		ALL	2	**1. BMT (donor sibling) 2. Salivary gland transplant**	1. 9.5 yrs 2. Approx. 7 yrs			
Wiebke	Mother							
Werner	Father							
Wido	Recipient					1. 23 yrs 2. 26 yrs	Did not participate in interview	Recipient: GvHD (arthritis, knee joint prostheses, failure of lacrimal gland), depression Recipient refused to take part in interviews.
Wilke	Donor					1. 20 yrs 2. 23 yrs	29 yrs	
Zucker		Hemophagocytic lymphohistiocytosis	2	**2 × BMT (donor-sibling)**	1. 1.5 yrs 2. 0.5 yrs			

(continued)

Family (members)	Role/ function	Diagnosis	Number of transplants	Kind of transplant	Time since transplant/ donation	Age at transplant/ donation (children)	Age at interview (children)	Notes
Zara	Mother							First BMT failed; second BMT successful so far;
Zlatko	Father							recipient: many – partially life-threatening –
Zedrick	Recipient					1. $3^9/_{12}$ yrs 2. $4^{10}/_{12}$ yrs	$5^4/_{12}$ yrs	infections, sepsis, failure of liver and spleen, dwarfism
Zorro	Donor					1. 9 yrs 2. $10^1/_{12}$ yrs	$10^7/_{12}$ yrs	
Zola	Grandmother							Donor: behavioural "problems" (e.g.
Zelda	Grandmother							aggression, anti-social behaviour

ALL acute lymphoblastic leukaemia, AML acute myeloid leukaemia, BMT bone marrow transplant, PBSCT peripheral blood stem cell transplant

About the Contributors

Jutta Ecarius is Professor of Social and Educational Science in the Faculty of Human Sciences at the University of Cologne. Her research interests include families and socialization, the changing situation of youth in late modern societies, dynamics of violence, transformation of education, and learning. She is author or co-author of seven monographs, has edited a handbook on family research (*Handbuch Familie*, VS Verlag 2007), and coedited a book on the methodology of qualitative education research. Currently, she is working on a longitudinal study of familial education over three generations in the context of historical changes.

Tim Henning is Professor of Practical Philosophy at the University of Mainz. He works on metaethics, normative ethics, applied ethics, and the philosophy of language. His work covers a broad range of topics, from foundational issues in normative and moral theory (e.g., the nature of reasons and the structure of reasoning) to specific problems in applied ethics (e.g., the role of lotteries in allocation conflicts, or the moral issues involving the creation of so-called "savior siblings").

Madeleine Herzog is a medical anthropologist and practicing relationship and sex therapist. Her research interests include anthropology of family and kinship, medical anthropology, sociology and anthropology of the body and of emotions, and praxeology. She was researcher in the project "Stem cell transplantation between siblings."

Martina Jürgensen (PhD) is a sociologist at the University of Lübeck. She has broad expertise from a series of projects in the field of medical sociology, health services research, childhood- and family studies, and qualitative methodology. Her current research focuses on children with diversity of sexual development (DSD). She was lead researcher in the project "Stem cell transplantation between siblings."

© The Author(s) 2022
C. Schües et al. (eds.), *Stem Cell Transplantations Between Siblings as Social Phenomena*, Philosophy and Medicine 144,
https://doi.org/10.1007/978-3-031-04166-2

Amy Mullin is Professor of Philosophy at the University of Toronto. Her research interests include family ethics as well as relationships characterized by mutuality, reciprocity, and asymmetry, more broadly speaking. She focuses in particular on questions about children and autonomy as well as connections between hope, gratitude, autonomy, and trust. She also has expertise in aesthetics on questions relating to connections between moral, political, and aesthetic value.

Christoph Rehmann-Sutter is Professor of Theory and Ethics in the Biosciences at the University of Lübeck in Germany and Honorary Professor of Philosophy at the University of Basel, Switzerland. He has widely published in philosophy and ethics of biomedicine. Research interests include philosophical foundations of bioethics and phenomenological philosophy of biology. With a hermeneutic approach to ethics and often with qualitative empirical methods, he has been working about ethical issues of genetic engineering, of prenatal genetics, transplantation, stem cell medicine, and palliative care, currently also on the ethics of climate change.

Lainie Friedman Ross is the Carolyn and Matthew Bucksbaum Professor of Clinical Ethics; professor in the Departments of Pediatrics, Medicine, Surgery and the College; associate director of the MacLean Center for Clinical Medical Ethics; and co-director of the Institute for Translational Medicine at the University of Chicago. Her research focuses on pediatric ethics, transplantation ethics, genetics ethics, and research ethics. Her fifth book, *The Living Organ Donor as Patient: Theory and Practice* was co-authored with Dick Thistlethwaite and published by Oxford University Press in 2021. Her work on this project was funded in part by a National Library of Medicine (NLM) G13LM013003 grant entitled "Sibling Obligations in Health Care."

Christina Schües is Professor of Philosophy in the Institute for History of Medicine and Science Studies at the University of Lübeck, and also Adjunct Professor of Philosophy in the Institute of Philosophy and Sciences of Art at Leuphana University of Lüneburg. Coming from classical and post-classical phenomenology, she is especially interested at the interface between epistemology, anthropology, and political ethics. Her research interests concern the relationality of the human condition in light of biomedical practices and anthropo-technologies; thereby, her focus includes the politics of the body, the power of time, and peace studies.

Margrit Shildrick is Guest Professor of Gender and Knowledge Production at Stockholm University and Adjunct Professor of Critical Disability Studies at York University, Toronto. Her biophilosophical research covers postmodern feminist and cultural theory, bioethics, critical disability studies, and body theory. Her publications include several single-author books and edited collections and many journal articles. Her new book, *Visceral Prostheses: Somatechnics and Posthuman Embodiment*, about the biophilosophical and embodied conjunction of microchimerism, immunology, and corporeal anomaly will be published in early 2022. She is currently engaged on a project entitled @The Meaning and Workings of the Gift.

Claudia Wiesemann is director of the Institute for Medical Ethics and History of Medicine at Goettingen University Medical Centre, Germany. She is a medical ethicist and has been working in the field for more than 30 years. Her research interests include the ethics of family, reproductive medicine, child rights in healthcare, and sex and gender issues. Her last book *Moral Equality, Bioethics, and the Child* deals with the child as a moral actor in healthcare. Currently, she is leader of a research group called "Medicine, Time, and the Good Life" funded by the Deutsche Forschungsgemeinschaft.

Literature for Study Description and Sample

Alderfelder, Melissa A., and Anne E. Kazak. 2006. Family issues when a child is on treatment for cancer. In *Comprehensive handbook of childhood cancer and sickle cell disease. A biopsychosocial approach*, ed. Ronald T. Brown, 53–74. New York: Oxford University Press.

Alderfer, Melissa A., and Caroline M. Stanley. 2012. Health and illness in the context of the family. In *Handbook of health psychology*, ed. Andrew Baum, Tracey A. Revenson, and Jerome E. Singer, 2nd ed., 493–516. London: Routledge.

American Academy of Pediatrics. 2010. Children as hematopoietic stem cell donors. *Committee of Bioethics Policy Statement Pediatrics* 125 (2): 392. https://doi.org/10.1542/peds.2009-3078.

Beverley, John, and James Beebe. 2018. Judgement of moral responsibility in tissue donation cases. *Bioethics* 32 (2): 83–93. https://doi.org/10.1111/bioe.12412.

Björk, Maria, Berit Nordström, Thomas Wiebe, and Inger Hallström. 2011. Returning to a changed ordinary life: Families' lived experience after completing a child's cancer treatment. *European Journal of Cancer Care* 20 (2): 163–169. https://doi.org/10.1111/j.1365-2354.2009.01159.x.

Hendrischke, Askan. 2010. Niemand ist alleine krank. Perspektiven der Systemischen Familienmedizin. Psychotherapie im. *Dialog* 11 (2): 134–139.

Herzog, Madeleine, Martina Jürgensen, Christoph Rehmann-Sutter, and Christina Schües. 2019. Interviewers as intruders? Ethical explorations of joint family interviews. Journal of empirical research on human research ethics. *Special Issue on "Research Ethics in Empirical Ethics Studies: Case Studies and Commentaries"* 14 (5): 458–461. https://doi.org/10.1177/1556264619857856.

Rehmann-Sutter, Christoph, Sarah Daubitz, and Christina Schües. 2013. "Spender gefunden, alles klar!" Ethische Aspekte des HLA-tests bei Kindern im Kontext der Stammzelltransplantation. *Bioethica Forum* 6 (3): 89–96.

Schoors, Van, Jan De Marieke, Hanne Morren Mo, Lesley L. Verhofstadt, Liesbet Goubert, and Hanna Van Parys. 2018. Parents' perspectives of changes within the family functioning after a Pediatric cancer diagnosis: A multi family member interview analysis. *Qualitative Health Research* 28 (8): 1229–1241. https://doi.org/10.1177/1049732317753587.

Schües, Christina, and Christoph Rehmann-Sutter. 2013. Hat ein Kind eine Pflicht, Blutstammzellen für ein krankes Geschwisterkind zu spenden? *Ethik in der Medizin* 25 (2): 89–102. https://doi.org/10.1007/s00481-012-0202-z.

———. 2014. Retrospektive Zustimmung der Kinder? Ethische Aspekte der geschwisterlichen Stammzelltransplantation. *Frühe Kindheit. Die ersten sechs Jahre* 2: 22–27.

© The Author(s) 2022
C. Schües et al. (eds.), *Stem Cell Transplantations Between Siblings as Social Phenomena*, Philosophy and Medicine 144,
https://doi.org/10.1007/978-3-031-04166-2

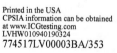

Printed in the USA
CPSIA information can be obtained
at www.ICGtesting.com
LVHW010940190324
774517LV00003BA/353

9 783031 041655